365 DAYS OF AYURVEDA FOR LIFELONG RADIANT HEALTH

365 DAYS OF AYURVEDA FOR LIFELONG RADIANT HEALTH

❖

Daily Wisdom & Simple Tips for Physical, Emotional & Spiritual Well-Being

RHONDA EGIDIO, PHD

365 Days of Ayurveda for Lifelong Radiant Health © 2019 by Rhonda K. Egidio

All rights reserved. No part of this book may be reproduced, stored in a retrieval system, or transferred by in any form or by any means—electronic, mechanical, photocopy, recording, or otherwise—without the express written permission of the publisher, except for brief quotations in printed reviews.

Radiant Life Press

ISBN: 9781707646340

Ayurveda information shared here is for general educational purposes and is not intended to substitute for medical or psychological advice. Please consult with a qualified health care provider in these matters and particularly if you are pregnant, nursing, ill, and/or on medication. In particular, some herbs are contraindicated for particular conditions and medications.

FOREWORD BY
PAUL DUGLISS, MD

It is with great pleasure and with great awe that I write this. It is a pleasure to see a former student embracing this timeless wisdom and taking it beyond her teachers. It is with awe that I view the comprehensiveness and practicality of what Dr. Rhonda Egidio has put together in this work.

Ayurveda—being such a comprehensive body of knowledge—can be full of abstract concepts and complex principles. Here Dr. Egidio has done a great service in making Ayurveda accessible to the Westerner.

Ayurveda is full of treasures, but a need exists to make it simple and modern. This book does both. *365 Days of Ayurveda for Lifelong Radiant Health* makes it practical and, most importantly, allows you to experience the principles of Ayurveda in your own awareness. It grounds it in easy-to-do daily practices.

What also makes the book so valuable is that you will have the supportive voice of the author through each and every day of your exploration of this wonderful knowledge. Drawing on her experience, she is able to offer authentic guidance and support you in the changes you are wanting to make.

Finally, the book is packed with valuable information that not only teaches you Ayurveda but gives you down-to-earth tools to aid your health and well-being.

I hope you will enjoy this book and reap its rich rewards.

Paul Dugliss, MD
Director and Academic Dean,
New World Ayurveda School

FOREWORD BY
DR. SUHAS KSHIRSAGAR

WE ARE ON the cusp of a major paradigm shift in medicine, where prevention means taking responsibility for your own health and well-being. People often say they know what to do to be healthier, but some may lack the discipline and motivation to learn, train, and empower themselves to change habits and simply change their life. Many people worldwide are turning to Ayurveda for answers and assistance.

Ayurveda is the science of life, and the language of Ayurveda is easy to understand and even easier to follow if you live in accordance with the laws of Mother Nature. As a practicing Medical Astrologer, I know that Sun is the biggest influencer for the life on planet Earth. Sun travels 365 days in 12 zodiac signs, which creates seasonal changes, day-and-night cycles, and lunar tidal rhythms. Our birth dates and times are influenced by Sun Return. And our own circadian clock is constantly responding to the changes happening in our near and far environment. We must take care of our health on a daily basis with mindful awareness towards diet, sleep, exercise, and many other rituals that bring us in harmony with Nature's flux and flow.

365 Days of Ayurveda cultivates that awareness towards a positive health habit one day at a time. It will empower you to apply the change and the inner cellular intelligence will synchronize itself with the master natural clock. This entrainment is the need of the hour (no pun intended). This attitude takes more words to express, but it simply links self-awareness with self-care. Prevention is truly based upon your inner transformation, which is deeply embedded in your consciousness. The Self-referral feedback loop of consciousness influences its own expression in more abstract and unpredictable ways and in the process, consciousness becomes intelligence. This is the very reason that these new habits will reprogram your lifestyle.

There are many valuable pearls of wisdom in the book that are time tested and scientifically validated. It brings together the insights of ancient Ayurveda with what we know about the workings of nature through the window of the latest science.

Rhonda Egidio, PhD, has written this remarkable and heartfelt book. She is an acclaimed Ayurvedic Practitioner who specializes in transforming the style of education. The book is also her own journey and discovery of the spiritual basis for everlasting changes in habits, attitudes, and a personal belief system.

Rhonda has designed a valuable companion for those wishing to understand and apply holistic concepts of health to real-life challenges. She has developed a novel way to deliver information on Ayurveda, which is a perfect blend of East and West. *365 Days of Ayurveda* is your companion in moving towards health, happiness, and enlightenment.

Dr. Suhas Kshirsagar, BAMS, MD (Ayurveda, India)
Director, Ayurvedic Healing Inc.

Author of *Change Your Schedule, Change Your Life*
and *The Hot Belly Diet*

http://ayurvedichealing.net

*With gratitude to all on the path of awakening.
The teachers and the seekers are the same.*

ACKNOWLEDGEMENTS

WRITING A BOOK seems like a metaphor for composing a life. You cannot do either without meaningful relationships and wise consult. Karyn Boatwright, my soul connection in life, has always supported my adventures with encouragement, deep presence, honesty and joy. I am grateful and blessed every single day because of her presence on this earth...in my life.

My sister Sandy Cole has been one of my most enthusiastic supporters. She wins the award for most referrals to sign up for my newsletter! Our family love goes deep and is a comfort in lifelong, peaceful knowing.

And then there are my teachers. Dr. Paul Dugliss has been my Ayurveda and meditation teacher since 2008. His heart and deep wisdom of the nature and fabric of consciousness astound me. Forever my teacher. I also acknowledge Karina Mirsky, my teacher of the consciousness of yoga and my precious friend. Her playfulness and skillfulness with titles and book covers made this process so much more fun and effective just as she makes life both deeper and more playful! What a mix.

Vicki Berglund, the general editor of this book is extraordinary. How does she do it? I know this whole book was in my head as I kept reviewing it, but how did she get the wholeness of it into her head. Her edits were abundant and strategic. She guided me through the components that I needed to address to write my first book. Her commitment to excellence and thoroughness and her pleasantness throughout this demanding process astounds.

Maren Showkeir did a first round of copy edits and it was a massive piece of work for such a voluminous manuscript. She brought tightness and alignment to my, sometimes wandering, words that benefitted this final outcome immeasurably.

Drs. Suhas and Manas Kshirsagar did an Ayurveda content review of the book. Like any practiced science there are different views of knowledge pieces. I wanted a second perspective and they provided this check. Dr. Suhas Kshirsagar is an Ayurvedic physician and an esteemed Ayurveda educator with many books of his own. He also provided shaping to the book that was a significant upgrade. Dr. Manas S. Kshirsagar, AD, is an esteemed certified Ayurveda Practitioner with broad and extensive training.

My thanks to the very special ones who provided thoughtful reviews of my early manuscript and continued with ongoing faith in my capacity to successfully complete this endeavor. Deep bow to you. You have no idea how meaningful your words of encouragement were. Likewise, all the folks who provide good cheer and honest camaraderie along the way—deep gratitude—my life is composed with you.

SPIRAL LEARNING TO EMBED NEW HABITS

Repetition is what forms habit. Spiraling back to key ideas and practices you learn here will reinforce the inspiration and learning needed to make changes and grow. Over time, you will be able to sustain new habits without effort. They will simply become part of who you are.

The dedicated purpose of *365 Days of Ayurveda for Lifelong Radiant Health* is to turn the knowledge of Ayurveda into your own personal wisdom. My commitment here is to help you make intelligent personal choices and form lasting healthy habits.

In this book you will learn the ancient and modern wisdom of Ayurveda combined with evidence-based Western science to support your confidence in trying out new behaviors to support the life you desire. Over the year, you will be introduced to short, digestible bits of knowledge which you will revisit, in some cases multiple times, (i.e., with the big tip, drinking hot spice water).

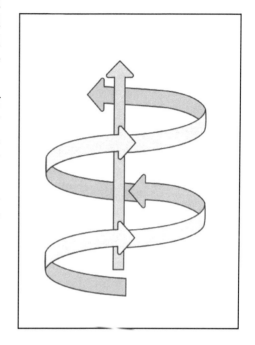

However, my commitment to your awakening is not enough. A healthy *Ayurveda-informed lifestyle* is achieved by taking action on your part. You can incorporate new good habits one-by-one until they become part of your new identity. As you see the benefits of the new behaviors, old habits will become inconsequential as they will no longer hold your interest.

But new habits do not form quickly. You'll need to experiment with the tools and techniques here and see the positive results for yourself. Only then will a new habit take hold and integrate into your emerging identity.

Returning to the individual tools you learn here time and time again is the spiral of integration. May this book be your companion to create a better life.

WELCOME TO 365 DAYS OF AYURVEDA
FOR LIFELONG RADIANT HEALTH, ONE DAY AT A TIME

A RE YOU SIMPLY accepting your health limitations? Or are you ready for a way of living that supports the well-being of every part of you—physical, emotional, and spiritual? Are you ready to shatter the illusions of who you think you are supposed to be, and discover exactly who you are? How do you establish the right conditions to elevate your current state of being?

As Dr. Gabrielle Cousins, author of Spiritual Nutrition, says: "When the vessel of the body-mind complex is strengthened, the body turns into a luminescent vehicle of Light."[1] You can achieve radiant living.

The arc of timeless Ayurveda wisdom, which goes back thousands of years, has never been more relevant for the modern world. Simply put, we must live in the Nature that holds us gently, which is, in fact, us. For our sake and the sake of our planet, we must find our way home as being a contributing and receiving part of Nature, not as ruling over Nature. I believe Ayurveda's time-tested knowledge and practices offer a superlative guide for lifelong radiant health.

When reading a book, one comes into relationship with the author. I offer to be your coach as you make your way through *365 Days of Ayurveda*. This book is designed to build self-knowledge and Ayurveda knowledge through daily wisdom and tips for one calendar year. After a year, you might be surprised to behold the wise progress you have made. Ideally, you will continue for many years to lean into the practices that clean you up and strengthen your good, radiant energy life force.

WHAT IS AYURVEDA?

AYURVEDA (PRONOUNCED EYE-YOUR-VAY-DUH) comes from the Sanskrit language and translates as "the wisdom of life."

"Ayus" means living or longevity, and "Veda" is science or revealed wisdom. A message of higher-consciousness living is the core, time-tested purpose of the science of Ayurveda—to strengthen and purify body, mind, emotions, and spirit so you can foster enlightenment and blissfulness.

As the science of life, Ayurveda includes, well—*everything*. It helps us understand that we are of Nature and the need to align with its pure vibration, our deepest source. Nature will guide us if we sit within her and listen.

About 5,000 years ago, the great seers of ancient India, called rishis, gathered for many years to contemplate the nature of the Universe. These seers elevated their consciousness and received special healing wisdom, which was compiled into the Vedas, the earliest literary record. Two of the books of sacred knowledge, the Rig Veda and the Atharvaveda, contained detailed knowledge of healing, surgery, and longevity. Their intent was to help people rid themselves of suffering. These books became the foundational knowledge for Ayurveda. Yet, Ayurveda is still profoundly relevant to our lives today.

CONNECTIONS WE'VE LOST

The world has seen much progress and many changes—not all of them good. People used to live closer to Nature, and some still do. But plenty of people feel disconnected. There are concrete reasons why.

- Only a few generations ago, most people ate what was grown locally. Today, convenient, nutritionally empty, processed foods are everywhere. While grocery stores can offer fresh foods from around the world, transporting them pollutes our environment and removes us from the seasonal cycles that gave us a measure of time close to Nature. Many diseases are primarily born of stress and an unwell body that can't process the constant diet of "unreal" foods. We have forgotten what and how to eat.
- Previous generations grew up around family and friends. They worked in the town in which they lived, and found meaning in relationships with those who lived nearby. Today, many people don't know their neighbors. Some work online with colleagues they never meet in person. People judge and separate themselves from those with differing political opinions.
- Whether we live in rural or urban areas, technologies keep us in light long into the evening. Blue light from mobile phones and computers messes with our circadian rhythms and melatonin production, disrupting sleep.
- The current, "state-of-the-art" medical system is oriented to treat disease with drugs and surgery and to manage the rising costs of healthcare, and simply put, separates body from spirit and Nature. According to the U.S. Centers for Disease Control & Prevention, chronic diseases are responsible for 7 in 10 deaths each year, many of which can be prevented with good health habits.[2]

Many people experience generalized anxiety, and feelings of being ungrounded. Anxiety disorders affect more than 18% of the U.S. population, and this number is on the rise.[3] In the U.S., for the first time, we have a generation that is not expected to live as long as their parents. Even with all the goodness in life, people know something is wrong.

Everywhere around the world, it is time to do something radical to save ourselves and our planet—and we know it. It's imperative to return to the great relationship within Nature. This is how we can step away from the despairing side of life and renew our hope for a better future, one that aligns us with our proper, healthy, radiant, truthful life within the arms of Nature.

TUNING OURSELVES WITH THE INTELLIGENCE OF NATURE

Pragya aparadh is a primary concept in Ayurveda. This is defined as being out of a balance with Nature, along with losing sight of our own divine nature.

Pragya means intellect, and aparadh means mistake or ignorance. Combined, the meaning is about doing the wrong things even though we know the negative effects. And as we learn about Ayurveda, we increase our knowledge about what serves us well, and we strive to align our behavior to what we know is good for us.

Ayurveda's central belief is that Nature is a grand, intelligent life force that, when we get in tune, helps us operate with great ease. As we live closer to the laws of Nature, we entrain to that intelligence. Its holistic system promotes health and well-being on all levels—physical, emotional, mental, and spiritual. Ayurveda treats the person as a whole, not as a collection of parts.

While Ayurveda does not treat disease per se, the person is always at the center. Its strategies are used to restore balance, returning the individual to a healthy alignment with Nature. Ayurveda serves to remove the conditions for disease, not fight the disease. For instance, people with diabetes likely have different dosha imbalances that led to that condition, and so require different approaches to heal.

But beyond being free of disease, Ayurveda offers promise of spiritual unfoldment and bliss. Though not a religion, Ayurveda is grounded and emerges from cosmic intelligence, which is why this path of vibrant health allows you to tap into universal energy and intelligence. You then reap the reward of feeling good, which is wonderful in itself. And feeling good may inspire you to serve others as you connect with the unity of all. And that is key to radiant living.

George Bernard Shaw says it well:

> *"This is the true joy in life, the being used for a purpose recognized by yourself as a mighty one; the being a force of Nature instead of a feverish selfish clod of ailments and grievances complaining that the world will not devote itself to making you happy. I am of the opinion that my life belongs to the whole community, and as long as I live, it is my privilege to do for it whatever I can. I want to be thoroughly used up when I die, for the harder I work, the more I live. I rejoice in life for its own sake. Life is no 'brief candle' to me. It is sort of a splendid torch which I have a hold of for the moment, and I want to make it burn as brightly as possible before handing it over to future generations."*

COMPREHENSIVE STRATEGIES

AYURVEDA IS INCLUSIVE and lively. It operates from the most subtle elements of well-being (intangible) to the most gross (tangible). Common Ayurveda strategies include:

- healthy eating
- good digestion
- restful sleep
- connecting to cosmic intelligence with meditation
- mood-shifting aromas
- massage for detox and alignment
- astrology for life context
- yoga for energy and balance
- herbs and spices for intelligence

ESSENTIAL TERMS

FOR OUR DIVE into Ayurveda, let's begin with common language. It can sometimes be a challenge to know where to start in explaining the concepts and principles because one term may be needed to define another. Each of these concepts gets more detailed discussion throughout the book, but a good starter vocabulary provides a foundation.

5 Elements

Panchamahabhutas, which are earth, water, fire, air, and space/ether. The five elements form the building blocks of Nature at all levels—physical, energetic, emotional, mental, and spiritual.

3 Doshas

Vata—energy of action, transportation, movement; composed of elements air and space; qualities are light, dry, rough, changeable/moveable, subtle

Pitta—energy of transformation and metabolism of food and experiences; composed of fire and some water; qualities are hot, sharp, light, mobile, flowing (but grounded)

Kapha—energy of structure, strength (immunity), lubrication; composed of earth and water; qualities are cold, wet, unctuous, and heavy.

Vitiated

When a dosha has become abnormal or spoiled or imbalanced.

3 Gunas

Rajas—quality of motion and energy, dynamism

Tamas—quality of inertia and resistance to energy, ignorance, darkness

Sattva—the stabilizing cosmic intelligence force, purity, clarity, evolution

Vikruti

Your current doshic state represented in pulse readings from Ayurvedic practitioners, where 2 is considered typical. For example, a pulse reading of Vata 1, Pitta 3, and Kapha 2 shows the Pitta excessive and Vata deficient. You can also get Vikruti self-report results from taking dosha inventories (see Assessment 1 at the end of this book).

Prakruti

Your doshic ratio from birth, which never changes. You might be predominantly Vata, second influence Pitta, and least Kapha. Your Prakruti can be determined with birth information used with Jyotish or Ayurveda astrology. You can also get an idea of your Prakruti from self-report assessments (also see Assessment 1 at the end of this book) or by consulting with an Ayurveda practitioner.

Dhatus

These are the seven tissue layers. Each layer of tissue evolves to the next, and the health of each is based on previous layers. The layers and their Sanskrit/Ayurveda terms are: Plasma (*Rasa*), Blood (*Rakta*), Muscle (*Mamsa*), Fat (*Meda*), Bone (*Asthi*), Bone marrow and nerves (*Majja*), and Reproductive fluids and seed (*Shukra*—male, *Andartava*—female).

Ama

A form of unmetabolized waste from food and experiences that results in physical and emotional toxins.

Agni

Digestive fire and capacity. Although each cell has agni, this term is most often associated with the stomach and duodenum.

Malas

Wastes from food, i.e. urine, feces, sweat, and waste products from tissues.

Ojas

The most refined and subtle essence of the body. It is the product of perfect digestion and metabolism, resulting in radiant energy, a healthy body, and a blissful mind.

Underlying Field

A unified field out of which all the laws of nature arise, all energy and all intelligence. This is a field of pure consciousness.

Ayurveda and My Story of Transformation

For months, I had been losing weight and experiencing frightening episodes of heart racing. In 2008, I was diagnosed with hyperthyroidism. My overactive thyroid gland sped up my body systems, resulting in a serious health threat. My primary care doctor offered me three treatment options to consider: remove my thyroid, irradiate it, or be on medication the rest of my life. None felt right, but the doctor said I was in a "danger zone," so I agreed to start with the medication. It would buy me time to take responsibility for my own health.

Within a month after the diagnosis, the term "Ayurveda" began clamoring for my attention. I attended an Ayurvedic workshop hosted by my yoga studio. I read several articles in yoga magazines and online. Finally, Elena, the creator of a natural skincare line, described the influence of Ayurveda in the products she had developed as she gave me a facial. She thought Ayurveda might help with my hyperthyroidism and referred me to Paul Dugliss, an MD and Ayurvedic physician.

Dr. Dugliss described an Ayurvedic approach to restore my health and balance, and I knew this was it. I wanted to learn all I could, and the timing was fortunate. His New World Ayurveda school [4] was starting a new class in a month. He invited me to join. Yes, yes, yes! I immediately integrated Ayurvedic practices into my daily routine as I began training to become an Ayurvedic practitioner.

Dr. Susan Carlson, my wonderful primary care doctor, worked with me as I engaged in this process of natural healing. Every three months, I would get new blood tests, and we slowly reduced the medication. After two-and-a-half years, I was off medication, and the hyperthyroid condition has never returned. My health is better than ever. Not only do I feel clean and healthy in body, this practice has supported the cleansing and settling of my mind. I ruminate less, and I have the energy to create neural pathways that serve higher consciousness. Just as wonderful: My capacity for compassion and love has increased.

HOW AYURVEDA HELPS: SUCCESS STORIES

Ayurveda transformed my health and my life, and it has helped many people with whom I have worked over this past decade. When you are in pain or suffering, it can be challenging for the best in you to shine through. Healing helps bring out the best version of you, and your presence can become healing to those around you.

My Ayurveda clients tell me about conditions that have caused them suffering for years, sometimes since childhood. I have worked with people across the full spectrum of age including those in their 20s and early 30s, newly on their own, who want to take responsibility for their health. As they look ahead, they want to avoid suffering throughout their adulthood. Other clients find me in their 50s and 60s, hoping to prevent unhealthy conditions from following them into their golden years. A health crisis, at any age, can create a sense of urgency to find a better way to live.

I love also working with those who feel that vibrant health is their birthright. Often, I consult with people who already have many healthy habits and are curious about what Ayurveda can offer. They appreciate the customized approach Ayurveda provides—it's for all ages, but isn't one-size-fits-all.

Each stands on a threshold of hope for a better life. Because Ayurveda is deep, time-tested, and customized, I have seen remarkable healings for those committed to learning, changing, and growing.

Cory: Difficult Digestion

Perfect digestion is a core goal of Ayurveda, considered the primary building block for improving health. Cory, a woman in her late 20s, described a history of digestive disorders. She experienced gas and pain when she strayed from eating mild and bland foods. Her diet had made her anemic. We worked to calm her excessive Vata and build her digestive agni (fire) with strategies such as hot spice water {xvi}, and using ginger in her cooking. She replaced salad meals with warm, cooked food. Within six months, her digestion had stabilized and her daily digestive pain ended. Cory was able to eat a variety of nutritious foods, had more energy, and her mood improved.

Jason: Arthritic Stiffness

Ayurveda views arthritis {Dec 9–11} predominantly as an issue of toxins that settle in damaged and/or vulnerable parts of our bodies. Joint pain slows you down and limits activity. This was the issue presented by Jason, in his early 60s. We arrived at an agreeable protocol to avoid new toxins by eating cleaner, more digestible foods. We worked to clear the ama (toxins) already in the body with detox strategies that you will find throughout this book.

Once a good bit of ama was cleared, he took an herb called ashwagandha, known for pacifying Vata, clearing ama, and rejuvenating tissues. Jason used another herb, triphala guggulu, at bedtime. Guggulu is known for pulling deep-seated toxins out of joints. Frequent abhyanga, a warm oil self-massage, also helped, especially in the affected areas of his body. Finally, Jason significantly reduced his sugar intake, which is the primary contributor to inflammation.

This is a typical healing path: cleanse toxins, then build and rejuvenate with diet, herbs, and lifestyle adjustments. Jason's goal was to stop arthritis from progressing. His condition halted, and he reported less pain and drastically reduced inflammation. He is back on his bicycle, something he had not imagined being able to do again.

Sarah: Spiritual Awakening

SOME PEOPLE MEET with me to learn how Ayurveda can help support general health. Once we get into their story, I often discover they want more than physical health. They are seekers, looking to evolve their consciousness. Ayurveda is ideally suited to support this.

Sarah was among many on this path. She did yoga, ate fairly well, and was active. But she felt an emptiness that was hard to name. After a few sessions, we talked about the practice and benefits of meditation, and I offered her a custom meditation mantra based on Jyotish Ayurveda astrology. We went deeper into the nature of food, discussing how to balance the doshas through diet and how food emerges from an underlying field of energy and information, just as humans do. The ability to receive and hold this energy is how we heal. This notion of food as transmitter of energy and operating information from the Underlying Field motivated her to be more conscious of what she ate, and the kind of environment in which she ate. Sarah did things such as play soft music during meals and she put living plants in her dining room.

I suggested Ayurvedic herbs noted for promoting higher consciousness, including ashwagandha to tone the nervous system and brahmi to invite blissful states. She was able to align deeper to her soul's journey through the blessings of Ayurveda.

Your Story

YOUR MOTIVATIONS FOR traveling the enlightened path of Ayurveda will be your own. Perhaps you want to resolve a health problem, or you want more energy, or you want to be more grounded, or to detox, or to discover deeper spiritual connection. Your desires might be pragmatic or ethereal. These needs and more are held in the promise of Ayurveda. It will serve you well. With time and steady progress, you will be enjoying a radiant, healthy life before you know it.

MORE ABOUT DOSHAS: ALL AROUND US AND IN US

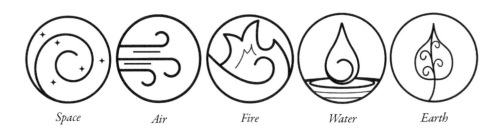

Space *Air* *Fire* *Water* *Earth*

Doshas are particularly important in Ayurveda, and to this book. The concepts and specifics of Vata, Pitta, and Kapha are relevant in many ways, which you will see as you progress through *365 Days of Ayurveda for Lifelong Radiant Health*.

- Doshas arise from the five basic elements: space, air, fire, water, and earth. Kapha is earth and water, Pitta is fire and water, and Vata is air and space.
- Doshas affect our individual nature and proclivities, as all of us have a mixture of the three in our constitution, with usually one predominating.
- Doshas correspond to—and provide useful guidance for—the phases of your life and even times of the day.
- Doshas are integral to the Ayurvedic seasons: Vata, Pitta, and Kapha. This book, for example, begins toward the middle of Vata season, which is the windy, cold season. That falls about November through February in many parts of the United States. Kapha is the wet spring season, and Pitta the heat of summer, again in many parts of the U.S. You can adjust for your locale.

The wonderful wisdom about doshas spirals in throughout this book. Some day entries are labeled "Kapha" for example. Even if your individual dosha is Vata or Pitta, read this information to understand the Kapha part of you, and enjoy learning about the characteristics of Kapha family members (perhaps your own children), friends, coworkers, and anyone in your life.

HOW TO USE THIS BOOK

INITIALLY, AYURVEDA MIGHT seem overwhelming. Just keep leaning in. Improving your health is a virtuous cycle. Each time you take a step, you have a stronger foundation for good choices, and the next step becomes easier.

The 365 readings (and one bonus for leap year) are organized around major themes for understanding the foundation of Ayurveda—how it applies to life and health—and include a daily Ayurveda Action. Some topics relate to the Ayurveda doshic season, and some are general.

Important topics will be revisited because they are just that large. Also, your understanding of concepts or strategies will change as you advance through the book. Building over time is important, and I purposely circle back to topics to keep them active in your thinking.

- You can read by calendar date.
- You can use the index to home in on a topic.
- If you like, visit the two Assessments and Dosha Chart at the back of the book first for a jump-start on personal understanding.
- Once you've gone through the year, start in again or simply use this book as a convenient reference to deepen your understanding and success.

I DIDN'T GET MY BOOK UNTIL JULY—DO I JUST START THERE?

Sure! Just read the beginning of the book and then dive right in.

I don't live in North America so the Ayurvedic seasons are different—can I still use this book?

Simply adjust to follow your seasons more closely. For example, if you are in Australia, your January is more like June in North America, so start there.

Be kind with yourself as you explore and learn. Ayurveda helps you see the reality of yourself more clearly as it offers custom balancing strategies. Keep in mind that backsliding is natural—it also can be healthy to let go. Have that pizza and a beer with friends and enjoy the moment! Joy is a health habit, too.

Open your mind, and you will discover the many gems in *365 Days of Ayurveda for Lifelong Radiant Health*. Here's to a great year of ever-improving, radiant health with the ancient wisdom of Ayurveda applied to your modern life.

BEST AYURVEDA ACTION FOR THE YEAR
DRINK HOT SPICE WATER

THIS BOOK WILL give you many Ayurveda health strategies. However, if you start only one new habit, this is the one. I recommend you begin now and continue every day. You will see this powerful tip reinforced throughout *365 Days of Ayurveda for Lifelong Radiant Health*. Small new effort, huge impact!

HOT SPICE WATER:

- 1/2 tsp organic fennel seeds
- 1/4 tsp organic cumin seeds
- 1/4 tsp organic coriander seeds

Add seeds to a thermos with 1-2 cups of boiled water. Steep at least 15 minutes. You may strain after brewing if you wish. Hot water on your tongue signals your body to digest. If you have just eaten, that will be the focus for digestion. Between meals, your body will pull out ama-laden (toxin) fat cells to burn. Plain hot water is great, but the three digestive spices kick it up a notch.

Hot spice water should be sipped about every 15 minutes through the day—not consumed all at once. With a meal, drink less than 1/2 cup of spice water, so you do not dilute the proper concentrations of digestive juices. Also, stop drinking 30 minutes before and 30 minutes after meals.

FENNEL

Best for strengthening agni without irritating Pitta
Relaxes digestive tract
Increases fat burning
Moves lymph

CUMIN

Slightly heating so pacifies both Vata and Kapha
Stimulates agni so dispels ama/toxic waste
Decreases gas
Soothes mucous membranes

CORIANDER

Pacifies Pitta
Improves digestion and absorption
Reduces inflammation
Relieves indigestion and gas

VATA SEASON

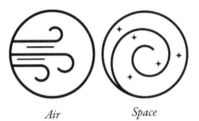

Air *Space*

JANUARY 1
CONSCIOUSNESS FIRST

LIKE WAVES ON an ocean, your individual consciousness is part of a vast sea of energy and intelligence. When you lose awareness of the ocean, each wave is seen as separate, unique, and isolated. But the ocean is always a part of each wave. A limited experience of consciousness can lead to an assumption that we are not the ocean. This is a mistake of understanding. We all have a body, thoughts, and emotions—but these things are not who we are. We are part of a universal whole that nurtures our cells, our thoughts, and our energy with sophisticated organization and intelligence. Ayurveda teaches us how to connect with the underlying field and gives us robust health for the journey.

> *"The Unified Field is what the ancients referred to as the Absolute. It is the sum total of all energy and potentials—all creativity and all intelligence. When it stirs within itself, it creates the relative, manifested creation. The term 'relative' means that something has manifested from the Unified Field that no longer demonstrates all the qualities of the Absolute and can be known relative to other aspects of creation."*[5]

—PAUL DUGLISS, *CAPTURING THE BLISS*

AYURVEDA ACTION
Engage the Unified Field

BE IN NATURE. Walk in silence outdoors or, if weather alerts prevent that, peer outdoors. Notice the nature of Nature at this time of year.

A Japanese ritual called *"shinrin-yoku"* translates to "forest bathing." This practice has likely existed for millennia, but was officially proposed by the Forest Agency of Japan in 1982.[6] Bathe in universal wisdom through a connection with trees. Even cities have parks with trees.

While outdoors, really see a tree: What is the texture of the bark to your eyes? And to your touch? What are the sounds of the leaves and inhabiting creatures? Look closely *and* look from a distance. See *and* feel.

Resist the urge to power walk or add steps on your Fitbit. Let go of effort—just walk mindfully, absorb, and feel your connection with something limitless. Reflect on your gratitude for how Nature provides. Strengthen your identity to the part of you that is limitless and connected with everything.

JANUARY 2
ONE SOUND, FIVE ELEMENTS, THREE DOSHAS

According to the founders of Ayurveda, from pure consciousness arose the sound of OM. In turn, the five great elements that comprise the universe—SPACE, AIR, FIRE, WATER, AND EARTH—were born. From those elements emerged the three doshas—VATA, PITTA, and KAPHA.

Ayurveda teaches that humans contain the five elements and the Soul. The character and qualities of the five elements is present in everything in an infinite variety of proportions.

Earth is in the substance of your body, including the bones and minerals needed for survival. More than two-thirds of your body is water, which supports movement and cell growth. Digestive fire breaks down food and transforms it to energy. Air is inhaled and blood carries oxygen, nourishing all aspects of your body. Space (aka ether) is the hollow cavities of the body and the vessel for spiritual receptivity. The elements combine in a bio-energetic form to create the doshas.

The essence of Ayurvedic healing is understanding your constitutional dosha balance from birth and your current dosha imbalance—the ways you are out of balance with your constitution. Through diet, meditation, massage, herbs, yoga, purification and other Ayurveda practices, you can restore balance to become a receptive vessel for healing from the underlying field of consciousness.

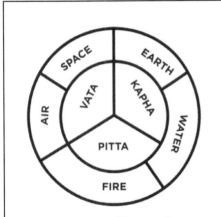

Vata is represented by air and space
Pitta is represented by fire and water
Kapha is represented by earth and water

AYURVEDA ACTION
Add a Slice of Ginger

Power up your hot spice water {xvi} this time of year. Add a slice of fresh ginger to add more heat to pacify Vata and Kapha. You can continue with this addition through Kapha season, which in many locations goes until June. When Pitta arrives in July, stop the ginger add-on and let your spice water cool to room temperature.

JANUARY 3
START IN YOUR IMAGINATION

What is your highest hope for life? Create a clear vision in your mind. Hold this image lightly now and let it change and evolve through the year. As you imagine a desired future, make small daily decisions that align with your vision. As the image finds a home in your subconscious, sometimes you're unaware you've made a decision toward alignment. These daily readings can keep your vision active as a new you takes root.

What is the desired state of being for Ayurveda? The revered state is a life emerging from the luxurious foundation of physical, emotional, and spiritual "ojas"! See {May 19} to find out more about it now.

As you move on a path of vibrant health, the reward is tapping into universal energy and intelligence and feeling good. That is wonderful, but health isn't the only goal. You want what good health provides—better moods to enjoy your loved ones, more energy to accomplish work, more joy to be a blessing to others, more excitement for the day, and falling asleep at night feeling fulfilled. We all want happiness. Those on a spiritual path also want enlightenment. Ayurveda is creation and Nature's beauty springs from the underlying field of possibilities.

AYURVEDA ACTION
Explore Your Highest Hope

Want to resolve a particular health challenge or make a specific change in your life? Why wait? Explore this book to find Ayurveda guidance that feels important to you.

Getting knowledge and support for your pressing issue will motivate you to more fully receive the vast knowledge of Ayurveda. You'll become hungry for it. Check out the index and explore a few ideas to improve your health and happiness today.

JANUARY 4
WHAT MOTIVATES YOU?

IMAGINE A LIFE of dynamic health and radiant vitality. Many people, maybe even you, are unable to find themselves in that beautiful life. It is natural to be interested in change and also be *tamasic*, resistant to change. Consider why.

FIRST:
You may need custom knowledge of yourself and specific strategies that work for you. Even with a general idea of healthy habits, you may not know what distinct foods are best for you, which herbs to take, and what kinds of activity can keep you healthy. Ayurveda begins with a constitutional assessment, including your current state of imbalance. From this start you, or you together with an Ayurvedic practitioner, can then develop an improvement plan that is customized and holistic—and based on more than 5,000 years of science and practice.

SECOND:
You've read articles and online posts about healthy habits. You know plenty of things you could do to be healthier, but maybe you are not doing them consistently enough to have a significant, sustained impact that leads to an elevated state. The right system can help you find the committed, focused energy to effectively do the things that will sustain you in a state of radiant health. You need momentum to break the mind and body habits that keep you down or stuck.

THIRD:
You might not have a vision for radiant health. You might even believe, at some deep level, that it is impossible or that you are not worthy. It is possible! You are worthy! You need to believe you can make that quantum leap to another orbit of reality. What will fuel this propulsion? What are the obstacles? Fear is a factor. Many people fear death less than painful or lackluster senior years. Recognizing this fear may provide motivation and commitment to sustain significant actions.

As you begin to drop weight and blockages you've been carrying, more energy becomes available for healthier attitudes, strength, and physical capacities. It is a virtuous cycle that supports your vision for radiant health. Begin in some small way and then notice and be inspired by results. Ayurveda will help you take the first steps toward restored health and will nourish and sustain you in full radiance.

AYURVEDA ACTION
Break Through with Custom Knowledge

TAKE ASSESSMENT 1 at the end of this book. There are many online Ayurveda assessments as well. Once you identify your Prakruti (constitution), and your Vikruti (current imbalance), you can keep these in mind as you learn more about Ayurveda. More on how to work with these as we go.

JANUARY 5
REASON ENOUGH

LET'S LOOK DEEPLY into the "why" of your exploration of Ayurveda.

- Are you having more frequent colds and flu, or just learned you have some other serious illness?
- Has an important relationship collapsed? What emotional patterns have come to the forefront?
- Is the energy of youth wavering? Does it take longer to recover from strains and events?
- Do you wish to maintain robust health as you age?

Shattering experiences can bring you to the brink of change and yet still, you hesitate. Maybe you no longer feel authentic. Or perhaps devastation isn't what inspires change, but rather a higher calling. Often, a call to change comes from incongruence with a new life that is trying to manifest on the planet.

Your reason is both unique and shared by others–and here you are. Regardless of how you have come here, your choices can spiral you upward to a higher, radiant, more integrated stage of consciousness.

AYURVEDA ACTION
Start One New Healthy Habit

A GOOD WAY to form a good habit is to intercept one that exists. Associate the timing with something you are already doing. Here are examples to consider:

- I will scrape my tongue {Apr 20} in the morning to remove ama.
  What is the first thing you do in the morning? Wash your face or brush your teeth? Set a tongue scraper or a spoon next to the items you use first—your washcloth or toothbrush, for instance.
- I will walk three mornings a week.
  Put walking clothes, socks and shoes by your bed, and don't let your feet touch the ground until you are dressed for the walk.
- I will drink hot spice water daily. {xvi}.
  Make up a batch of spices weekly. Consider putting the spices in your teapot or thermos as you turn off lights for the night.

Get the idea? There is a whole science to habit change. One book I recommend is *The Power of Habit* by Charles Duhigg.

JANUARY 6
QUALITIES ON A SEESAW

AYURVEDA USES 20 qualities, appearing in 10 pairs, to help us understand the fundamental nature of everything in our world. By understanding the qualities of manifest items—such as food or the furniture in our home, as well as energetic existence like emotions or thoughts—we can make intelligent choices for healing.

Ayurvedic knowledge and progress are experienced as a mixture or balance of these qualities. An excess or deficiency of one can lead to an imbalance—so eat food, engage in lifestyle activities and take herbs activated with opposite qualities to balance the seesaw.

Heavy—Light
Unctuous/Oily—Dry
Stable—Mobile
Slimy/Smooth—Rough
Gross—Subtle
Cold—Hot
Slow—Sharp
Soft—Hard
Dense—Liquid
Cloudy—Clear

Invoke opposite qualities to create harmony. For instance, mustard greens have hot and light qualities. Strawberries are cold and light. Acorn squash has a heavy quality. Emotions also have qualities that need to be balanced. Anger is hot and sharp. Cool and soft foods and experiences balance anger and pacify Pitta. One of my favorite sources of information about the qualities of food is the joyfulbelly.com website.

AYURVEDA ACTION
Notice the Qualities in Food

PAY ATTENTION AS you prepare food. Is the dish heavy or light? Is it hot or cold, regardless of temperature? Is it dense or light? As you begin to see the qualities of your food, you will learn how to consume a dosha-balancing diet by introducing foods with the opposite qualities from those that are currently excessive.

What are the qualities of adding peppers to your food? Do you need heat to balance Vata or Kapha cold? If you have too much heat, how about eating cucumbers? As you understand the nature of food, you'll develop the ability to make changes by thinking it through rather than memorizing what you should eat for balance.

JANUARY 7
YOU ARE WHAT YOU EAT *AND*...

"You are what you eat" is a reminder to consume what nourishes and avoid junk food (and thoughts) for the reward of good health. Ayurveda expands on this: You are what you eat *and* what you do not eliminate.

Fresh, clean food, prepared with love, influences consciousness and feelings. It can fortify every cell with natural, birthright intelligence. In this state of heightened cellular intelligence, your energy is vital and your health radiant.

Spices, often used in seed form, contain concentrated forms of Nature's intelligence. They rise up from the underlying field of consciousness, also known as the quantum field. Most foods begin to deteriorate when they are picked. Seeds hold their potency and productive blueprint for more than a year to enable planting and new growth.

Ayurveda is the science of life. The approach is to support a person's return to a balanced life close to Nature. Food intake can throw you off, and the Western diet has become dangerously poor. Detox cleansing comes first if you need it, and then diet is a good place to focus your daily efforts for big improvements.

AYURVEDA ACTION
Add Intelligent Digestive Spices

Adding spice seeds to your daily diet will sound a healthier tuning fork in your physical and emotional body. Feel the resonance of intelligence and life force. Enjoy the bliss of fine-tuning through the easy practice of adding herbs and spices to your diet.

Top Digestive Spices:

- Coriander seed is among the most cooling of five digestive spices and eases excess Pitta heat.
- Cardamom seed makes foods easier to digest. A member of the ginger family, it reduces extreme acidity of food and coffee and supports a healthy liver.
- Cumin seed is a powerful digestive spice. It detoxifies and boosts agni (digestive fire), even though it cools the digestive system.
- Fennel seed combats gas and bloating and serves all three doshas. Fennel is very sattvic (pure) and is great for digestion.

JANUARY 8
GUIDING PRINCIPLES

One way not to be overwhelmed about what is helpful and what is destructive in an Ayurveda lifestyle is to understand its underlying principles and apply them to think through your choices. Here are three principles to guide your engagement with Ayurveda.

PRINCIPLE 1: RESTORE AND MAINTAIN BALANCE

When your three doshas are balanced to your original constitution, when digestion and metabolism are strong, when your seven-tissue layers are nourished, when you have proper elimination of wastes, when your mental-emotional state is balanced and you have a contented soul, radiant health follows.

PRINCIPLE 2: INTRODUCE LIKE/UNLIKE

Like (similar) increases like. Unlike (opposite, dissimilar) decreases like. To reduce excessive qualities, introduce the opposite. To reinforce strong qualities, do more of the same.

PRINCIPLE 3: CONNECT WITH SOURCE OF CONSCIOUSNESS

Connect with the tremendous power of the source of consciousness—the energy and intelligence of the underlying field—to re-create wholeness and health.

Your life is always in the state of movement. It is dynamic, and a multitude of processes are happening as you navigate your daily experiences and emotions. Even when sleeping, great activity of body and mind—sometimes dramatic and sometimes quiet—is happening. These Ayurvedic principles can guide you to make effective, continuous course corrections.

In the next few readings, we will explore each principle one at a time.

AYURVEDA ACTION
Understand the Principles to Guide Your Decisions

UNDERSTANDING AND APPLYING these principles is a navigation system. Without understanding, your option is to try to memorize everything to make choices—not good. Slippages and breakthroughs will happen. Be kind to yourself as you learn. Ayurveda is a lifestyle, not a quick fix. Lifestyle changes are slow-moving and long-lasting. That is why I wrote this book, to offer you a supportive voice every day for a year. For a more constant reminder, copy the three principles into a form you can put on your refrigerator or bathroom mirror, or take along with you anywhere.

JANUARY 9
PRINCIPLE 1—BALANCE LEADS TO RADIANT HEALTH

PRINCIPLE 1

When your three doshas are balanced to your original constitution, when your digestion and metabolism are strong, when your seven-tissue layers are nourished, when you have proper elimination of wastes, when your mental-emotional state is balanced and you have a contented soul, radiant health follows.

Hmmm...maybe read that again. This is the big picture of how health at all levels works to integrate and balance well-being. Every day you react to change to find a new balance. The body uses doshas to buffer changes to prevent disease. When you maintain a ratio similar to your original constitution, you have good health.

When the weather changes, or stressors erupt, or you eat unhelpful foods or eat them in a way that is unsettling, or you are thrust from your comfort zone, the doshas are the first responders. They can become aggravated or elevated. With small changes or strong resilience, the doshas accommodate the daily dynamics without noticeable effect. However, if the body's capacity to deal with change is overextended, or life's demands agitate you mentally or emotionally, or if you are already depleted, then imbalances lead to problems, and possibly, disease.

AYURVEDA ACTION
Determine Your Vikruti Imbalance and What It Means

Review your Assessment 1 results. The goal is to restore balance to your Prakruti (P for primal). However, your current imbalance, Vikruti (V for variable), is of greater interest and will be the focus. When Vikruti is tamed, Prakruti is restored.

The doshic column total with the highest number for your "Current Doshic Balance/Imbalance –Vikruti" indicates the one most out of balance. If two are high, like Vata and Pitta, choose where to start. Look at the attributes in the assessment, and if one has items that feel critical to your well-being, start with that dosha. If you cannot decide, and Vata is one of the doshas, choose Vata. Vata is responsible for more than half of presenting health conditions and is the easiest to go out of balance and will often bring other doshas back into balance when restored.

Review the guidance in this book on what happens when your dosha is out of balance. Review the Three Doshas At-A-Glance Chart at the end of this book. Check out the index and look other places as well. What if a particular dosha is out of balance? What qualities will get agitated, what results from that imbalance, and what can you do about it? Doshic balancing will be revisited throughout the book. These readings and actions are most helpful when you know which dosha is out of balance.

JANUARY 10
PRINCIPLE 2—LIKE ↑ LIKE VS. UNLIKE ↓ LIKE

PRINCIPLE 2

Like (similar) increases like. Unlike (opposite, dissimilar) decreases like. Principle 2 says that to reduce excessive qualities, introduce the opposite. To reinforce strong qualities, do more of the same. To find the balance noted in principle 1, apply the principle of similar and opposites.

THIS PRINCIPLE IS the lever for balancing actions in Ayurveda. Excessive doshas are brought into balance by eating foods and doing activities that draw the opposite to us, digesting and integrating the quality to restore balance. For example, if Vata is excessive with dryness, add moisture through warm, cooked, moist foods or abhyanga (warm oil self-massage). If Pitta is excessive with heat, cool it with walks in the moonlight or eat foods with cooling effects, such as watermelon. If Kapha is excessive, we are sluggish. Find balance by exercising and adding pungent spices to foods.

Become observant of the qualities within yourself and what you are taking in from the world. Look for the qualities of foods and activities. By recognizing what is out of balance, you engage the law of similar and opposites to activate and increase the opposite quality. Balance results. Low doshas tend to rise when balance is restored to the excessive one.

AYURVEDA ACTION
Introduce Foods that Balance

WITH A DOSHA to balance identified, go to the Three Doshas At-A-Glance Chart at the end of this book and find the row "Foods that Balance." The list offers opposite qualities to the dosha it pacifies. Choose three vegetables, two spices, and one grain to introduce to your diet this week. If your dosha is Kapha, wet and heavy, select foods on the list that bring dryness and light. Opposite qualities pacify. Makes a lot of sense, doesn't it?

JANUARY 11
PRINCIPLE 3—CONNECT WITH THE SOURCE OF CONSCIOUSNESS

PRINCIPLE 3

Connection with the tremendous power of the source of consciousness—the energy and intelligence of the underlying field—re-creates wholeness and health.

HEALTH IS WHOLENESS—WHOLE with the source of healing. Healing is organized and intelligent. We are energetic beings who utilize energy and information contained in the underlying field. Once connected to the underlying field of consciousness, a smooth flow of consciousness or energy to and through your physical, emotional, and spiritual body is available for nourishment, to release blocks, and to move natural intelligence into all aspects of your being. This is the radiance. This is the Nature of Ayurveda.

Clearly, this is not a quick process. It is a lifestyle path. Rewards and challenges accompany the path. In the journey is the beauty and reward. It is a cake that can be baked.

Everyone has moments of connecting with this underlying field. Being in love, witnessing a baby's birth, enjoying a breathtaking view of Nature, being moved by a celestial piece of music—things like these connect you to the life-giving energetic field. These blissful moments can motivate you to be in that connection more frequently. Regular meditation is one of the best-known ways for cultivating an experience of the great underlying field.

AYURVEDA ACTION
Find Your Sweet Spot

WHERE, WHEN, AND how do you connect with the Underlying Field of Consciousness? Think about this as your "sweet spot" in life. You may have many ways to be in this sweetness. Find them often.

How can you choose to spend more time in this field? Meditate regularly? Plan time in Nature, play in your garden, create art, or share your love more? Perhaps make a gentle shift in awareness about what you eat. Whatever connects you to the Underlying Field, do more of it today!

JANUARY 12
PANCHABHUTAS—FIVE ELEMENTS

In Ayurveda, the five elements are called the Panchabhutas. Pancha means five, and bhuta means elements or living entities. The three doshas as well as life, Nature, and the entire universe arise from these elements. The panchabhutas are space, air, fire, water, and earth. Space is most subtle, and earth is most dense.

Each element has an associated sense organ for receiving and experiencing the element and also a seat in the body, the first place the element may go out of balance. You will learn which organ goes with which element in subsequent entries.

Let's recall how the doshas and elements relate to each other. Doshas are balanced by applying the principle of opposites to the qualities that have become excessive. The qualities come from the elements that shape the doshas:

- Vata is created of air and space.
- Pitta is created of fire and water.
- Kapha is created of earth and water.

The next five entries will advance your foundational knowledge of the elements.

AYURVEDA ACTION
Be Mindful of Your Senses

Honoring your senses can relax and ground you and restore your connection to Nature, especially when you are overwhelmed or stressed. Try this five-senses mindfulness activity:

1. Sit in a comfortable upright position.
2. Notice your breathing: in—out—inhale—exhale.
3. Bring awareness to each sense for about one minute.

    a. Hear—Notice sounds around you, near and far. Try not to judge, just notice. Are you hearing more than you would normally?
    b. Smell—Shift attention to odors. Can you detect food, plants, or even paper?
    c. See—Observe colors, shapes, movements, and textures.
    d. Taste—What can you taste even without food? Run your tongue around your mouth. Does your saliva have a flavor?
    e. Touch—Notice where your body touches the chair or where the air touches your skin. You might also pick something up to feel it.
    f. Do you feel differently from five minutes ago?

JANUARY 13
PANCHABHUTA – SPACE

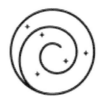

SPACE (OR ETHER): Akasha in Sanskrit. This is the first and most subtle element, from which all things come and to which all things return. It is the essence of emptiness, like a limitless container holding the other elements. This emptiness has a dynamic quality of aliveness and potentiality. It is the space the other elements fill.

Space (or ether), unlike the other elements, comes from the absence of qualities. For instance, ether is cold because it "lacks" the warmth of fire. Ether is light, immobile, subtle, omnipresent. It has no forms or boundaries. Ether is contained in all other elements. Winter is the season of ether.

Ether is sound in its primordial form. Sound and ether are inseparable. The ear is the sense organ. This is how we receive and offer sound.

Ether is expressed in the body's empty spaces—bladder, blood vessels, intestines, lungs, and the mind, which is formless and limitless. When ether is impaired in the body, space increases where there was once structure. Parkinson's disease is an example of increased emptiness where structure once was. Vata is comprised of ether and air, so disturbance in these elements disturbs Vata.

A Sattvic (undisturbed) mind is the greatest expression of ether.

AYURVEDA ACTION
Keep Your Life Richly Filled

ONE WAY TO keep Vata healthy is to keep ether from increasing. You can do this by filling your life. It's not about keeping busy, but rather attending to proper nourishment physically, emotionally, and spiritually. This can mean moist, heavy, nutrient-rich real foods for physical health. The highest form of emotional nourishment is love. Honor your spiritual path. Ether element practices are ripe with devotion and meditation. Serving your path serves you. Can you identify one area where you are uncomfortably "empty?" This is Vata. Reflect on how to fill this particular void. Hint, it may not be food.

JANUARY 14
PANCHABHUTA—AIR

Air: Vayu in Sanskrit. Air evolves from ether and is responsible for all forces, movement, and kinetic energy. The origin of air is sparsha, which is the unmanifest, primordial form of touch. Touch and air are inseparable—skin is the primary sense organ. Dysfunction of the air element results in tactile issues or grasping physically or emotionally. The influence of the air element is seen in the seasonal changes, in the movement of the nervous system and mobility, and the autumn.

Air qualities are subtle, cool, light, mobile, dry, rough, flowing, sharp, hard, and clear. The concept of vayu (air) is synonymous with prana (life force). The ancient rishis described the five directions of the vayus or prana: inward (prana); outward (vyana); upward (udana), downward (apana). The force that pulls toward the center and balances these movements is samana. These directions are the subdoshas of Vata. More on that in later day entries.

The force of movement is air, which activates blood flow, breathing, nerve communication, joint movement, and thought flow. Excess movements cause hyperactivity, for instance, or heart racing. When air is deficient, movement forces are dull and sluggish, as in constipation or joint immobility. Positive air qualities are sustained through steady, healthy routines.

Vata is made of air and ether, and is vitiated, or impaired, when either is imbalanced. When the motion of air is controlled yet flowing, Vata is at its best.

AYURVEDA ACTION
Stay Grounded

Steady routines and healthy, grounding food keep air element in good form and Vata happy. A heavier diet of nourishing foods, like winter squashes, is perfect for maintaining stability. Air flows freely in a body and mind that has cultivated surrender and attention to the Self and the divine.

A yoga practice that is gently mobile, light, cool, and grounding will keep the air element in check. A devotional practice with pranayamas (breath work) also will lift spirits yet ground energy.

JANUARY 15
PANCHABHUTA—FIRE

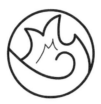

Fire: Tejas in Sanskrit. Tejas evolves from ether and air. The fire element is responsible for all transformation and generates energy for us and for the universe. The essence of the fire element is rupa, which means form or color, associated with perception, light, understanding, luster, energy, and vision. The eyes are the associated sense organ.

The fire element promotes digestive activity, and the primary fire for that is pachaka agni. Digestive fires exist in all systems and in each cell. The fire element, for instance, stimulates our neural synapses at the minute level as well as our larger transformations, including mental and emotional shifts. Summer is the season of fire.

The qualities of fire are hot, light, dry, rough, subtle, flowing, sharp, clear, and soft. Excess fire results in a build-up of heat, causing inflammation, skin rashes, intense emotions, or fever. Lack of fire results in loss of skin luster, poor digestion, or a sluggish mind.

When fire is right, we are focused and energetic, and we digest food and ideas more easily.

AYURVEDA ACTION
Fire Up Agni

Weight gain or sluggishness might indicate low fire. Increase digestive fires with hot and spicy foods and avoid heavy and cold foods. Make the diet spicier and lighter until digestion returns to normal. Healthy digestion is characterized by minimal gas, along with a daily bowel movement in the morning and perhaps one more later in the day.

Hot, energetic yoga and particularly kundalini yoga will increase the fire element.

JANUARY 16
PANCHABHUTA—WATER

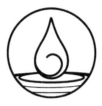

WATER: JALA AND apas in Sanskrit. Water evolves from ether, air, and fire. The origin of water is rasa or taste. The tongue is the sense organ of water. Without water in our mouth, we cannot taste. Spring is the season of the water element.

A bit of water is found in Pitta, but mostly in Kapha. Water element is cool, stable, fluid, heavy, moist, smooth, gross, dull, cloudy, and soft. Water is responsible for the initial connection of egg and sperm, thought to emotion, and the magnetism of love. Water is connection, cohesion, and protection.

Too much moist or oily food and water can build up to douse digestive fire, which slows the digestive process. Signs of this are reduced appetite or heaviness in the stomach. When digestion is sluggish, water can seep out from our digestive system into our tissues, with a possible result of edema or obesity.

Water deficiency results in dehydration, dry skin, dry mucus, decreased urination, or weight loss.

Water cools our fires so they do not rage out of control, and it keeps us moving, at ease, and connected to others.

AYURVEDA ACTION
Increase the Water Element

THE SWEET TASTE is the primary source of water in our diet. If you are feeling too warm, inflamed, dehydrated, emaciated, ungrounded, irritable, thin, sharp-tongued, immobile, or your heart has hardened, increase the water element. Try eating more cooked grains, oils, raw nuts, fatty meats (if you eat meat), and juicy fruits. These are the sweet taste in Ayurveda. Remember, it's not about eating sugar.

Of course, be sure to hydrate with water. Most people need to drink more water every day. Hot water is more hydrating than room temperature water, and you should avoid iced water unless you are seriously overheated. Pittas may need to stick with room-temperature water.

Issues around loss of appetite, a feeling of heaviness after eating, overweight, or signs of chronic swelling in the body mean too much water element. Decrease watery foods.

Try a flowing yoga or sensual yoga practice to fortify the water element.

JANUARY 17
PANCHABHUTA—EARTH

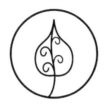

Earth: Prithvi in Sanskrit. Earth evolves from and contains the essence of all the elements. Earth is responsible for the physical form, structure, and the development of body tissue and all of creation. It is the most gross, the least subtle. Though you tend to identify with your body, it is the furthest from who you really are.

The primordial origin of the earth element is the sense of smell, called ganha. The nose is the sense organ, processing scents and impressions of all creation. Earth element is kept in balance through consumption and defecation. Too much earth released results in diarrhea and your structure weakens. Too little earth released creates constipation. The Kapha dosha is made of earth and water. When water is vitiated, Kapha is out of balance.

Earth is cool, stable, heavy, dry, rough, gross, dense, dull, clear, and hard. Earth is prevalent in the seasons of late winter and early spring, and we should eat lighter, high-quality foods in these times.

If you are feeling too warm, chaotic, emaciated, vulnerable, stressed, or ungrounded, you need the cool, stable qualities of earth. Deficiencies in the earth element result in weaknesses in body tissues and bones, and muscle mass is replaced by fat. You might often feel cold and get pushed aside because you cannot "hold your ground."

AYURVEDA ACTION
Eat for Earth

Feed and nourish your earth element by eating real food that comes from the earth and by spending time in Nature. The earth element is the structure of all foods but is especially found in grains, nuts, root vegetables, meats, and moderately in dairy. You can consume more of these to increase the earth element.

When there is too much earth element, such as with overeating, the body tissues get too much raw building material. Tissues become bigger and thicker, which results in pressure and possibly inflammation. Excess raw materials can get stored as fat. In this case, reduce grains, nuts, meats, and dairy.

A yoga earth practice calls on your capacity to build strength and stability.

JANUARY 18
SEVEN DHATUS

Fully digested food nourishes the tissues (dhatus) beginning with plasma and working its way to the more sophisticated reproductive fluids. Agni, digestive fire, ignites this transformative process as nutrients move from one tissue level to the next. What we eat and the experiences we have nourish even our most complex tissues. Complete seven-layer nourishment can take six days to a month or more. An imbalance within any tissue affects tissue nourishment down the line. More on these topics to come.

SEVEN LAYERS OF TISSUES—THE DHATUS

1. Plasma (Rasa)
2. Blood (Rakta)
3. Muscle (Mamsa)
4. Fat (Meda)
5. Bone (Asthi)
6. Bone marrow and nerves (Majja)
7. Reproductive fluids and seed (Shukra—male, Andartava—female)

AYURVEDA ACTION
Stay Hydrated for Healthy Plasma and Blood

Plasma is the liquid that holds blood cells in suspension. Staying hydrated is an important action for keeping plasma healthy and nourishment flowing to the next tissue level, blood. You learned about drinking hot spice water to promote digestion, and it's extremely hydrating as well. When boiled water is drunk warm, or even cooled to room temperature, the air and fire quality drives hydration further into the tissue layers.

Coconut water also is ideal for hydration because of its excellent electrolyte composition. It has an ideal composition ratio of sugar, sodium, potassium, and other electrolytes. In World War II, it was used as IV (intravenous) hydration. It has a slight laxative effect. Coconut water is especially helpful if you are dehydrated from being sick or if you have been cleansing, exercising, or sunning. Your action of the day is to try coconut water. I like the organic version that has bits of coconut in it. If you like coconut water, it is a great addition to your daily hydration.

Just one serving of coconut water per day during Vata season is enough, because even though it is hydrating for imbalanced, dry Vata, it is also cooling.

JANUARY 19
THREE MALAS FROM FOOD AND TISSUES

MALAS ARE THE body's waste products. Our body processes food and breaks down nutrients in our tissues, which creates waste. It is important to get rid of wastes easily and regularly.

Ahara Malas—waste from food

- Urine
- Feces
- Sweat

Dhatu Malas—waste from tissues

- Secretions of the nose, eyes, ears
- Lactic acid, carbon dioxide, and other metabolites of cellular respiration
- Exfoliated hair, skin, and nails

Just as it's important to build tissue with good, nourishing food, it is equally important to eliminate waste efficiently. Without good elimination, you will retain ama, which can lead to disease. My Ayurveda teacher, Dr. Paul Dugliss, taught that constipation is the first thing to deal with when looking to improve health. This makes sense. If we don't get rid of wastes, they can be reabsorbed, which blocks the process of complete digestion. Consider the actions below, but see what is right and safe for you.

AYURVEDA ACTION
Encourage Healthy, Regular Bowel Movements

NOT HAVING A daily bowel movement? Try these Ayurveda approaches.

- Upon arising, drink a glass of warm or hot water with lemon.
- Hot spice water to the rescue again—it has a slight laxative effect.
- Increase your intake of healthy organic oils like coconut and avocado oil for cooking and room-temperature olive oil.
- Eat juicy fruits like grapes, strawberries, mangoes or water-soaked raisins and dates; or drink prune or pineapple juice.
- Make a tea of 1/2 tsp powdered triphala in a cup of hot water at bedtime. Some people take 1–2 triphala tablets at bedtime, which is not as effective but more convenient.

JANUARY 20
VIBRATING WITH THREE GUNAS

The three gunas—sattva, rajas, and tamas—are the fundamental vibrations that weave the cosmos. They are irreducible and operate at the most subtle levels of the universe. Our state of mind is reflected in the presence and strength of the gunas. As in all of Ayurveda, the goal is to balance the gunas and enliven the helpful functions that contribute goodness to our lives.

People interested in Ayurveda have influences from all the gunas, but rajas typically is the most out of tune for us and often more sattva has been cultivated. Increasingly, fear and lack of judgment are being stimulated in our global society, which brings out the tamasic qualities that lower vibration. Tamas is present when you experience grief or exhaustion.

Tamas is the quality of inertia and resistance. It primarily influences the Kapha dosha. Tamas means darkness in Sanskrit—it is absent the movement of rajas and the light of sattva. In excess, tamas produces apathy, sloth, destruction, passivity, chaos, and confusion. It is a heavy quality. Tamas might sound totally negative, but sometimes we need the force of destruction to let go of what no longer works. The chaos or confusion of tamas can be a good sign—that you're releasing old patterns.

Rajas is the quality of motion and energy, and often characterizes the Pitta dosha. In excess, it can produce physical and emotional pain, nervousness, restlessness, thoughtless change, addiction to activity, and hyperactivity. Healthy rajas is mobilizing and energizing and stirs us to bold action and passionate living.

Sattva is the stabilizing cosmic intelligence force and a strong influencer of the Vata dosha. Sattva is expressed as luminosity. Its qualities are harmony, goodness, balance, purity, pleasure, contentment, truthfulness, and peacefulness. When your mind is sattvic, you have access to inner wisdom and the light of the spiritual path. To live radiantly, focus on increasing your sattvic nature and leaning toward the "good sides" of rajas and tamas.

Use Assessment 2 at the end of this book to understand your guna state.

AYURVEDA ACTION
Add Light

Light is the symbol of sattva, so burn a candle or walk in the moonlight. A salt lamp, with its soft, warm-pink tone, is especially helpful in the bedroom, inviting rest by signaling to your circadian rhythm center that the day is ending. Mine is on a timer and is set to come on at 6 a.m. to 7 a.m. and 9 p.m. to 10 p.m. each day.

JANUARY 21
OJAS—SANSKRIT FOR VIGOR

THE THREE VITAL essences—prana, tejas, and ojas—are the positive forms of Vata, Pitta, and Kapha doshas, respectively. Ojas is both a concept and a substance. In Sanskrit, ojas (oh-jas) means "vigor" and relates to our physical, emotional, and spiritual well-being—all one in Ayurveda. Ojas gives rise to vitality, immunity, radiance, sound sleep, physical tone, happiness, compassion, cohesion, resilience, contentment, and spiritual strength. As a concept, ojas represents radiant health and a bioscience of high-level functioning. Ojas as a substance is an expression of consciousness that leads to this state of vitality.

Ojas is the ultimate refined product of the most subtle level of proper and complete metabolism, digestion, assimilation, and absorption of food and experiences. Through healthy agni (digestive fire) and balanced digestion, we create ojas. It is the fundamental energetic essence of food—a "cosmic glue" that engages cells to function in organized wholeness resulting in radiance and bliss. Ojas, the juice of life, pervades all tissues, cells, and spaces and connects mind, body, and consciousness. If food transforms quickly into ojas, it is good for immunity. If our experiences are interpreted with gentleness and an open heart, ojas is added to our consciousness.

In Western medicine, ojas would be connected to peptides and small protein molecules. Certain peptides are neurotransmitters that control our immunity and hormones, plus our digestive and nervous systems.

How do we get more ojas? The answer is simple. Perfect digestion of food and experiences equals ojas. Also—drink Hot Date Nut Milk to build ojas. It pacifies all doshas but especially Vata. This drink is revered for ojas boosting.

AYURVEDA ACTION
Drink Hot Date Nut Milk for Ojas

---

1. Soak 10 raw organic almonds and 2-3 organic Medjool dates overnight.
2. Peel almonds in morning (or alternatively-quick peel by soaking in boiled water for about 2 minutes then drain and rinse with cold water and pop out the almonds).
3. Boil 1 1/2-2 Cups organic raw whole milk or milk alternative like coconut milk.
4. Put peeled almonds in a blender and add:
    - Peeled and pitted dates
    - 1 tsp ghee (or up to 1 Tbl)
    - Ground spices-about 1/4 tsp or to taste—mix of cardamom, cloves, and cinnamon (can fresh grind every few weeks)
    - 1/4 tsp green spirulina powder. Can add Chyawanprash or herbs like ashwagandha

JANUARY 22
PRAKRUTI/PRIMAL AND VIKRUTI/VARIABLE

Let's review.

Vata is created of air and space.

Pitta is created of fire and water.

Kapha is created of earth and water.

These doshas play and interact within you to create your state of health. Ayurveda looks at two levels of this interplay: Your Prakruti and your Vikruti.

Prakruti (P for primal)

Prakruti is your unique, primal constitution, or doshic makeup, from birth. It never changes except by rare transformation. A person might have more Pitta, modest Vata, and a little Kapha in his or her Prakruti, for instance. Prakruti can be assessed by looking at lifelong qualities and attributes. Jyotish—Ayurveda astrology—can definitively determine your Prakruti using your birth time, location, and date.

Vikruti (V for variable)

Vikruti is your current doshic ratio that varies with circumstance and state of imbalance. Prakruti shows what is strongest for you, which gives clues as to what might go out of balance in Vikruti. Your strongest dosha might not always be the most imbalanced. Vikruti is assessed by looking at current symptoms and issues. An Ayurvedic practitioner typically will determine Vikruti through a pulse and tongue assessment and an in-depth health interview. The inventory in Assessment 1 is a start to understanding your current imbalance.

AYURVEDA ACTION
Know Your Prakruti and Vikruti

LOOK AT YOUR results from the Prakruti/Vikruti in Assessment 1. Whatever is strongest in your constitution, known as your Prakruti, often is susceptible to going out of balance, but that might not be the case for you. However, it is worth watching your strong, constitutional doshas. Vikruti is what to work with first—know the current imbalance and restore to balance. When your Vikruti is fairly balanced, you will be able to live more fully in the Nature that is your Prakruti. But first things first. Know your constitution, but work with your Vikruti, imbalances that can be affected by diet, lifestyle, environment, season, and stage in life.

JANUARY 23
THREE DOSHAS: VATA, PITTA, KAPHA

Understanding the doshas is foundational. We will continue to revisit them, looking at different layers of doshic influence. Ayurveda's primary strategies for doshic balancing are:

1. Determine your out-of-balance dosha, meaning that which is excessive.
2. Understand the dosha's qualities.
3. Introduce the opposite qualities to bring the dosha to balance.

	VATA	*PITTA*	*KAPHA*
Function	Movement, transportation, communication	Digestion, metabolism, and transformation	Strength, structure, immunity, lubrication
Keyword	Changeable	Intense	Relaxed
Elements	Air & Space	Fire & Water	Water & Earth
Physical	Thinness	Medium sized, good muscle tone	Strong frames, strong immune system
Governs	Colon, nervous system, bones	Small intestines, stomach, liver, skin	Structure, lubrication in body/mind
Qualities	Light, dry, rough, dark, changeable, movable, subtle	Hot, sharp, pungent, intense, flowing (but grounded)	Unctuous (oily), cold, heavy, sticky, slimy, moist, stable, strong, soft, slow, steady
In Balance	Enthusiastic, creative, spirited	Strong digestive fire, goal-oriented, successful, smart, analytical	Good-natured, sweet, loving, calm, loyal
Out of Balance	Tire easily, gas, anxious, fearful, dry, constipated	Excessive digestive fire, heated emotions, sensitive to heat/light	Slow moving, slow digestion, lethargic, depression, mucus, colds, overweight

AYURVEDA ACTION
Go for Understanding

Aim to understand the Nature of each dosha rather than memorize all its components and influences and which foods to eat. Which dosha was most out of balance when you took Assessment 1? Study that column in the chart above and consider how the descriptions relate to the dosha. For instance, Vata is made of air and space with associated qualities: light, dry, rough, dark, etc. To balance Vata, eat warm, moist food, do warm-oil massage, and spend time in warm environments.

JANUARY 24
DOUBLE AND TRIPLE DOSHAS

Everyone has a constitution composed of all three doshas, and often one dosha has the greatest influence. However, you might be strongly influenced by two doshas: one dominant and the second close to it. In rare cases, the three doshas show up nearly equally in a person's constitution.

Certainly, more than one dosha can be imbalanced in your Vikruti, which creates a challenge when bringing the doshas in balance. In work with clients, I have found that when all doshas are out of sorts, the issue is ama (toxins), and the first step is to cleanse. Support for cleansing can be found in various entries. {See index.}

Dual and triple dosha influences are tricky because balancing one could introduce the qualities that imbalance another. For instance, introducing warm and moist foods to pacify Vata might aggravate the heat of Pitta and the wetness of Kapha.

But you need to find a place to start. When in doubt, always start with cleansing practices. Sometimes one stronger doshic imbalance will emerge. Or perhaps a serious issue demands attention. Too much heat might leave you with disturbing skin eruptions and inflammation, for example. Pacifying Pitta might be the place to begin. An Ayurvedic practitioner would take your pulse, do a tongue analysis, and conduct an in-depth interview to determine a good starting place.

In the case above, a stronger Vata imbalance may be fanning Pitta's flames and causing irritations. If you are unable to work with an Ayurvedic practitioner, do the best you can using self-assessments. Analyze results to create an action plan. If you notice symptoms and issues getting worse, look at the data again and explore a different route that could also fit with your results. If it is really confusing on where to start, Vata pacifying is often a good call, as this dosha is about movement and so is frequently the first to go out of balance. Vata is aggravated by stress, and it can affect the other doshas.

AYURVEDA ACTION
Determine Your Secondary Doshic Influence

Return to your inventory results from Assessment 1. What is the second highest number for your Vikruti? How much influence does this imbalance have on your health? Look for ways to mitigate effects from balancing the highest dosha on this second one. For instance, if you want to balance Vata, you want to add heat. But if Pitta is running a close second, too much heat isn't good. Consider introducing warm, cooked food, maybe with a light sprinkling of black pepper, but avoid the jalapenos (and hot yoga).

JANUARY 25
DOSHA TIME AND SEASONS

DURING THE SEASONS, the indicated dosha is more easily pressured out of balance. For instance, Vata is more likely to fall out of balance in the fall and early winter's colder weather, which has Vata qualities.

Below are general guides for climates with hot summers and cold winters. But the length of time of the doshic season will be affected by the climate in your location. If you live in a rainforest, Kapha season seems to last forever. Adjust for your locale.

Likewise—the designated dosha also corresponds to the time each day that is most active, and so might be more likely to be out of balance. Work with this knowledge to maximize the influence of that dosha time. Finally, there are doshic times of life.

	VATA	PITTA	KAPHA
Season	fall, early winter	Summer	Winter, early spring
	November—February	July—October	March—June
Clock Time	2-6am & 2-6pm	10am-2pm & 10pm-2am	6-10am & 6-10pm
Life time	About 55-60 +	Middle Age 20-55	Youth: birth to about 20

AYURVEDA ACTION
Know the Best Time of Your Doshas

Let's put a little bit together here. Look at Three Doshas At-A-Glance {Appendix}, which gives an overview of the doshas' qualities, and the chart above. Think on these questions:

- When is the best time to go to bed?
- When is the best time to arise?
- When is the best time to eat your largest meal of the day?

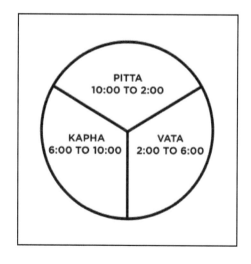

For example. Kapha time is best for sleep because of the qualities of slow, steady, and heavy. By checking the chart above, Kapha time is from 6 p.m. until 10 p.m. The heavier elements predominate in Nature in these hours and favor being in bed before 10 p.m. The best time to eat your largest meal of the day is midday, Pitta time, when digestive fire is the strongest. These are general guidelines, but remember you are the expert on you. Always see what works for your nature and your demands.

JANUARY 26
AMA (TOXINS)

Ama is the Ayurvedic term for the toxins our bodies produce. These toxins build up due to incomplete or improper digestion of food and experiences. In a physical sense, ama is plaque-like and sticky, a white, thick, mucous substance that gunks up the system and inhibits organ function. The thick, white coating on your tongue in the morning is ama and should be scraped off with a spoon or tongue scraper {Apr 20} each morning. Ama is sometimes referred to as "Kapha gone bad." The earth and water qualities of Kapha can get muddy and sluggish—conditions for ama to form.

Digestion transforms inputs from the environment into something useful for your physiology. Inputs include food, pollution, sensory experiences, emotional stimuli, and so on. When physical, emotional, or mental digestion is not strong enough to transform inputs, toxic waste is deposited as ama. We are what we take in and what we do not eliminate.

Emotional ama may take the form of Vata anxiety and fear, Pitta anger and jealousy, and Kapha attachment and depression. Emotional ama interferes with physiology and can lead to physical ailments. Unresolved anger, for instance, can lead to blood-pressure issues as the heart and vessels get restricted. Ever had a sugar rush followed by a letdown? What we eat can affect our emotions and moods.

When digestion is weak or overloaded with the wrong foods, or when food is eaten under the wrong conditions, sticky ama builds up in the digestive tract. If ama continues to accumulate, it can leave the digestive tract and circulate throughout the body. The evolution of disease, or samprapti, begins with digestive toxins. They block the intelligent life force from manifesting and flowing through the body. It is important to eliminate them—and even more important to prevent them.

AYURVEDA ACTION
Detox Daily

Here is a simple Lemon Detox Drink that can be taken and enjoyed every day.

- 1 1/2 cups boiled water
- 1–2 slices of lemon, squeezed
- 1 slice ginger

When dining out, ask for hot water and lemon, a good detox even without ginger. Limit yourself to about 1/2 cup of water with a meal unless your food is very dry.

JANUARY 27
FORMATION OF AMA

FOOD AND EXPERIENCES both nourish you, and Ayurveda considers them equally important. Let's focus on food for now. Here is the ideal:

- Food should be completely and perfectly digested.
- About half of what is eaten is absorbed as nutrients that are delivered throughout our body, so what remains should be eliminated as waste.

But this ideal 50:50 ratio of nourishment to waste can be thrown off course by stress or by consuming improper foods in improper ways. When food is not fully digested, the lump left behind leads to the formation of toxins or ama. So, then you have 1/3 nourishment, 1/3 waste, and 1/3 ama—and you have introduced this third category that is not good for you.

Fat-soluble ama accumulates in the body's fat cells. When under stress, your body reacts to the "emergency situation" and sends a message to store fat for energy in the future. Stress-fat laden with toxins is mostly stored around our bellies and lower bodies. It can provoke a craving for stimulants, sugar, and carbohydrates.

You can prevent ama from collecting by practicing good eating and lifestyle habits (including daily tongue scraping). You can eliminate ama with purification strategies. Even small changes will reward you with more energy, clarity of expression, and strengthened immunity.

AYURVEDA ACTION
Drink Lemon Detox/Weight Loss Tea

HERE'S AN UPGRADE for yesterday's tip:

- 1/16 tsp cayenne pepper
- 1 cup boiled water
- 1/4 lemon, juiced
- 1 tsp raw honey
- 1/8 tsp raw apple cider vinegar (ACV) with the "mother" (i.e. unfiltered)

Mix all ingredients, adding honey when the water has cooled enough to drink. This morning drink clears ama from overnight digestion. You also can sip slowly 30 minutes or more before or after a meal to boost fat digestion and metabolism and stimulate the flow of bile from the liver and gallbladder to your gut to digest fats. Note: Using ACV in larger quantities (>2 tsp) and for more than 30 days without a break is not advised as it can have a negative effect on bone density. ACV is contraindicated for low bone mineral density or osteoporosis.

JANUARY 28
AMA, AMAVISHA, GARAVISHA

How does ama (from internal and environmental factors) become disease? There are three types of toxic progression: ama, amavisha, and garavisha.

Ama often first disturbs the dosha in its home or seat. The seat of Vata is the colon, Pitta the small intestines, and Kapha the stomach. If you see the imbalance in this early stage and address the causal factors, you can clear the ama.

If ama accumulates, it begins to move. Ama on the move accumulates in weakened parts of the body or our weakest emotional states. This second type of toxin is referred to as AMAVISHA, a more reactive, toxic type of ama that begins to manifest in the physiology and appears as disease.

For Vatas, accumulation can be in the joints. Kaphas tend to accumulate ama in fat cells, causing weight gain. Pittas tend to have less ama as their agni (digestive fire) tends to be higher. Pittas can be susceptible to imbibing toxins like alcohol.

The third type of toxin is GARAVISHA, which is external. Environmental toxins increasingly affect our health, including chemicals and pesticides used in agriculture as well as the preservatives and additives used in food production and genetically engineered foods. Food spoiled with harmful bacteria also is considered garavisha. Environmental toxins exist in the home, such as lead, asbestos, arsenic, chemicals in household supplies, and in our clothes, furniture, and carpets. The harmful elements form air and water pollution. Chemical environmental disasters are also garavisha.

AYURVEDA ACTION
Use Environmentally Friendly Cleaners

Using homemade products could reduce garavisha in your home, and you may find you feel better. It's also satisfying to know you are doing your part to protect Mother Nature from assault by harmful chemicals. Try this formula for a simple home cleaning product.

All-Purpose Cleaner

1. Add 2 Tbsp distilled vinegar and 1 tsp liquid castile soap (like Dr. Bronner's) to a glass spray bottle.
2. Add 2 Tbsp baking soda. Wait until foaming stops, then add 2 cups warm water; shake gently.
3. Use on kitchen and bathroom surfaces.

JANUARY 29
AMA BUSTERS

Everyone has ama. Stressful demands, fast food, rushed meals, and lots of change—wanted or not—invite it. Here are nine ways to give ama the boot.

1. Use ginger—in all forms. Cook with minced fresh ginger. Add fresh ginger to boiled water for tea.
2. Sip hot spice water throughout the day: Add 1/2 tsp fennel, 1/4 tsp cumin and 1/4 tsp coriander seeds to a quart of hot water in a thermos.
3. Balance your out-of-balance dosha.
4. Spend time in the arms of Nature, the great rebalancer.
5. Practice meditation and deep breathing.
6. Chew fennel seeds after a meal to improve digestion.
7. Soak in a hot Epsom salt bath. Use 2 cups of salt per bath and enjoy for 20 minutes.
8. Good sleep is essential. Be restful in late evening and go to bed by 10 p.m. Drink a cup of warm coconut or almond milk with fresh ground nutmeg or ashwagandha at bedtime.
9. Clean your home with natural products.

AYURVEDA ACTION
Drink Ama Busting Tea

Here is another tea recipe to try.

- 4 cups boiled water
- 1/2 tsp cumin seeds
- 1/2 tsp coriander seeds
- 1 tsp fennel seed
- 1/2-inch slice ginger
- 5 black peppercorns
- 3 cloves
- 1 shard from cinnamon stick

Add boiling water to dry ingredients. Pour into a teapot or thermos flask. Strain spices before drinking. Sip throughout the day.

JANUARY 30
DINACHARYA—DAILY ROUTINE

Dinacharya is Sanskrit for "daily routine" or "daily ritual of self-care." Occasional dramatic, healthful events don't serve you as well as daily routines that maintain the powerful circadian forces and cycles of Nature. Circadian rhythm is your natural body rhythm, set to an approximately 24-hour clock.

According to Dr. Suhas Kshirsagar, author of *Change Your Schedule, Change Your Life*, the "rhythm directs the body on when to digest food, how to prepare for sleep, and how to regulate everything in your body including blood pressure, metabolism, hormone production, body temperature and cellular repair. Your skin cells, too, repair and regenerate on a daily schedule. Even the population of microbes in your intestinal tract changes on a daily schedule."[7]

What sets this rhythm? Morning light starts the rhythm, and diminished light calms and slows physiology for nighttime rest. Circadian rhythms operate best on natural light, and new research that aligns with the arc of ancient Ayurveda wisdom speaks to the importance of daily habits.

"The body can use social cues, such as timing of meals, sleep, and exercise, as a substitute when light signals are absent."[8] Light entrainment is preferred to set your circadian rhythm, but maintaining daily habits is a secondary support. In our world of artificial light, ubiquitous technologies, and a life pace out of sync with Nature, dinacharya—a daily routine—is your best strategy to keep on track.

Body cells have their own clock and also are engaged or disrupted by the rhythms or the arrhythms of life. When you eat regularly and well, when you get good rest and sleep, and when you experience a liveliness in your daily life, your cells entrain to these rhythms for optimal health. As we learn more about rogue, inflamed, and malfunctioning cells being central to disease, the importance of living in natural light and maintaining good daily habits for cellular health comes into focus.

AYURVEDA ACTION
Eat Early

Many people eat a quick, light lunch and a late, heavy supper. This messes with the circadian rhythms and eons of Ayurveda wisdom. Move toward eating your large meal at midday with rest time after. Load up with nutrient-rich, fresh food and you won't need to overeat. Finish the day with an early, light dinner such as a brothy vegetable soup. Don't snack until morning, when you "break the fast." This schedule is aligned with natural, circadian rhythms.

JANUARY 31
RECAP AND WHAT'S AHEAD

Your Ayurveda year has begun. I hope that the first month of *365 Days of Ayurveda for Lifelong Radiant Health* has been a useful launch. Ayurveda's science of well-being supports a healthy lifestyle that is physically, emotionally, and spiritually radiant. It takes time to learn new ways. Small steps are important.

This month you learned that Ayurveda is born of, and sustained by, consciousness. A connection to the underlying field is your lifeline to well-being. We covered the five elements that emerge from the underlying field, how they form the three doshas, and your doshic ratio. Vata is created of air and space. Pitta is created of fire and water. Kapha is created of earth and water

Early in the month, readings were designed to stimulate reflecting on your motivation to learn about Ayurveda and to make useful changes for your health.

We spent time with three foundational principles:

1. Balance leads to radiant health.
2. Like (similar) increases like. Unlike (opposite, dissimilar) decreases like.
3. Connection with the source of consciousness re-creates wholeness and health.

WHAT'S NEXT?

Next, we will introduce Vata. Its season is generally November through the end of February. We will explore more about agni—the digestive fire and the six tastes. Be patient. It will come together a little at a time.

MONTHLY REFLECTION TIME

What actions did you try? What was your experience? Did you have positive or adverse reactions? What new actions feel worthwhile? Put a check in the third column for actions you plan to incorporate, whether daily, weekly, monthly, seasonally, or on occasion.

What New Actions This Month?	*Your Experience?*	*Habit Worthy?*
		☐
		☐
		☐

FEBRUARY 1
ALL ABOUT VATA

Your combination of three doshas is unique, like a fingerprint. Everyone has Vata influence in their constitution. Vata dominant constitutions tend toward thinness. Even if you are overweight now, if you were thin in youth and most of your life, it could indicate a Vata constitution/Prakruti.

Vata qualities are:

- Dry
- Light
- Cold
- Rough
- Mobile
- Subtle
- Clear

Balanced Vata is enthusiastic, creative, and spirited. Dancers and those who move gracefully on their feet are representative of a Vata constitution. Nicole Kidman, Fred Astaire, and Bruno Mars are classic Vatas. Many artists and spiritual figures have the best of Vata.

The Vata dosha controls the nervous system and body movement functions. Strong Vata constitutions, Prakruti, are most bothered by issues of anxiety, fears, and sleep challenges. Physical issues from excessive dryness in the system can result in digestive issues like constipation, and for women, menstrual cramps. Vatas are light in physical substance, with little reserve from which to draw, so can tire easily. Vatas need sufficient rest and to not overdo it. They do best by eating warm, cooked foods. Because Vatas can be "flighty," a regular lifestyle routine will maintain balance.

You don't have to have a Vata constitution (Prakruti) for your Vata Vikruti to become out of balance. Vata tends to be the first dosha to go out of balance and lead other doshas astray. It is responsible for more than half of the current imbalances. Stress is a major factor in Vata imbalance, so Vata balancing is something everyone needs to do. When Vata is in balance, the other doshas tend to stay in balance.

AYURVEDA ACTION
Check November Readings for More on Vata

We will dive deep into Vata in November, which is the start of the Vata season. Skip ahead to November readings if you are curious about Vata now.

FEBRUARY 2
RITUCHARYA—SEASONAL ACTIONS FOR VATA

February closes Vata season, which generally runs from November to February in cold-winter, hot-summer climates. Leaves blow wildly, the wind howls, the earth has hardened from the cold, and we feel the chill against our skin. People tend to spend more time indoors, which for many people means warm, dry, forced-air heat. This exacerbates Vata.

At this time of year, you should change some seasonal rituals. We will revisit this in November when Vata season begins, but here are ideas for now.

Look at the qualities of Vata season, as these external forces will affect you: dry, rough, light, cold, subtle, and mobile. Even if you do not have a Vata imbalance, Vata will be pushed on in this season and can easily fall out of balance. Remember Principle 2: Like (similar) increases like. Unlike (opposite, dissimilar) decreases like.

Engage practices, activities, and foods with Vata's opposite qualities to prevent imbalances or to restore balance. These form your Vata riticharya or your Vata seasonal routine.

Vata quality	*Balancing quality*	*Example*
Dry	Unctuous	Hydrate with more liquids, watery soups, healthy oils.
Rough	Slimy	Try abhyanga massage to soften skin.
Light	Heavy	Eat grounding foods such as winter squash. Try a heavy comforter on your bed.
Cold	Hot	Eat warm cooked food. Enjoy a sauna.
Subtle	Gross	Build something. Manifest a goal/desire.
Mobile	Stable	Meditate, eat more slowly. Try a grounding yoga practice.

AYURVEDA ACTION
Add Routine to Balance Vata

Establish regular times for daily activities to keep Vata grounded and balanced. In Vata season, consider actions that are warming, stable, and moistening and make them a regular habit. Eat, go to bed and arise, and meditate at regular times. Reflect on the past few days. Are there ways to introduce more regularity in your daily life? Life happens, of course, but try to find your way back to regularity. The Vata in you will be happier.

FEBRUARY 3
WAYS TO PACIFY VATA

You want to eat warm, grounding and moist foods to pacify the cold, dry, and mobile qualities of Vata season. Also, drink warming liquids to help your body keep its temperature in the toasty zone—such as raw cow's milk or milk alternatives with ghee and honey at bedtime. In your warm cooked meals, favor sweet, sour, and salty tastes. More on that later, but here's a preview.

Sweet—fruits, most grains, nuts, seeds, root vegetables, raw milk, ghee

Sour—sauerkraut, kimchi, cheese, sour fruits like grapes, lemon, pineapple, and grapefruit

Salty—natural mineral salt to get trace minerals

AYURVEDA ACTION
Add in Sour Taste with Lemon—Easy!

You probably get enough sweet and salty tastes by choice, so focus on sour. Start the day with hot lemon water, using organic lemons, and add a spritz of lemon juice to your foods. The sour taste enlivens physiology, sharpens senses, moistens food, and calms the air quality. I always order a cup of hot water with lemon when eating out. Actually, 1/2 cup of water is the most helpful amount with a meal.

FEBRUARY 4
THREE POWERHOUSE VATA ROOTS

HERBS ARE MESSENGERS of consciousness. Most foods begin to lose their liveliness once picked, but dried herbs maintain their aroma and most of their essence for years. That is some kind of powerhouse. Shatavari, ashwagandha, and ginger root are highly revered in Ayurveda and are particularly useful for pacifying Vata.

As you read about the attributes of each, consider if these herbs might be helpful to add to your routine in Vata season. An Ayurveda practitioner can help you to assess if these herbs are for you. A general dosage is 1/4 to 1/2 tsp once or twice daily.

SHATAVARI translates to "she who possesses 100 husbands," and it is rejuvenating. It is particularly advised for women but also serves men and is a reproductive and vitality tonic for both. Although shatavari is cooling, it also is unctuous, which pacifies Vata dryness. Because of the cooling effect, this herb is often combined with heating ashwagandha when used for pacifying Vata. The moisture effect of shatavari supports memory, reproductive fluids, libido, and sperm count. It also counters dryness, hot flashes and irritability. The cooling quality soothes inflammation. Shatavari is an ojas builder. It calms the mind and promotes love and devotion.

ASHWAGANDHA translates to "smell of a horse," a testament to its strengthening qualities. It helps tone muscle and bone, calms the nervous system, focuses the mind, and is prized as an adaptogen, a nontoxic plant extract that supports the body's ability to resist the damaging effects of stress. It particularly supports adrenal function, reproductive health, and overall vitality. Ashwagandha is particularly advised for men but is also helpful for women. Avoid taking with any other sedatives as it may be too calming and lower blood pressure.

Ashwagandha has a heating quality and sweet taste that are helpful for pacifying Vata. Even though ashwagandha is vitalizing, it also provides a calming energy that promotes sleep. It is helpful in arthritis, diabetes, and chronic stress.

GINGER is heating—a great quality for pacifying Vata. Ginger improves digestion and relieves gas and cramps. Regular consumption reduces the pain and swelling of arthritis. Fresh ginger is better than dried. Caution: Ginger is a blood thinner, so consult your doctor for any contraindications.

AYURVEDA ACTION
Add Ginger to Your Spice Water

TO ENJOY THE benefits of ginger, add a slice to your hot spice water.

FEBRUARY 5
AGNI—OUR LIVES ARE SACRED FIRE

Agni can be thought of as the enzymes and endocrine factors governing digestive and metabolic functions. In Ayurveda, it is our "digestive fire." Agni digests food to nourish the body's billions of cells with energy and intelligence. Jathara agni is the most typical meaning when people talk about agni and resides in the stomach and duodenum. However, Bhuta agnis govern the five basic elements, and Dhata agnis are present in each of the seven dhatus. Agni is also in every cell of the body. Interference in healthy agni is the root of illness, and healthy agni leads to perfect digestion and radiant health. Through healthy agni and balanced digestion, we create ojas.

Ojas is the fundamental energetic essence of food, the "cosmic glue" helping cells function in organized wholeness and resulting in radiance and bliss. We want ojas so we want strong agni.

The doshas govern digestive activity, which may become excessive or deficient when a dosha is out of balance and our agni suffers. Excess Vata produces weak, irregular digestion and causes gas. Excess Pitta burns food too quickly and may cause burning sensations, thirst, and acid indigestion. Too much Kapha in the digestive tract results in low digestive fire, making it difficult to digest food. You may feel dull and lethargic, and you may gain weight.

AYURVEDA ACTION
Use Detoxing Spices When Preparing Food

Clearing out toxins supports toned and effective agni. Ginger, turmeric, coriander, cumin, fennel, and fenugreek help open the srotas, the energy channels of the body, to support flushing toxins via the skin, liver, urinary tract, and colon.

First sauté spices in ghee, coconut, or avocado oil to release their intelligence. These three oils are the only ones I recommend for cooking, as their qualities remain unaltered and healthy when heated. Good-quality olive oil is healthy but should be used only at room temperature, not heated.

Put a few of these spices on your shopping list and start clearing the toxins and stirring your agni today.

FEBRUARY 6
FOUR TYPES OF AGNI

What is your agni type?

Vishama agni—Vata. This agni is characterized by irregular digestion due to vata coldness dampening agni. Hunger may be insatiable or, you could go all day without eating. Vishama agni leads to bloating, gas, and constipation. You might have dry skin, dry mouth, cracking joints, receding gums, anxiety, and/or fear.

Tikshna agni—Pitta. This agni is hot and sharp. You cannot skip meals without irritation and great hunger. Your digestive fire is hot and high, but the fierce fire can mean everything passes through too quickly, with insufficient time to extract nourishment. Tikshna agni, or hypermetabolism, can result in diarrhea, heartburn, acid indigestion, skin conditions, and an intense craving for sweets. Tikshna agni can trigger jealousy, hate, and judgment. Pittas get used to eating a lot.

Manda agni—Kapha. This agni is dull and sluggish. With manda agni, you would have low appetite. Kapha types might eat a lot for emotional reasons, even when they are not hungry, leading to ama and weight gain. Dull agni means more time and energy to digest, leaving you feeling tired and lethargic. With manda agni, you might experience frequent colds, congestion, and sinus issues. Emotionally, manda agni can lead to feelings of boredom, lethargy, attachment, and greed.

Sama agni—Balanced, tri-doshic agni is what we want. Food is digested in a timely fashion. With sama agni, you can eat a wide range of foods without discomfort. Sama agni allows a clear and contented mind and a healthy body.

AYURVEDA ACTION
Correct Your Agni Imbalance

Correcting Vishama (Vata) agni

Increase warmth and stability in diet and lifestyle. Consider daily yoga. Use good amounts of healthy oils like ghee for cooking or olive oil at room temperature. Eat a "ginger pickle" {Mar 19} 30 minutes before a meal—slice of ginger the size of a quarter with lemon or lime juice dripped on and a sprinkling of salt.

Correcting Tikshna (Pitta) agni

Add cooling herbs to your diet like coriander, cilantro, cardamom, and fennel. Eat cooling foods such as asparagus and cucumbers. Avoid hot, spicy foods. Eat at regular times and focus on your meal.

Correcting Manda (Kapha) agni

Eat warm, cooked, spicy foods. Use spices like cayenne pepper, ginger, cinnamon, and cumin. Avoid cold drinks. Enjoy hot spice water daily. Avoid overeating. Eat in a peaceful environment. Move.

FEBRUARY 7
MORE AGNI, PLEASE

Spices enliven digestion and create more ojas (juice of life). In Vedic fire ceremonies, spices, oils, seeds, and nuts are offered to the fire. It is a practice of devotion and reverence to the elemental energies of life. Such practices invoke the subtle energies of the elements and call forth blessings.

Likewise, think of your daily eating as ritual: offering food, spices, seeds, and the like to your digestive fire. As you take in earth's bounty, think about the energy and intelligence with which you are nourishing yourself. Your daily nourishment will transform from eating for calories and quick energy to eating for healing, cosmic intelligence, and deep nourishment.

Vata season is a good time to pacify the pressure created by seasonal influences like wind and dryness. When cooking with the spices listed below, first honor the spices and bless them for your nourishment. Then sauté on low heat in a little ghee, coconut, or avocado oil. Offer to your digestive fire and feel the full experience.

Caution: Vata spices are often heating. If you know Pitta is a significant imbalance for you, be careful.

AYURVEDA ACTION
Use Stimulating Spices in Cooking & Teas

Vata-balancing and agni-stimulating spices are warming and grounding and can easily be added to everything from simple vegetables and rice to soups and stews.

- Cardamom
- Cayenne
- Ginger
- Cinnamon
- Cloves
- Cumin
- Mustard seed
- Salt
- Turmeric

Also, stimulate agni by sipping lots of warm water, especially hot spice water, or teas throughout the day.

FEBRUARY 8
FIRE UP YOUR AGNI!

AGNI IS THE inspiring flame that arises from our innermost being. It is the force of transformation and digestion. Fire always moves upward. Keeping agni strong and toned is essential for maximum health.

In Vedic literature, Agni is major, the god of fire. Agni is spoken to in the first verse of the Rig Veda:

"O Agni, I adore Thee,
O priest, O divine minister
Who officiates at the divine Sacrifice,
Who is also the invoker, the Summoner,
Who most bestows the divine wealth upon us."

Agni is conceptualized as the messenger between heaven and earth and represents energy and the knowledge of transformation. At least 40 types of agni are at work in your body. "Agni" most often refers to jathara agni, the primary agni for transforming food to nourishment. Every cell has agni intelligence for transforming nutrients to food.

Agni becomes sluggish when we eat the wrong foods, or eat them at the wrong time, or eat them with the wrong attitude. These habits lead to ama accumulation, which is like putting a wet blanket over our digestive fire. To maintain maximum health:

1. Stoke agni by cleansing ama.
2. Build digestive agni.
3. Keep your system clean and moving.

We will explore these three ways to build agni in the entries ahead.

AYURVEDA ACTION
Take Advantage of Your Midday Agni

YOUR AGNI IS strongest during the Pitta time of the day, which is 10 a.m. to 2 p.m. As you have more digestive fire at this time, ideally your midday meal should be the largest.

FEBRUARY 9
STOKE AGNI BY CLEANSING AMA

Cleansing ama should be ongoing, even if you eat well. Organic food is cleaner, but even organic crops pick up toxins from the air. Consider doing a seasonal cleanse, a weekly cleanse, a situational cleanse, or you can cleanse daily (see April 1-5 for more on cleansing).

Situational Cleanse—Did you eat poorly last night or over a long weekend holiday? Are you feeling blah? Try a digestive reset. It's not officially a cleanse, but it helps enkindle agni and clear recent ama. A reset allows you to catch things in the early stages of unwellness to correct imbalances.

A simple mono-diet for a day can reset your digestion. Just eat kitchari—the Ayurveda staple—for every meal. See {Mar 19} for a recipe. Enjoying three simple, easily digestible meals in a row allows agni to reboot. You will restore your light, subtle, and clear qualities. A liquid-food day also is good. Throw a light lentil soup in the blender or drink vegetable juices for the day. Or just eat fresh fruit. Note: Fruit juice is too concentrated with sugar to be an effective cleanse.

Seasonal Cleanse—Do a 1- or 2-week cleanse at least once a year in the spring and perhaps also in the fall. The season change from Vata to Kapha is the most important time to do a seasonal cleanse. For many people this would be late February through April. The dry toxins from Vata winter begin their move with mucus and fluids that come with the Kapha spring. You want them to move out, not redeposit in the body.

Working with an Ayurveda practitioner during your cleanse is best. However, online guidelines are available to support a substantial cleanse. These have comprehensive resources:

Banyan Botanicals—banyanbotanicals.com
John Douillard's Life Spa—lifespa.com

AYURVEDA ACTION
Cleanse Daily

First, avoid forming ama. Then try daily cleansing rituals, such as:

- Scrape your tongue each morning (Apr 20).
- Sip hot spice water daily—This supports digestion and cleanses toxins primarily stored in fat cells.
- Add fresh ginger (Feb 4) to food or spice water.
- Consider taking triphala, 1–2 tablets or 1/4–1/2 tsp powder, in hot water at bedtime. Triphala supports digestion.

FEBRUARY 10
BUILD YOUR DIGESTIVE AGNI

Strong agni, or digestive fire, helps break down the food and drink we ingest so the body can assimilate what is useful and eliminate the rest. Strong agni is essential to build and fortify healthy tissues with nutrients and to support the body's elimination of wastes. Strong agni produces ojas, that subtle substance that gives radiance to your appearance and expression. On the flip side, impaired agni is the root cause of every imbalance that leads to disease.

Agni is most commonly thought of as digestive fire, but it is also the fire of your intelligence and your transformative processes. Agni transforms food to consciousness. Agni connects lower consciousness to higher consciousness and links us to the cosmos.

Agni has the qualities of hot, sharp, mobile, subtle, light, and dry. Foods and activities that nourish these qualities build agni. Agni is sacred fire—we enable it by honoring it.

AYURVEDA ACTION
Build Strong Agni Daily

Building strong agni is a daily lifestyle. Here are tips to kindle it:

- Eat real, living foods, not processed foods with digestive inhibiters.
- The majority of your immune system lives in your gut, so keep it healthy.
- Don't overeat—aim for 75% full.
- Eat three meals daily and avoid snacking (unless you are hypoglycemic), to allow your digestive system to relax after eating and inspire agni to build.
- If you are not hungry, don't eat. Learn to distinguish between hunger that is satisfied by eating modestly and hunger caused by boredom, exhaustion, or addiction.

FEBRUARY 11
SPIRITUAL LOVE

Are you ready for a radical notion of love? Allowing your ideas and experience of love to evolve is essential, especially for those on a spiritual path. With Valentine's Day approaching, let's consider the question, what is love? Left to default, love might be defined by wrapping it in the illusion of safety, which formed in your unconscious mind mostly before you were six years old...hmmmm.

The spiritual journey is often conceptualized as a singular, vertical experience requiring detachment from daily life. People think it is sitting on a meditation cushion hoping for enlightenment, or at least movement in that direction, to reduce angst and suffering. While meditation is important, it is a tool. The "householder path" spiritual adventurer grows through engagement in everyday life, and isolation does not serve this path. Your horizontal connections—your efforts to love and appreciate others—lead to the real spiritual adventure.

In their book *Evolutionary Love Relationships*, Andrew Harvey and Chris Saade recognize that we are living in a world in dire need of social, political, and economic healing.[9] They call us to a radically new vision of love based on passion, authenticity, and sacred activism, which enables us to hold sufficient energy, truth, and action to lift consciousness and heal the world. Does this beckon you?

Evolutionary love is not just about intimate partnerships. The call includes all significant connections: our community tribal members, inspired work relationships, deep friendships, benevolent revolutionaries, and spiritual partners.

One example is couples. When they share sacred activism, the nature and content of the relationship shifts. Rather than building a case against the other, a couple could engage sacredly in the evening by talking about mutual interests in volunteering, by serving food together at a homeless center, or by sharing details about an upcoming rally. Serving others and larger causes releases the addiction to someone else making us happy. Sacred relationships exhibit great care, compassion, vulnerability, and active attention to the well-being of your partner, but as an offering of love—not a demand.

AYURVEDA ACTION
Appreciate Another

Ayurveda has a principle—add and squeeze. As attention is placed on authenticity, expansion of one's consciousness, and appreciation of each other, complaints and expectations are squeezed out for lack of space. Try it today with a significant other or even with someone in the line at the grocery store. See another through soft eyes of appreciation.

FEBRUARY 12
THE 6 TASTES & HOW HUNGER WORKS

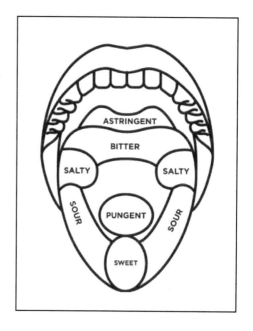

It's on the tip of your tongue. Ayurveda recognizes six tastes, called Rasas, which is Sanskrit for "essence." The six tastes are sweet, sour, salty, bitter, pungent, and astringent. Including all six in every meal, or at least every day, provides a natural guide to proper nutrition and also brings a feeling of satisfaction in eating. Without all six tastes in your diet, the brain calls for more food because the body's nutritional needs are not satisfied. You keep eating, take in too many calories, yet remain malnourished.

Taste buds identify tastes, of course, to give us an experience of food—you're attracted to some tastes and repelled by others. But taste does more than help us enjoy eating; it unlocks food's nutritive value and provides a spark for digestion.

When the brain senses a need for energy and information, it sends hunger signals. As you eat, taste buds alert the brain that you have ingested foods that provide energy and information. The six tastes provide coded information about a meal's nutritional content to your nervous system.

Though you want a supply of all six tastes each day, emphasizing three in a meal can pacify an imbalanced dosha. The next day entry contains examples of foods containing the six tastes. Subsequent entries will explore each taste one at a time.

AYURVEDA ACTION
Learn to Discern Taste

Eat slowly to see if you can discern which taste, or which combination of tastes, are in each food. Some might be easy: sweet, salty, pungent (hot, spicy), and sour. Others may take more attunement: astringent and bitter. Where are you experiencing the taste on your tongue? Reflecting on your food in appreciation is a way of slowing down to promote complete digestion.

FEBRUARY 13
BALANCING THE DOSHAS WITH TASTE

Tastes correct out-of-balance doshas. Essentially, you ingest two of the elements with each taste. By consciously introducing tastes, you add the qualities of those elements to the digestive/nourishment process. With taste, the strengths of doshas are supported to fortify the good qualities of stable doshas and balance out-of-whack doshas. Effect on dosha: + means increases/aggravates, - means decreases/pacifies.

Taste and Element	*Effect on Dosha*	*Qualities*	*Examples*
Sweet = Water & Earth	Vata – Pitta – Kapha +	Grounding, nourishing, heavy, oily, moist, cooling builds tissue	Grains-rice, dairy, ghee, dates, pumpkin, licorice root, sweet fruits, almonds, cashews
Sour = Water & Fire	Vata – Pitta + Kapha +	Stimulates appetite and saliva, light, heating, oily	Sour fruits-lemon, vinegar, yogurt, pickles, fermented food, wine
Salty = Earth & Fire	Vata – Pitta + Kapha +	Grounding, hydrating, heating, adds taste, cleanses, increases absorption of minerals	Salt, sea vegetables black olives
Pungent = Fire & Air	Vata + Pitta + Kapha –	Stimulates digestion, clears sinuses, stimulates blood, think clearly, critical	Chili peppers, ginger, onions, hot spices
Astringent = Air & Earth	Vata + Pitta - Kapha -	Cool, dry, firm, mentally purify, mentally strengthen	Legumes, green grapes, pomegranates, cranberries, sprouts
Bitter = Air & Space	Vata + Pitta – Kapha –	Cool, light, detoxifying, removes waste, mental purification	Leafy greens, turmeric, green and black teas

AYURVEDA ACTION
Balance Imbalanced Doshas With Taste

Look at the chart above. You need all six tastes, but which tastes should be emphasized to lower your excessive dosha? Recall your most imbalanced dosha from your assessment or other source. Choose those with a "-" effect on your imbalanced dosha, as that means it will reduce or pacify the excessive dosha. Circle 3–5 foods to add to your diet this week.

FEBRUARY 14
THE SWEET TASTE

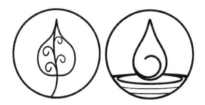

BALANCES
Vata and Pitta

AGGRAVATES
Kapha

PRIMARY ELEMENTS
earth and water

ENERGY (VIRYA)
cooling

POST-DIGESTIVE EFFECT*
sweet

QUALITIES
heavy, cold, moist, unctuous,

BENEFITS
grounding, nourishing, building, satisfying, promotes growth of tissues/skin/hair, rebuilds weakness

EFFECT IN EXCESS
unhealthy cravings, attachment, greed, diabetes, obesity, laziness, excessive sleep, swelling, loss of appetite, weak digestion

BALANCED EMOTIONS
love, joy, compassion, bliss, happiness

IMBALANCED EMOTIONS
attachment, greed, possessiveness

LOCATION ON TONGUE
front tip

FOODS
most grains (especially wheat, rice, barley), dairy, ghee, corn, carrots, coconut, dates, maple syrup, eggs, nuts, most oils, root vegetables, bread, starchy vegetables, dairy, meat, fish, sugar, honey

HERBS/SPICES
licorice root, basil, cardamom, cinnamon, coriander, fennel, mint, nutmeg, saffron

SOME FOOD TASTES are obvious. You know honey is sweet. Did you know grains also have a sweet taste? Next time you eat a grain, try to find the sweet taste in it. Moderation is key: sweet is one of the most overdone tastes in the modern Western diet. It has led to a host of health issues like excessive weight gain, diabetes, and inflammation.

AYURVEDA ACTION
Add Licorice Root to Spice Water

ADD LICORICE ROOT slices or pieces to hot spice water to add a sweet taste without sugar's effects. Licorice is sweeter than sugar, so you don't need much. It helps liquefy Kapha and break up ama. This root slightly increases heat, and often is used to decrease Pitta ama. It does not increase acidity, which heating herbs often do. It also reduces HCl (hydrochloric) acid in the stomach. Licorice moistens Vata and cools Pitta. It tones the adrenals while calming the nervous system and invites contentment. Licorice strengthens the body and maximizes the effects of other herbs, so it's a great enhancer. That is one special herb!

---

*VIPAKA, OR THE post-digestive effect, is the final taste of a food after exposure to digestive enzymes or the final outcome of the transformation of the rasa (taste).

FEBRUARY 15
THE SOUR TASTE

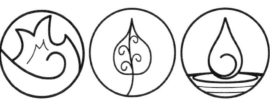

BALANCES

Vata

AGGRAVATES

Pitta and Kapha

PRIMARY ELEMENTS

fire, earth and water—in that order

ENERGY (VIRYA)

heating

POST-DIGESTIVE EFFECT

sour

QUALITIES

hot, unctuous, liquid, light

BENEFITS

cleanses tissues, promotes adventurousness, stimulates appetite, sharpens mind, strengthens sense organs, stimulates digestion and assimilation. Increases absorption of minerals. Causes secretions and salivation, increases blood circulation, purifies, moistens other food, lessens flatulence

EFFECT IN EXCESS

increases thirst, toxifies blood, edema, heartburn, itching, irritation, fever, muscle weakness, diarrhea

BALANCED EMOTIONS

understanding, perception, receptivity, enhanced mental activities

IMBALANCED EMOTIONS

selfishness, criticism of self and others, irritation

LOCATION ON TONGUE

front edges

FOODS

sour citrus fruits, butter, cheese, sour cream, yogurt, alcohol, vinegar, sauerkraut, pickles, kimchi, tomatoes

HERBS/SPICES

amalaki, bringaraj, pomegranate seeds

AYURVEDA ACTION
Drink a Cup of Hot Lemon Water Each Morning for Sour Taste

SQUEEZE A SLICE of fresh lemon into your water. Drink in the early morning. Lemon cleans the mouth and reduces bad breath. Lemon also stimulates agni and increases digestive power. It can help to clear mucus, especially excess Kapha mucus in the stomach.

Bonus tip: Keep green grapes on hand for the sour taste.

FEBRUARY 16
THE SALTY TASTE

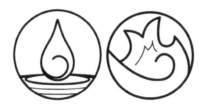

BALANCES
> Vata

AGGRAVATES
> Pitta and Kapha

PRIMARY ELEMENTS
> water and fire

ENERGY
> (virya) heating

POST-DIGESTIVE EFFECT
> sweet

QUALITIES
> hot, unctuous, heavy

BENEFITS
> stimulates appetite and digestion, promotes salivation, helps retain moisture, supports proper elimination, improves flavor of foods, and is antiflatulent, slight laxative effect, maintains the electrolyte balance (particularly important in summer and at change of seasons). Salt provides energy, and aids growth of bodily tissues.

EFFECT IN EXCESS
> hypertension, hyperacidity, kidney stones, skin problems, stagnation of blood, excessive thirst and can cause wrinkles.

BALANCED EMOTIONS
> confidence and zest for life

IMBALANCED EMOTIONS
> greediness, addiction, attachment, irritability, overambition

LOCATION ON TONGUE
> rear edges

FOODS
> kelp, seaweed, also most watery vegetables like cucumbers, zucchini, black olives, and tomatoes in small amounts

HERBS/SPICES
> various salts

AYURVEDA ACTION
Use Moderate Amounts of Mineral Salt

DEFINITELY AVOID PROCESSED foods, which are loaded with salt. Sea salts have been trendy but can also contain high levels of mercury. I prefer a land-mined mineral salt, a great way to get trace minerals. Check out your source for salt and make sure it includes iodine, especially if you do not eat a lot of fish.

FEBRUARY 17
THE PUNGENT TASTE

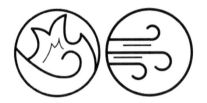

BALANCES
Kapha

AGGRAVATES
Pitta and Vata

PRIMARY ELEMENTS
fire and air

ENERGY (VIRYA)
very heating

POST-DIGESTIVE EFFECT
pungent

QUALITIES
hot, sharp, light, dry

BENEFITS
kindles agni, purifies, thins, and moves blood, promotes seating and detoxification, improves metabolism, relieves muscle and nerve pain, stops itching, reduces gas

EFFECT IN EXCESS
thirst, depletion of bodily fluids (too much is drying)

BALANCED EMOTIONS
zeal, excitement, focus, clarity, vim, vigor, vitality, opens mind and senses

IMBALANCED EMOTIONS
aggression, impatience, rage, anger, competitiveness, selfishness, envy, irritability

LOCATION ON TONGUE
center

FOODS
chili peppers, radishes, wasabi, leeks, onions, turnips

HERBS/SPICES
various peppers, garlic, cloves, ginger, mustard, asafoetida (hing), cinnamon, cloves, coriander, cumin

AYURVEDA ACTION
Upgrade from Black Pepper to Trikatu

Plain black pepper is an important cleansing, healing spice. It is a bioavailablity enhancer because it transports the benefits of other herbs to targeted locations in the body. Black pepper stimulates oxygen flow to the brain and circulatory system, enhances digestion, is warming, and supports the joints.

Mix this great spice with two others and you have a powerful triumvirate called trikatu. Equal amounts of black pepper, ginger, and long pepper, also known as pippali, magnify the effects of each. This triumvirate has its primary effects in the upper gastrointestinal tract, where it enhances agni to break down food and allow absorption of nutrients.

Replace the black pepper in your shaker with trikatu for upgraded effects. You can find trikatu from Ayurveda herb providers.

FEBRUARY 18
THE ASTRINGENT TASTE

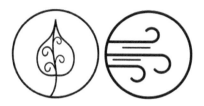

BALANCES

Pitta (from coolness) and Kapha (from dryness)

AGGRAVATES

Vata

PRIMARY ELEMENTS

earth and air

ENERGY (VIRYA)

slightly cooling

POST-DIGESTIVE EFFECT

pungent

QUALITIES

dry, heavy, cold, rough

BENEFITS

reduces inflammation, cools excess heat, reduces diarrhea and sweating, tones tissues, lightens body, mentally purifies, cleans the mouth, and strengthens

EFFECT IN EXCESS

dries tissues, slows digestion, causes flatulence

BALANCED EMOTIONS

cools anger, stabilizes scattered thoughts, grounds, unifies

IMBALANCED EMOTIONS

fear, nervousness, attachment, rigidity, judgmental, depression

LOCATION ON TONGUE

center back

FOODS

dried and fresh beans, legumes, lentils, figs, teas, green apples, green bananas, green grapes, pomegranates, cranberries, alfalfa sprouts

HERBS/SPICES

amalaki, haritaki, arjuna, manjistha

ASTRINGENT MAY BE the most challenging taste to discern. Astringent taste is the flavor of dryness. We find it in beans and some vegetables. The astringent taste makes us want to pucker.

AYURVEDA ACTION
Add Sautéed Hing to Bean Dishes

BEANS ARE A great source of the astringent taste, but they have a high air quality. Asafoetida, also known as hing, effectively reduces the gaseous effect of beans. Sauté asafoetida in ghee and add to your beans while cooking. It has an extremely strong aroma—I keep mine in a jar inside another jar. Once sautéed and added to food, however, it settles down and adds a good taste. You only need a pinch.

You can also find organic hingvastak churna—a combination of herbs and containing hing—at Ayurveda herbal suppliers. This is a good way to get your hing and you can be assured of the other ingredients. When you buy something just labeled hing, there could be fillers you might not want. Check your ingredients when buying.

FEBRUARY 19
THE BITTER TASTE

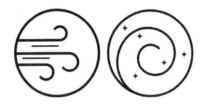

BALANCES

Pitta and Kapha

AGGRAVATES

Vata

PRIMARY ELEMENTS

air and space

ENERGY (VIRYA)

very cooling

POST-DIGESTIVE EFFECT

pungent

QUALITIES

cold, dry, light, rough

BENEFITS

reduces fat, cleanses, detoxifies, stimulates nervous system, anti-inflammatory, anti-viral, relieves thirst, helps manage food cravings, tones the liver, kindles agni, firms skin

EFFECT IN EXCESS

inhibits sexual energy, gas, upsets stomach, depletes tissues

BALANCED EMOTIONS

clear thinking, independence, self-awareness, clear senses and emotions

IMBALANCED EMOTIONS

boredom, isolation, bitterness, spaciness, anxiety, fear, insomnia

LOCATION ON TONGUE

middle

FOODS

bitter greens (kale, dandelion, collards), coffee, bitter melon, eggplant, chocolate

HERBS/SPICES

turmeric, fenugreek, sesame seeds, cumin

AYURVEDA ACTION
Try Fenugreek to Regulate Blood Sugar

Exciting new research on fenugreek (see greenmedinfo.com) has shown a capacity to significantly lower blood glucose. The seeds contain fiber and other components that may slow the body's digestion and absorption of carbohydrates. All dosages in Ayurveda are personal to your situation, but you could start by adding 1/4 tsp to your daily hot spice water.

If you take regular blood-sugar readings, watch your numbers to see how this works for you. When taking Ayurveda herbs, pause once in a while to let the body adjust. Often six weeks on an herb and two weeks off is recommended. This allows the body to adjust to the herb effect and rise up to meet the intelligence without relying on the herb forever. Stop and check how you feel. If the adjustment is complete, you could stop taking the herb. Again, ideas offered here are never a recommendation to go off medicines prescribed under a health provider's care.

FEBRUARY 20
PUTTING THE SIX TASTES TOGETHER

Here is a quick reference for using taste to balance your doshas:

	Balance with	*Aggravated by*
Vata	sweet, sour, salty	pungent, astringent, bitter
Pitta	sweet, astringent, bitter	sour, salty, pungent
Kapha	pungent, astringent, bitter	sweet, sour, salty

Foods for each taste:

- Sweet—whole grains, starchy vegetables (peas, lentils, corn, potatoes), dairy, meat, poultry, fish, sugar, honey, molasses, mangoes, melons, almonds, cashews, coconut, basil, cardamom, cinnamon
- Sour—citrus, berries, plums, dough breads, tomatoes, pickled foods, vinegar, alcohol, cheese, yogurt, most fermented foods
- Salty—soy sauce, seaweed, salted meats, fish, food with added table salt
- Bitter—bitter greens, endive, chicory, spinach, kale, romaine lettuce, leafy greens, celery, broccoli, sprouts, beets, turmeric, coffee, dark chocolate, sesame oil
- Pungent—peppers, chilies, onions, garlic, cayenne, black pepper, cloves, ginger, mustard, salsa, paprika, raw spinach, radishes
- Astringent—lentils, dried beans, green apples, grape skins, cauliflower, figs, pomegranates, tea, popcorn, potatoes, most raw vegetables, chickpeas

AYURVEDA ACTION
Shop for Six Tastes

Pick one food item from each taste to add to your shopping list. Emphasize those food items to reduce your excessive dosha.

FEBRUARY 21
A DAY OF SIX TASTES

Want to get all six tastes in your meals in one day? Try incorporating these menu ideas.

Breakfast:
Steel-cut oats with dry pan-roasted shredded coconut and sesame seeds—a sweet dish to start your day—all three ingredients have a sweet taste.

Or try a half grapefruit (sour and bitter) with cardamom (pungent) and ginger (pungent) powder—this gets you going with sour, bitter, and pungent tastes. Top with a bit of raw honey if you wish.

Lunch:
Sweet potato (sweet) with kale (bitter and astringent), rice (sweet), and fresh ginger (pungent). Add a bit of salt (salty).

Dinner:
Carrot (sweet) soup with ginger (pungent) and black pepper (pungent).

AYURVEDA ACTION
Gather Ayurveda Recipes

Joyfulbelly.com is an amazing site for dishes focused on Ayurveda benefits. It offers remarkable, free support for creating a dosha-balancing diet. The recipes are great, and the tastes and qualities are identified for each ingredient. Highly recommended.

Other good dosha-balancing recipes can be found at mapi.com/ayurvedic-recipes.

Consider getting an Ayurveda cookbook. I recommend one that gives the dosha that each recipe primarily balances. Otherwise, you will need to analyze ingredients to see if the recipe is balancing the dosha to which you are attending. A note on recipe books: If the recipe says it is good for Vata, for instance, it means the recipe will pacify or lower Vata. This can be confusing. If there is a recipe that will increase a dosha, it will typically say that. If nothing is said, the default is that the dosha named is reduced.

FEBRUARY 22
SPICES AND HERBS—CHETANA PRANA

I can't say enough about the benefits of spices and herbs, which in Ayurveda are sometimes called chetana prana. Chetana means living intelligence, while prana means life energy. Spices and herbs are concentrated forms of healing, with both energy and intelligence. Unlike most foods, herbs and spices are designed to hold their intelligence over time. Herbs and spices are also referred to as yogivahi—meaning they enhance delivery of nutrients to the body's cells, tissues, and organs. They also enhance the bioavailability of nutrients in the body.

SPICE FOR PERFECT DIGESTION

Selecting and eating healthy, wholesome food does little good if your body cannot absorb the nutrients to build healthy body tissue. The beej-bhumi theory {Feb 27} of disease in Ayurveda states that poor digestion is the root cause of most disorders. Improperly digested food creates ama, or toxins, which clogs physical and energetic microchannels of the body. This blocks nutrient flow to the body, weakening the immune system and hampering elimination of wastes. The results create an environment where disease and infection can take hold and disease manifestation begins. Ama will move and deposit in your most vulnerable areas, such as your digestive process or joints.

SPICES ARE AMA-FIGHTERS

Most spices enhance digestion and make the food more delightful. Spices also remove accumulated ama. Spices have a fat-soluble portion and a water-soluble portion. Often spices are sautéed in ghee or other fat to release their intelligence before being added to dishes. Ghee thus helps transport the therapeutic value of the spice throughout the body. Combining spices offers the benefits of synergy and balance, an important focus of Ayurvedic cooking.

Spices are best taken whole as they appear in Nature, especially through eating, rather than to take isolated nutraceuticals, where the so-called "active" ingredient is isolated in pill form.

AYURVEDA ACTION
Start the (Digestive) Fire!

Here's a reminder on great agni fire spices. Add agni-stimulating spices to your cooking or drink these spices in teas. These are some of the best agni stimulators: ginger, peppers (especially cayenne), fennel, cumin, cinnamon, and cardamom.

FEBRUARY 23
HEAL-THY SELF FROM A COLD

The word "healthy" is made up of the words "heal" and "thy." Now that I see it, it feels like finding a hidden object in a child's activity book—boom—got it!

Colds, coughs, and the flu are common at this time in winter. Despite your best efforts, sometimes you just get sick. It happens to everyone. This is not failure. It can even be good for us, because as the immune system responds to bacterial and viral intrusions, it builds memory and fortifies against more formidable future challenges.

One of the best cold preventions is to stay moist. You might do this with a humidifier in your home, by using nasya oil {Sep 28} in your nose passages, by doing warm oil self-massage (abhyanga), and by eating warm, moist food. Also, drink plenty of fluids, especially hot teas.

If you do get a cold, move through the illness as quickly and as best you can. Here are DIY "medication" recipes, starring ginger, to be prepared.

- Mix equal amounts of ginger powder, turmeric, and black pepper. Take 1/2 tsp of the mixture with raw honey or warm water and honey daily.
- Mix 1/2 tsp of fresh ginger juice with 1/2 tsp raw honey and take on an empty stomach up to three times daily.
- Mix equal amounts of powdered ginger, clove, cinnamon, cardamom, turmeric, and black pepper. Take 1/2 tsp of this mixture with raw honey or make into a tea.

AYURVEDA ACTION
Eat Light, Simple, and Warm

When your immune system is fighting back, give it a fighting chance with helpful foods. Eat simple soups with clear broth as well as light, warm food in general. Avoid raw, dry, or frozen foods and dairy, which are hard to digest. Focus your strength on recovery. If you have mucus, gargle with salt water.

FEBRUARY 24
HEAL-THY SELF FROM A COUGH

A COUGH OFTEN accompanies a cold or could show up on its own. You might have a wet cough, with mucus, or a dry cough. In winter, it's easy to get dry from breathing heated forced-air and eating sugary, drying foods for energy and pleasure. When cilia in the back of the nose (small, sweeping, hair-like projections) get too dry, it irritates the mucous membranes and signals the body to balance by making more mucus.

Some mucus comes out of the nose, resulting in sniffles. Some drips down the back of the throat into the bronchioles, which can tickle the throat and trigger a cough to expel it. Catch the cough early. Lubricate the sinuses and throat with herbs to soothe your scratchy throat. Prevent the thin, reactive mucus from thickening and dripping into the bronchioles, which is a more serious condition.

When mucus is substantial and the cough is productive, a breeding ground for bacteria and viruses is created. Prevent coughs, colds, and allergies by staying moist (drink hydrating beverages and use a humidifier, for example). Or if they show up, use an herbal cough remedy to prevent the cough from becoming more serious.

AYURVEDA ACTION
Make Your Own Cough Syrup

- 1 quart pure water
- 1/4 cup freshly grated ginger root (or 1 Tbsp ginger powder)
- 1 Tbsp cinnamon
- 1 Tbsp slippery elm bark
- 1 Tbsp horehound bark
- 1 Tbsp marshmallow root
- 1/4 cup lemon juice
- 1 cup raw organic honey
- For a cough with heavy mucus, add 1 Tbsp wild cherry bark, which is drying.

Add the herbs to boiling water. If you don't have them all, just include the ones you can find and increase the amount so you still have 5-6 Tbsp of herbs. Simmer until the volume of water is reduced to less than half. Strain the herbs and when cooled, add the lemon juice and honey. Never add honey to boiling water. Excessive heat changes honey's composition to be unhealthy.

Adults dosage is 1 Tbsp two or three times a day. Children under 12 could have 1 tsp two or three times a day. Babies under 1 year old should not consume honey. Consider substituting grade B maple syrup.

FEBRUARY 25
STRONG LIKE BULL IMMUNITY

Ayurveda immunity is not against specific infectious agents or diseases in the way Western medicine provides "immunizations" or treatment after disease sets in. Ayurveda immunity is avoiding the loss of integrity, relationship, and homeostasis among the individual's doshas, dhatus (tissues), and mind. Your immune system might be more unstable at the change of seasons. Agni can fluctuate dramatically and ama (toxins) can build—especially in spring when ama accumulated over the winter melts and moves through the physiology.

Immunity-Boosting Foods

Consume organic raw milk and yogurt, fresh vegetables, fresh fruits, whole grains, ghee, warm home-cooked meals. Avoid commercially processed foods, canned and frozen foods, old food/leftovers, cold foods and beverages, and alcohol.

Immunity-Boosting Lifestyle

Choose abhyanga (self-massage), moderate exercise, yoga, pranayama, meditation, proper rest/sleep, time in nature, loving emotions, dancing. Avoid staying up late, working at night, eating at irregular times, exposing the body to stress and fatigue, wrong understandings of Nature, and overindulgences.

Immunity-Herbs/Rasayanas

These herbs are known to strengthen immunity:

- Herbs for body immunity—ashwagandha, shatavari, brahmi, amalaki, guduchi, licorice root, fresh ginger, turmeric, black pepper, cumin, fennel, coriander
- Herbs for protecting integrity of mind—shankhpushpi, brahmi, ashwagandha, guduchi, jatamansi

AYURVEDA ACTION
Boost Immunity 3 Ways

1. Foods—Cook with coconut oil, ghee, or avocado oil, which have a high flash point and can handle high temperatures without becoming unstable. These oils build ojas.
2. Lifestyle—Add more routine to your day. Go to bed by 10 p.m., which is still in Kapha time, to encourage deeper rest.
3. Herbs/Rasayana—Add fresh ginger to your spice water. Ginger is a gentle daily cleanser.

FEBRUARY 26
IMMUNE SYSTEM—
THE WESTERN VIEW

In Western medicine, the immune system is comprised of networked cells, tissues, and organs that protect the body. The cells in this defense system are white blood cells or leukocytes. Leukocytes are produced or stored throughout the body, including the thymus, spleen, lymph nodes, and bone marrow. Leukocytes circulate through the body between the organs and nodes by means of the lymphatic vessels. They can also circulate through the blood vessels. In this way, the immune system works in a coordinated manner to monitor the body for germs or harmful substances.

Two basic types of leukocytes have specific duties:

1. Phagocyte cells chew up invading organisms.
2. Lymphocytes are intelligent cells that allow the body to remember and recognize previous invaders and defend against them.

Here's how this works: A foreign substance, called an antigen, invades the body. When the body detects antigens, several cells work to respond by triggering lymphocytes to produce antibodies. Antibodies are specialized proteins that lock onto specific antigens. Antibodies and antigens fit together like a lock and key. Once lymphocytes recognize antigens, they develop antigen memory and immediately produce antibodies if the antigen enters a person's body again. That's why if someone has a certain disease, like chickenpox, they typically don't get sick from that again.

Antibodies can recognize antigens and lock onto them, but they can't destroy them without help. That is the job of T-cells, part of the system that destroys antigens tagged by antibodies. Antibodies can also neutralize toxins (poisonous or damaging substances) produced by different organisms. All of these specialized cells and parts of the immune system offer the body protection against disease. This protection is called immunity.

AYURVEDA ACTION
Build Your White Blood Cells

The Western view on immunity can add to the Ayurveda perspective. Healthy white blood cells, or leukocytes, are key to strong immunity. Fortify white blood cells by taking cat's claw and astragulus daily. In the fall and winter, I take 1/4 tsp of each herb daily. Take the powders on food such as oatmeal or in warm raw milk, coconut milk, or as a tea.

FEBRUARY 27
IMMUNE SYSTEM—AYURVEDA

The beej-bhumi theory, which means "seed and land," is the foundation for understanding the Ayurveda view on immunity. The body is analogous to the land. Infection, "bugs," and virus intruders are like seeds. A body that has accumulated ama and lacks ojas will be fertile ground for hosting and growing the seeds of infection. Strong digestion, resulting in stronger ojas, will create infertile ground for the seeds of infection. Pathogens (capable of producing disease) require essential conditions to take hold and flourish. In the absence of favorable conditions, the immune system can eradicate disease and sustain or rebuild a balanced condition. A seed will not propagate in unfertile soil, just as a fire without fuel or air cannot burn.

THREE LEVELS OF IMMUNITY

It's simple: Whatever weakens digestion weakens immunity.

- Hereditary (Sahaj)—innate level of immunity from birth; chromosomal level
- Seasonal (Kalaja)—fluctuating levels of immunity due to change of seasons, stage of life, environment (abundance of water and pleasant climate build immunity) and planetary cycles
- Acquired (Yuktikrit)—a balanced, permanent level of immunity that can be realized by following an Ayurvedic diet and lifestyle

In the winter, digestion is naturally high. You feel hungrier and can digest better in the winter. But this is the season we typically eat junk food, or rich foods that are hard to digest. People often eat improperly—perhaps on the run, or simply too much. We have the potential to nourish well in winter, but through unhealthy habits, we can create bad immunity.

AYURVEDA ACTION
Make an Immunity Spice Mix

Make a spice mix to and use it as your go-to for building immunity and adding flavor.

Add 3 parts turmeric and fennel powders to 1 part cumin, coriander, ginger, and black pepper powders. You can also add a bit of cinnamon to taste. I like to fresh-grind many of these with a dedicated spice grinder. Mix and store in an airtight container. Use about 1/2 to 1 tsp in your recipes. Sauté the mix first in ghee or coconut oil before adding to food to release the spices' intelligence and flavor.

FEBRUARY 28
BOOST YOUR IMMUNITY WITH FOOD

Back to basics! Let's concentrate on food. Here's what you can do to continuously boost your immunity.

1. Choose intelligent, easy-to-digest foods that are radiant with energy. Pick out the freshest, brightest, most colorful whole, organic foods.
2. Cook with intelligent, immune-boosting spices. Especially consider turmeric, which is revered in Ayurveda and has many proven benefits from Western research as well. Also use cumin and black pepper to detox ama. Sauté spices in a little ghee first to tap their intelligence.
3. Eat foods that build a strong immune system. Stewed apples {Nov 18} contain lots of fiber to clean the intestines. Sweet, juicy fruits eaten alone convert quickly to ojas, the great immunity fortifier. Bitter leafy greens like kale and Swiss chard also cleanse and fortify when cooked with spices. Whole grains provide fiber—more cleansing. Ghee and raw milk are ojas building and strengthen the immune system.
4. Eat warm cooked food but avoid overcooking—it diminishes the intelligence.
5. Eat your largest meal at midday, when agni is the strongest, to enhance immunity.
6. Overeating will overwhelm and suffocate your digestive fire. Eat to three-fourths of your capacity and sip a half-cup of warm water with your meal.
7. Choose foods that are in season and that can balance your imbalanced dosha.

AYURVEDA ACTION
"Pop" and "Stick" Daily Spice Water

Have you made a habit of drinking hot spice water? A thermos with a "pop-top" mechanism keeps everything warmer longer—and it's portable, too. Click to elevate the top for pouring without opening the thermos. However, if seeds get stuck in the pop-top, they can breed bacteria.

So here is a great tip for keeping your thermos top clean of seeds. Look for a slender tea infuser, sometimes called a stick infuser. Put your seeds in that and then in your thermos. A small muslin bag works too, but the metal stick infusers fit through the thermos opening and are easily cleaned for re-use. Drinking hot spice water daily is one of the best Ayurveda strategies because this mild (but necessary) daily detox supports digestion.

FEBRUARY 29
RECAP AND WHAT'S AHEAD

Here is your recap and look ahead on the Leap Year day. February was an introduction to Vata. The Vata season is generally November through the end of February in places where winters are cold and summers are hot. You can find more about Vata in the November and December readings.

Primarily Vata is dry, cold, and mobile. The most important way to balance excessive Vata is to moisten, warm, and stabilize. Eat warm cooked food that is grounding. Watery winter-squash dishes are ideal.

Spices to pacify Vata include ginger, cardamom, cinnamon, cloves, cumin, turmeric, peppers, and salt. The major Ayurvedic herbs to pacify Vata are ashwagandha, shatavari, and ginger—both dried and fresh.

You also learned more about agni, the sacred digestive fire. In the winter months we build tissue. We generally eat more to support this part of our natural cycle of health. The more you stoke a strong fire, the better for digesting the increased amount and heaviness of winter foods. If not, you can get that thing we call "winter weight." Keep your agni strong with fire spices and digestive spices like ginger, fenugreek, cumin, fennel, and turmeric.

You also learned about the six tastes: sweet, sour, salty, pungent, astringent, and bitter. Tastes signal your physiology about how to operate. Eating all six tastes daily assures that you are engaging the processes that you need to be healthy. A core principle is that food is the intelligence that ignites how we operate.

WHAT'S NEXT?

Next month the focus is Kapha. This season is generally March through June. Excess Kapha can lead to weigh gain, lethargy, and low emotions. Kapha is our strength and structure, so we want it to be healthy.

MONTHLY REFLECTION TIME

What actions did you try and what was your experience? What new actions feel worthwhile? Did you have any adverse reactions? Put a check in the third column for actions you plan to incorporate daily, weekly, monthly, seasonally, or on occasion.

What New Actions This Month?	*Your Experience?*	*Habit Worthy?*
....	....	☐
....	....	☐
....	....	☐

KAPHA SEASON

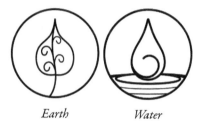

Earth   *Water*

MARCH 1
KAPHA SUPPORTS US

People who are mostly Kapha by constitution tend to have strong, substantial frames, strength and stamina. Think Beyoncé and Harrison Ford. Kapha is comprised of earth and water—the stuff of which bricks are made. This strength offers Kaphas robust immunity, unflagging energy, and a good nature. Balanced Kaphas are calm, loving, and loyal. They often enjoy good health.

Kaphas are affectionate and sweet; however, when out of balance they are often lethargic, lean toward depression, and retain ama. Kaphas move slowly, eat slowly, learn slowly (even though they are great at retaining), and speak deliberately.

Kapha constitutions need to keep moving or "couch potato" syndrome could set in. They may be slow to change and need to avoid attachment to the past. They need to be careful not to overeat, as they're prone to being overweight. Kapha's sweet, loving, and dependable nature can be great support to the other doshas.

Everyone has Kapha, so even if it's not your strongest dosha, it's important to keep Kapha in balance and healthy. Kapha dosha controls moisture, so Kapha excess may result in too much or too thick mucus, which becomes a breeding ground for colds and allergies. This is especially true in the cold and wet season of late winter and early spring. If Kapha is excessive, you might need the cold and cough formulas discussed on Feb 23 & Feb 24.

Kaphas know how to relax. When at the beach, they are at the beach and are not thinking about what needs doing.

Kapha qualities are:

- Unctuous/oily
- Slimy/smooth
- Cold
- Wet
- Heavy

- Stable/static
- Soft
- Cloudy/sticky
- Slow
- Dense

AYURVEDA ACTION
Determine Your Kapha Influence

Check your Assessment 1 results to see how strong your Kapha is. Most people need to do Kapha balancing during Kapha season. Consider the strength of your Kapha and how much balancing you should focus on over the next four months of the season. A little? Or a lot?

MARCH 2
KAPHA FUNCTIONS

KAPHA'S PRIMARY FUNCTIONS are strength, structure, immunity, and lubrication. The stomach is the seat of Kapha. Once Kapha accumulates in the stomach, it could flood into other tissues or organs.

Are you having any stomach issues? While it could be any of the dosha imbalances, because the stomach is Kapha's home, it is worth considering. This is especially true if digestion is sluggish and you are fatigued.

The Kapha bioenergy provides lubrication in the stomach and moistens food in initial stages of digestion. If, however, Kapha becomes excessive in the stomach, it will start to migrate, often in the form of mucus that gets deposited in weak areas—causing colds, coughs, swollen glands, or worse.

Kapha also shows up in other areas of the body that require moisture and lubrication to be at full function, including the heart, lungs, throat, sinuses, and joints.

AYURVEDA ACTION
Add Heat with This Tea

MUCUS CAN GET gooey and thick. Bringing heat to your daily routine adds softness and mobility so that mucus can move out of the body more efficiently. Try this recipe for Mucus-Softening Tea.

Boil the following organic ingredients in a cup of water; strain and cool enough to drink:

- 1 tsp black peppercorns
- 3-5 whole cloves
- 1 inch ginger root, peeled

MARCH 3
KAPHA PHYSICAL TRAITS

Kaphas typically have a large frame, are thickset in the hips and shoulders, and have large, spherical faces. Kapha women are often curvaceous, and men often have a rounder physique.

Kaphas exhibit strong endurance and more stamina than the other doshas. Once begun, physical activity is steady and rarely draining—it's getting started that's the challenge.

Kapha skin is generally oily, smooth, and cool and can be pale. Kaphas often have thick hair, and it can be wavy and oily. Ancient texts describe Kapha eyes as "doe-like" as if "filled with milk." With a slower metabolism, their tendency is to be overweight. If Kaphas eat to past full, the excess gets stored. The metabolic processes cannot rally to deal with overeating.

Kaphas have a graceful walk. They have the cold quality, but good circulation, so typically do not have cold hands and feet.

Kaphas tend to have soft, regular stools.

AYURVEDA ACTION
Eat Warm Cooked Foods to Balance Kapha

Because of the cold quality of Kapha, warm cooked foods are best. Emphasize pungent, astringent, and bitter tastes. Keep meals light—include healthy fats but go easy. Beans are astringent, so are very good for Kaphas. Beans, especially large beans like kidney and garbanzo, are also drying, which balances Kapha's wet quality. If you are concerned with too much dryness, add a dab of ghee to your beans. Hot peppers are pungent and warm up the cool Kapha. Try cooked greens for the bitter taste.

MARCH 4
KAPHA SUBDOSHAS

Not Kapha dominant? You will still have Kapha operating in your subdoshas. Knowledge of subdoshas helps pinpoint where excessive Kapha may be causing issues and will give you additional language to understand what is going on in your system.

Bodhaka Kapha: Located in the tongue, mouth and throat, it governs taste perception, saliva secretion, and the first stage of digestion. Bodhaka Kapha imbalance leads to impairment of taste buds and salivary glands, obesity, food allergies, and diabetes. Taste buds lose sensitivity if abused by eating too much, too often, or compulsively.

Kledaka Kapha: Located in the stomach, it moistens stomach lining through gastric mucosal secretions essential for digestion. It is responsible for moistening food in the first stages of digestion, absorption, and assimilation

Avalambaka Kapha: Located in the chest, heart, lower back, and lungs, it is the moisture responsible for support. It is watery in constitution, distributed by the heart and lungs, and stores phlegm. Avalambaka keeps the heart, chest, and lungs strong. The imbalance of avalambaka Kapha leads to excess phlegm, chest congestion, wheezing, asthma, heart diseases, and low back pain. Smoking is particularly harmful.

Tarpaka Kapha: Located in the brain, sinus, and cerebrospinal fluid. Tarpaka governs nourishment and moisturizing of senses and motor organs. Prana vayu (movement of life forces) carries sensory perceptions to tarpaka Kapha. It is moisture for contentment and memory. Tarpaka Kapha imbalance leads to sinus congestion, hay fever, impaired sense of smell, and general dullness of senses.

Shleshaka Kapha: Located in joints as synovial fluid, it governs lubrication of joints holds them together while keeping them flexible. Shelashaka Kapha imbalance leads to loose, watery joints and causes joint diseases.

AYURVEDA ACTION
Try This for Bliss

Yoga practices are an uplifting influence on tarpaka Kapha by encouraging contentment and bliss (ananda). Bliss comes with stillness. Regular meditation is the best way to set the conditions for bliss. A regular practice, even five minutes a day rather than 20 or 30 minutes once in a while, offers the most benefit. Yoga asanas (poses) before meditating are enhancing. Many communities offer meditation classes—or look online. Guided meditations also are available from apps such as Insight Timer.

MARCH 5
KAPHA MIND

Remember, everyone has Kapha tendencies that likely need attending when the forces of Kapha season are here.

The Kapha mind is kind and forgiving. Kaphas are not easily shaken, remain steady in crisis, and tend to be tolerant. While Kapha nature has a strong sense of inner security, excessive Kapha can also lead to stubbornness, dullness, and lethargy. Kaphas are often slow to grasp new information but strong on retention. Good memory is another Kapha quality, which can be not so good if holding on hurts.

Kapha is most associated with the white matter and the adipose/fatty tissue layer in the brain and nervous system. White matter is brain tissue composed of connecting nerve fibers. The myelin sheaths around nerve fibers are the fatty layers that protect the nerves and become frayed when stressed or undernourished. Even Kaphas need healthy fats in their daily diet to tone the sheaths and keep them flexible and healthy.

The balanced Kapha mind is calm. "Keep calm and carry on" is a banner slogan for Kaphas, who are likely to anchor those around them. Too much density in one's lifestyle and diet aggravate Kapha and show up in a dull, dense, and slow mind as well.

Kaphas do not like cold, damp weather. They can respond mentally by becoming even slower and perhaps depressed. Kaphas can sleep long and heavily, sometimes oversleeping. They often snore when they sleep and feel rested upon awakening.

AYURVEDA ACTION
Try Brain Herbs

Consider the herbs gotu kola and bacopa for mental clarity. Both are tri-doshic, meaning they balance all three doshas. Each is referred to as brahmi even though they're two different herbs. Both boost brain function, memory, focus, mood, clarity, and learning—but unlike a stimulant, they also nourish and tone the nervous system. According to John Douillard, bacopa targets increased cerebral circulation, which washes and cleanses toxins from the brain. Gotu kola supports the brain's lymphatic drainage to eliminate toxins.[10] They work well taken together.

Dosage is best determined individually with the help of an Ayurvedic practitioner and in consultation with your doctor, especially if you are taking medications. You could consider starting with 1/8 tsp powder each day and increasing up to 1/4 to 1/2 tsp daily.

MARCH 6
KAPHA EMOTIONAL QUALITIES

KAPHA AND ITS Kapha influences are calm and self-contained. Kaphas are slow to react and especially slow to anger. They will withhold controversial views to keep the peace—they would rather enjoy your company than win an argument. The Kapha motto is "I'm OK, and you're fabulous." People love being around Kaphas for their sweet nature.

Healthy Kapha emotions include love, loyalty, regard, caring, kindness, stable security, and a general emotional sense of ease.

Kapha is the densest dosha, so excess density throws emotions out of balance. Kapha imbalances can lead to feelings of depression, complacency, stubbornness, greed, and excessive attachment.

AYURVEDA ACTION
Spark e-Motion

A SEDENTARY LIFESTYLE is a big factor in Kapha accumulation. Moving your body will help keep emotions flowing. Kapha nature does not like to move, but that is exactly what it needs. Let your Vata show your Kapha what to do. Even if your Vata is minor in your constitution or vikruti (see Assessment 1) honor it with movement and your Kapha will benefit. Remember, you have three doshas. By recognizing their roles and responsibilities, you can let a minor dosha take the lead to improve your health.

Kaphas are social, so it can be useful to exercise with a friend or join a group class. Those with strong Kapha are more likely to follow through when others are involved.

MARCH 7
KAPHA RITUCHARYA— SEASONAL REGIME

Kapha season is generally March through June for northern hemisphere climates that are cold in the winter and warm in the summer. Kapha starts with the rainy season and goes until summer heat and dryness kick in.

Adjust the timeline for seasonal doshas based on where you live. Kapha season could be one month long or six, depending on location and how long the rainy season lasts. If you live in Australia, for instance, your seasons are opposite of the United States.

Kapha season emphasizes and exacerbates the qualities of cool, moist, sticky, heavy, and slow. Plants and animals come to life in Kapha season and so should you, beginning with a lighter diet and more movement. What are the squirrels doing? What are the crocuses doing? What about the color of your grass? Mimic nature and the spirit of fresh new life.

When the Kapha qualities come rolling in, you might succumb to their influence and become even more sedentary. A Kapha balancing diet {Mar 13} is called for. Also eat lighter, wear brighter colors, and move around in the freshness of spring.

Kaphas respond to the world primarily through the sense of taste. Abusing the sense of taste by overeating or eating the wrong foods can cause compulsive eating. When taste is dulled, you can become attracted to dramatic, addictive tastes like sugar and processed foods that are formulated to dominate the taste sensation. Mindful eating helps restore a broad sense of taste.

AYURVEDA ACTION
Come to Your Senses with a Raisin

The classic mindful eating practice is centered on a raisin. Begin by holding the raisin in your hand. Look at it like you have never seen it before. Turn it with your fingers, noticing the folds and textures. Smell it. Bring it to your ear and squeeze it. As you slowly take it to your mouth, notice how your arm moves. Become aware of your mouth watering as you chew slowly. As you swallow, feel it pass down your throat.

You can try this with any food. Let this mindful practice influence how you eat. It can restore your sense of taste and reduce compulsive eating.

MARCH 8
KAPHA TIME OF DAY

KAPHA IS THE dominant dosha from 6 a.m. to 10 a.m. and 6 p.m. to 10 p.m. Kapha influence brings cool, moist qualities to these times of day. It's best to awaken and actually get out of bed before 6 a.m., otherwise the earth/water, heavy, sluggish qualities of Kapha can accumulate and decrease motivation for the rest of the day. Getting up early is especially challenging for Kapha types, but they benefit tremendously if they do. It is also best to go to bed during Kapha time, which means by 10 p.m.

Kapha influence contributes to a good memory. If you need to retain information, early morning Kapha hours would be a good time to learn. Because Kapha is calm energy, Kapha hours are also good for meditating.

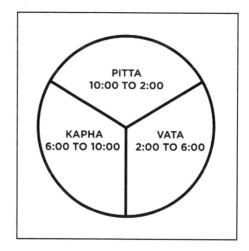

Kapha digestion is slow, so breakfast should be light and easily digestible. Likewise, dinners should be light. As discussed previously, the midday meal, at Pitta time, should be your largest. Overloading your physical and emotional digestion can occur if you eat cold, moist meals in morning and evening Kapha hours, especially during the Kapha season. The result can be weight gain or depressed emotions.

Call on Kapha strength and stamina to support an exercise regime. Exercising during the Kapha hours of 6 a.m. and 10 a.m. and early evening is great. Exercising during these hours helps keep Kapha excess moderated and motivates the day.

AYURVEDA ACTION
Go to Bed by 10 p.m.; Rise by 6 a.m.

IF YOU ARE sleeping well, great. Getting sufficient sleep eludes many. If you are having difficulties falling or staying asleep, align with Kapha timing for going to bed (10 p.m.) and getting up (6 a.m.). A late bedtime invites a second wind from Pitta influence and you may have difficulty falling asleep. If you're currently going to bed at midnight, adjust to an earlier bedtime by 15 minutes every day or two until you are in bed by 10 p.m. Or, just be in bed by then, even if you are reading or listening to guided meditations. Your body/mind needs time to adjust, so move slowly to the earlier bedtime.

The same applies to morning. Slowly adjust your getting-up time to 15 minutes earlier until you are stabilized at about 6 a.m. If you are not ready to jump out of bed and start your day, read in bed or do yoga stretches.

While these times put most people in sync with Nature's rhythm, see what works best for you.

MARCH 9
KAPHA TIME OF LIFE

THE DOSHA LIFE cycle also influences you, along with your constitutional dosha. In our youth to age 20 to 25, you're most influenced by Kapha qualities. At age 20 or so, Pitta asserts influence. At age 50 or 55 and beyond, Vata rules. These doshic qualities help you to attune to your engagements and responsibilities for the evolving stages of the life cycle.

So Kapha time of life is the beginning. "Baby fat" might stay with you for a few years, and you experience more carefree days. You get more sleep, take naps. Kapha issues such as greed and possessiveness can emerge as identity and a sense of self is formed.

Children make a lot of mucus. Dr. John Douillard, a noted Ayurveda leader and educator, says, "Kids make mucus for a living."[11] The wetness and lubrication of Kapha helps build tissues, but sometimes the mucus gets thick with ama and traps viruses and bacteria. This can result in a plethora of minor childhood illnesses.

Mucus production is fairly heavy in the first 12 years of life; then it slows down in teenage years. In the middle adult years, it remains fairly stable until our senior years, when we tend to dry out. Applying Ayurveda principles and strategies helps keep aging systems moist.

If you are caring for a child who seems to have excessive Kapha, consider doing some balancing. The right amount of mucus is important, so aim to reduce Kapha mucus only if it is excessive. When mucus is the right consistency, it collects and carries bacteria, viruses, and other threats out of the body.

AYURVEDA ACTION
Try Turmeric to Liquefy Mucus

TURMERIC IS GREAT for reducing excess mucus, and it also reduces inflammation in the sinuses and respiratory tract. A good way to take turmeric is to mix equal parts of raw honey (though generally not recommended for Kapha on a daily basis, okay on occasion) and turmeric into a paste and have 1/2 to 1 tsp daily. If you are treating a cold, take the paste every few hours throughout the day for up to 7 days.

MARCH 10
KAPHA OUT OF BALANCE

Because the body's moisture is a Kapha contribution, an imbalance will show up in the mucus membranes. Disturbed Kapha manifests as congested sinuses, allergies, colds, asthma, and sometimes, swollen joints. Kapha imbalances show up especially in late winter and in spring, at the start of Kapha season.

Emotionally disturbed Kapha can show up as greed or attachment. Your Kapha nature is the pack rat in you. Maybe you're hesitant to cut people out of your life. Sometimes even positive change takes a long time. Stagnation is an issue.

Too much Kapha? You might notice these signs:

- excess mucus in the sinuses or in stool
- lethargic, "couch potato"
- thick, slimy white coating on tongue
- dull thinking
- overly attached to people or things
- oversleeping
- feeling heavy, especially after eating and emotional overeating
- resistance to change, or stubbornness

Although diseases do not automatically emerge from a particular out-of-balance dosha, some diseases are more aligned with a specific dosha imbalance. Some excessive Kapha conditions to watch for are obesity, diabetes, high cholesterol, high blood pressure, edema, colds, congestion, asthma, allergies, low mood, and depression.

AYURVEDA ACTION
Cleanse Kapha Often

Kapha, in general, needs more regular cleansing than the other doshas. Daily spice water {xvi} helps. An all-liquid diet one day per week could be beneficial. You could have a light vegetable juice drink in the morning with kale, spinach, and sprouts plus a squirt of lemon or lime and water. For lunch, puree vegetables from the Kapha diet list {Mar 13} with water. Or, make a brothy soup and run it through a blender.

Do not mix fruits and vegetable juices, and never mix yogurt with other food. Digestion rates among these food items vary—it's better to stay with vegetables for your juice. Finally, unless you are very hungry, for supper have a cup of fresh ginger tea with a bit of raw honey or fresh fruit, such as an apple or berries.

MARCH 11
BALANCING KAPHA

KAPHA IS EARTH and water. Kapha influence provides lubrication, support, tissue development, and strength. In the fable of the tortoise and the hare, Kapha is definitely the tortoise—slow and steady wins the race.

In balance, Kaphas are sweet and loving—a joy to be with. They are dependable, nurturing, stable, relaxed, and loyal. Kapha is characterized by tissue growth, overall strength and stamina, and the strongest immunity. Kaphas are stand-up, solid folks. With their tolerance and patience, they are balancing for judgmental Pittas.

Recall that Kapha qualities are unctuous/oily, slimy/smooth, cold, wet, heavy, stable/static, soft, cloudy/sticky, slow, and dense. According to Principle 2 {Jan 10} you engage opposite qualities to balance, so do activities and choose foods that are dry, light, rough, subtle, mobile, and clear.

Regular, sustained detoxification is particularly called for to balance Kapha. Its naturally slower metabolism allows toxins to accumulate and pollute the body's tissues. Fatigue is a sign of toxin accumulation.

Even though it does not come naturally to them, Kaphas need stimulation. Without it, inertia can take over. They can cling to old possessions or relationships that no longer serve. Kaphas really need to move to stay in balance. As they like people, I recommend taking yoga or exercise classes with others or arrange to meet a friend for walks. The social connection may engage them when pure exercise does not.

A light, spicy diet is good for Kapha. Pungent spices are heating and stimulating. Kapha needs these to fight tendencies to accumulate ama. Beans are also good for Kaphas, because the drying quality counteracts Kapha's excess moisture. In fact, Kapha is the only dosha that can eat large, airy beans to balance.

AYURVEDA ACTION
Try a One-Day, Two-Part Reset

GIVE YOUR DIGESTION a chance to rest and to reboot with this one-day reset. First, eat kitchari {Mar 19}—the rice and mung-bean Ayurveda staple—for breakfast, lunch, and dinner. Second, sip hot spice water with a slice of fresh ginger throughout the day, but only 1/2 cup with your kitchari. Try to drink a total of 2 quarts hot spice water.

MARCH 12
KAPHA AND THE TASTES

KAPHA IS PACIFIED by pungent, astringent, and bitter tastes—PAB. Kapha is aggravated by the tastes that pacify Vata—the S trilogy—sweet, sour, and salty.

It's Kapha season, so conditions will likely aggravate and bring out excessive Kapha in everyone. Now is the time to favor PAB.

PUNGENT tastes are composed of fire and air, which can heat, dry, and eliminate Kapha. Think hot. Pungent ignites Kapha's sluggish qualities by increasing energy. The pungent taste kindles agni and improves digestion and elimination. Examples are chili peppers, mustard greens, radishes, onions, and spices like ginger, cloves, cardamom, cayenne, and especially, black pepper.

ASTRINGENT taste is composed of air and earth. It's the flavor of dryness, causing the mouth's mucous membranes to contract. If food makes you pucker, it is astringent. Kapha can pool dampness in the body, which often exhibits as mucus: astringency breaks it up. Astringency is good to tone tissues. It's also cooling—not always good for Kapha—so include pungent tastes along with astringent. Foods to favor include apples, green bananas, cranberries, pomegranate, avocado, cabbage, cauliflower, and especially beans. Astringent spices include basil, bay leaf, coriander, oregano, nutmeg, and poppy seeds.

BITTER is made up of air and ether—again, the qualities that lighten and move stagnant Kapha. Most people are not drawn to bitter, yet it is astoundingly beneficial for us. It promotes a healthy pancreas, liver, and spleen and is the paramount blood cleanser. Bitter is known for a capacity to break up fat and toxins. It tones the muscles and skin and relieves flatulence. Because bitter is drying, be cautious if your Vata is imbalanced as it may further dry your tissues. The best sources are lightly cooked greens such as kale, collards, and dandelion greens. And blessed be, dark chocolate is also a good source of bitter! Of course, your chocolate should not be accompanied by processed sugars, particularly high-fructose corn syrup. Sesame seeds and oil, fenugreek, turmeric, and saffron are also good sources.

AYURVEDA ACTION
Eat Toasted Sesame Seeds

NEED A LITTLE crunch in your diet? Add toasted sesame seeds to your dishes for bitter taste in a delicious way. Heat seeds in a dry skillet over medium heat for 3–5 minutes or until lightly browned. Sesame seeds strengthen bones and hair and are a known aphrodisiac.

MARCH 13
KAPHA BALANCING DIET

Favor warm cooked foods and eat lighter. Favor pungent, bitter, and astringent tastes.

Dairy
Heated raw milk is the best milk option but often it is not available. Most other dairy is not advised. Use alternatives such as almond milk.

Raw honey
In moderation, it is excellent for reducing Kapha. Do not heat, although you can add to tea when warm. Reduce white and brown sugars, as they will increase Kapha.

Grains
Most grains are fine, especially quinoa, barley and millet. Avoid wheat and rice (other than easily digestible white basmati); they increase Kapha.

Fruits
Lighter fruits, such as apples and pears, are better. Pomegranates and cranberries are also good and cleansing for Kapha. Reduce heavy or sour fruits such as oranges, ripe bananas, pineapples, figs, dates, avocados, coconuts and melons.

Legumes
All beans are fine, except tofu.

Vegetables
Most are good, except tomatoes, cucumbers, sweet potatoes and zucchini, which increase Kapha. Favor radish, asparagus, green leafy vegetables, beets, broccoli, carrots, cauliflower, pumpkin/squash, and celery.

Spices
All are fine, except salt.

Nuts
Reduce consumption of all nuts.

Meat for Non-Vegetarians
Chicken and turkey.

Oils
Small amounts only—almond, sunflower, ghee, olive.

AYURVEDA ACTION
Eat a Kapha-Balancing Diet

Eat foods that are light, dry, warm, and rough at every meal. Fruits and vegetables are generally light and should be lightly cooked. Even fruits such as apples are better for Kapha if stewed and spiced. Cook with lots of heating spices. Drying foods are good. Beans are an excellent example of a drying food, and they are a great source of protein. Avoid oily foods, nuts, and cheeses.

MARCH 14
KAPHA BALANCING LIFESTYLE

THE MOST IMPORTANT lifestyle practice to balance Kapha is regular exercise. When out of balance, Kaphas can be lethargic and may need to push themselves to get moving. Kaphas often need vigorous and longer-lasting exercise[12]. Engage your relational Kapha for motivation, by committing to exercising with friends and family or by taking a class.

Out-of-balance Kaphas often become shallow breathers. Deep breathing or kundalini yoga would be helpful. Deep breathing also stimulates metabolism, so should be a core practice of the healthy Kapha lifestyle—any dosha for that matter. With shallow breathing the air enters only your upper chest, which causes diminished oxygen to your blood vessels and strain on your heart and lungs. In deep breathing, you take in nearly seven times as much oxygen and prana.

Another good lifestyle habit good for all doshas, but particularly Kapha, is to eat the largest meal at midday when Pitta/agni is strongest, which helps you digest food more easily and completely. Thus, ama waste is less likely to form.

Hey, Kaphas: If your supper is not digested to the point where you are hungry in the morning, Ayurveda says "don't eat." Eating when you are not hungry leads to incomplete digestion—the primary condition that creates ill health. Wait until you are hungry to eat your breakfast or any meal for that matter.

AYURVEDA ACTION
Do Three-Part Breathing

DIRGA PRANAYAMA, OR three-part breathing, brings you into the moment, a good practice for Kapha, who tends to dwell in the past. Release your arms and soften as you go. Continue at your own pace, without pausing, for up to five minutes.

- Sit upright, with straight spine, in easy cross-legged pose or in a chair. Close your eyes and relax. Place your left hand on your abdomen below the navel and your right hand on your rib cage.
- Focus on breathing through your nose. Naturally, with relaxed breath, your belly will lift first, followed by your ribs, and finally the chest. On inhalation, feel the slight compression of your ribs, followed by your belly on exhale. Exhale, pressing gently on your abdomen to completely expel air. Exhale first from the chest, then the ribs, and lastly the belly.
- Next move your left hand to your chest just below your collarbone. Inhale, bringing air all the way up to this area.

MARCH 15
KAPHA AND WEIGHT MANAGEMENT

Ama (toxins) is the biggest factor in excessive weight for most people. Toxin overload slows metabolism, which leads to more ama—a vicious circle. Ama is more an issue for Kapha than any other dosha. Kaphas, and those with its strong influence, are prone to slow metabolism because of the heavy earth and water elements that form this dosha. Remember, these traits will be more likely to show up for everyone in the Kapha season.

Kaphas are structurally bigger, with bigger bones. Make peace with that—it's not advisable to be "skinny." A Kapha-balancing diet and lifestyle will help you find a healthy weight. The main principle for balancing Kapha weight management is to introduce the fire element to balance earth and water. Hot, spicy food is the way to go. Stay away from cold foods, especially cold desserts like ice cream. Avoid fried, oily foods. Eat light, clean foods (like fresh cooked vegetables) with peppery heat in them.

As noted in the lifestyle entry yesterday, exercise is important to keep Kapha in check and essential for maintaining an ideal weight.

AYURVEDA ACTION
Swap Out Grains to Manage Weight

If you like grains but also want to lose weight, consider quinoa and basmati rice. Quinoa is high in protein and zinc and is slightly drying. Quinoa also has the intelligence of the fire element, so it's great for pacifying excessive Kapha.

Next best is white basmati rice. It also has a slightly drying quality. If you don't desire the dryness, add ghee to these grains. Brown rice is sometimes touted as healthier because it offers more fiber; however, according to Ayurveda it is harder to break down and digest.

Be sure to mix some fire with your grains, such as cayenne or fresh ginger.

MARCH 16
KAPHA SPICES

Spices are intelligent. They hold power and influence long after being picked. So, adding spices to food is smart, especially for Kaphas. When Kapha is excessive, the body tends to produce thick, gooey, cold mucus that covers over our liveliness. How do we balance that? The gelatinous nature of excess mucus needs to be broken up. Heat helps because it is a vasodilator that opens up the blood vessels and heat stimulates vascular and energetic movement. So first, and most importantly, add heating, pungent spices to your diet to balance Kapha and break up the gooeyness. You will benefit from astringent and bitter spices. If you recall {Mar 12}, Kapha is balanced by the tastes of pungent, astringent, and bitter.

Here are pungent spices to balance Kapha:

- Cayenne pepper
- Black pepper
- Hot peppers
- Ginger
- Cardamom
- Mustard seeds

- Cinnamon
- Cumin—also bitter
- Clove—also bitter
- Turmeric—also astringent and bitter
- Fenugreek—also astringent and bitter

AYURVEDA ACTION
Keep Kapha Churna on Hand

A good way to get your spices is to make a Kapha churna (spice mixture) focused on Kapha balancing. Keep it ready to use in your cooking in an airtight container.

Mix together:

- 2 Tbsp fenugreek seeds
- 2 Tbsp whole coriander seeds
- 2 Tbsp whole cumin seeds
- 1 Tbsp ground ginger
- 1 Tbsp ground turmeric
- 1 Tbsp ground cardamom
- 1 Tbsp ground cinnamon
- 1 tsp ground clove
- 1/2 tsp cayenne pepper or 1 tsp ground black pepper or 1 tsp red pepper flakes

Pan-roast the seeds first if you wish. Then grind all ingredients in a spice/coffee grinder. You might change up this recipe for your preference in spices as well as what you already have.

MARCH 17
KAPHA CHUTNEY

CHUTNEYS ARE CONDIMENTS that not only add flavors to food, but also introduce a selection of the six tastes to support dosha balancing. Ayurveda chutneys often include four or more tastes, especially the sour taste. Sour draws attention to the food, causes salivation, and improves fat metabolism.

Kapha is balanced by pungent, astringent and bitter tastes. You will find those in this chutney along with sweet and sour. Overall, this chutney balances Kapha because the spices have a more powerful influence than their representative quantity.

- 4 cups apples (sour, sweet) or half apples & half pears (sweet, astringent)
- 1/2 tsp cumin seed (bitter, pungent)
- 1/2 tsp mustard seed (bitter, pungent)
- 1 tsp ghee (sweet)
- 2 pinch fenugreek powder (bitter, pungent)
- 2 pinches dried ginger (pungent)
- 2 pinches cayenne pepper (pungent)
- 1/4 tsp cinnamon (pungent, astringent, sweet)
- 1/2 tsp turmeric (bitter)
- 1/4 cup raw honey, or use less (sweet)
- 1/4 cup water or orange juice (sweet, sour)

Peel apples and chop into small pieces. Sauté the seeds in ghee for 2 minutes to release their intelligence, then add the powdered spice to the ghee for 1 minute. Cook the apples in water that you bring to boil, then simmer for about 15 minutes until just soft. Add the spice paste and raw honey (to taste) to the cooked apples.

AYURVEDA ACTION
Make an Even Quicker Chutney

IN A HURRY? This simple chutney recipe balances Kapha. Just combine these 5 ingredients in a food processor.

- 1 Tbsp lemon or lime juice
- 1/2 cup orange juice
- 3/4 cup chopped, peeled ginger root
- 1/2 cup raisins
- Pinch of cayenne pepper

MARCH 18
KAPHA BREAKFAST

Kaphas should only eat when hungry. It is fine to skip breakfast if the evening meal has not fully digested, or keep it light—a piece of fruit or freshly juiced fruit and/or a cup of tea. Good fruits to balance Kapha are apples, berries, lemons, limes, and pomegranates.

Hungry and ready for breakfast? Warm, cooked grains like quinoa, barley, rye, and basmati rice make an excellent hot breakfast cereal. Add spices like cinnamon and cloves to the cereal and perhaps soaked, peeled almonds and pumpkin or sunflower seeds. A small amount of raw honey is fine, but add only when cereal is cool enough to eat. Eggs are also good for pacifying Kapha, but hold the cheese.

Kaphas respond to the world primarily through the sense of rasa, or taste, and gandha, or smell.

Overeating or eating the wrong foods abuses the sense of taste and can lead to compulsive eating. When the taste is dulled, the attraction to dramatic and addictive tastes like sugar and processed foods is strong. Try mindful eating to restore a broad sense of taste.

AYURVEDA ACTION
Attend to Emotions to Avoid Overeating

Hunger signals a need for nourishment, but it can also occur when you are trying to pacify an emotion. Difficult emotions, or even boredom, can create a void that you're tempted to fill with food, especially sweets.

To stop a cycle of emotional eating, try to discern the emotion that triggers hunger. If you're feeling anxious, a warm bath with Epsom salts might better serve you. If you're sad, arrange to spend time with a friend or process the sadness by journaling or sitting quietly.

Emotional overeating is a habit of mind. When you know what is going on, you can make different choices.

MARCH 19
KAPHA LUNCH/DINNER

Kaphas especially need to eat their largest meal midday when the digestive fire is strongest between 10 a.m. and 2 p.m. Lots of steamed or very lightly sautéed vegetables like carrots, broccoli, peas, and cauliflower are great. Serve them over barley, millet or quinoa. Quinoa can help with weight loss. Add fresh grated ginger, cayenne pepper, or other hot pepper. Toasted sunflower or pumpkin seeds add crunch. For protein, add a boiled egg or a bit of healthy chicken. No fatty red meats.

Perhaps the ideal midday meal for Kapha is kitchari. It is easy to digest, with metabolism-boosting spices. Cloves enhance blood flow to the skin and stimulate the lymphatic system. Cardamom breaks down mucus and ginger stimulates the heart and circulation. Cumin and bay leaves ease water retention.

KITCHARI—THE AYURVEDA STAPLE

- 1/2 cup white basmati rice
- 1 cup mung beans/dahl (split yellow)
- 6 cups water
- 2 tsp ghee
- 1/2 tsp cumin seeds
- 1/2 tsp mustard seeds
- 1/4 tsp cardamom powder
- 1/2 tsp cinnamon powder
- 1/4 tsp clove powder
- 1/2 tsp cumin powder
- 1/2 tsp turmeric powder
- 1 inch fresh ginger, grated
- 1/4 tsp mineral salt
- 4 bay leaves

Optional: assorted vegetables such as greens, asparagus, Brussels sprouts, cabbage, cauliflower, or green beans

Pick out any stones from mung beans, rinse thoroughly, and soak several hours. Drain mung beans and rinse rice. Add 6 cups water, bring to a boil, and cook about 20 minutes. Scoop away any foam that forms. Clean and cut any vegetables into bite-sized pieces; add to the pot for about 10 minutes. Melt ghee and sauté spice seeds until they pop, then add spice powders for 20 seconds. Add spices and bay leaves to the pot.

AYURVEDA ACTION
Increase Agni with Ginger Pickle

Ginger pickle boosts agni by releasing the proper digestive juices in the mouth, activating metabolism, and stimulating digestion. Eat 10-15 minutes before a meal. Cut a slice of fresh ginger the size of a quarter. Squeeze fresh lime or lemon juice on it. Sprinkle with salt. Chew well. Options: Grate the ginger and add a small dab of raw honey. You can also make enough for three or four days. Store in a small glass jar in the refrigerator.

MARCH 20
KAPHA SUPPER

Supper should be light, which is not the norm in many cultures. Warm, clear-broth soups with vegetables and beans are recommended for pacifying Kapha. Add spices like cumin, fresh ginger, turmeric, and peppers. Kaphas should avoid cold foods.

A sweet potato, kale, and ginger soup would be lovely for Kapha balancing, or a mung bean soup with a few veggies would be pacifying and detoxifying, like the recipe below. Search for other recipes at joyfulbelly.com.

MUNG BEAN SOUP

- 1 cup whole green mung beans (soak at least 6 hours)
- 3 1/2–4 cups water
- 1 Tbsp ghee
- 1/2 tsp cumin seeds
- 1/2 tsp mustard seeds
- 1/2 tsp turmeric powder
- 1/4 tsp hing powder (aka asofoetida—not necessary for Kapha but for Vata & Pitta)
- 1 bay leaf
- 1 1/2 tsp ginger, chopped or grated
- 1 1/2 tsp lemon juice

1. Soak the mung beans overnight in water.
2. Drain and rinse beans and put them in pot with water.
3. Cook beans until they break apart, about 45 minutes.
4. Heat ghee in a separate pan. Add seeds and sauté 2 minutes; then add powders, bay leaf, and ginger.
5. Add ghee mixture to cooked mung beans and stir.
6. Add mineral salt and pepper to taste. Add lemon juice.
7. Add greens like kale or spinach if desired.

AYURVEDA ACTION
Eat Mung Beans for Big-Time Cleansing

Ayurveda extols mung beans for their cleansing action. Add them to other recipes or make the mung bean soup above. If you are feeling tired or bloated, eat mung beans for soluble and insoluble fibers that scrape the colon clean to help you feel better. They are small and easier to digest than large beans. Mung beans tone digestive organs and purge mucus from the bowels, moving out toxins and parasites in the process. Their astringent taste is pacifying for Kapha.

MARCH 21
KAPHA BALANCING DRINKS

Hot, warm, or room-temperature beverages provide the fire Kaphas need, and help digestion during this Kapha season for everyone. Avoid cold drinks, especially iced drinks.

Dairy is particularly difficult for Kapha to digest, so unless you can get raw milk, drink milk sparingly or avoid it. The traditional Indian lassi—made with yogurt, water, and spices—can be consumed in moderation because spices and fermented dairy makes this delicious drink more easily digestible.

Because Kapha digestion is sluggish, occasional days of liquid diet are advised. Kaphas can sustain energy even when eating light or skipping meals. Try a liquid diet one day a week. A mix of vegetable juices, including beet and carrot juice, is good. Or try fruit juice made with apple and pomegranate. Do not mix vegetables and fruits. They are processed at different rates which can confuse your system.

Here is a tasty tea to support Kapha balancing for detoxing, releasing mucus, and weight loss. Each measurement is a "part." Depending on how much you want to make, 1 part could be a teaspoon or a cup.

KAPHA BALANCING TEA

- 4 parts ginger powder
- 4 parts cardamom powder
- 1 part clove (the spice, not garlic) powder
- 1/2 part turmeric
- 1/2 part pepper
- 1/4 part saffron

Mix and take as 1/2 tsp per 1 cup boiled water. Adding a bit of raw honey also pacifies Kapha.

AYURVEDA ACTION
Drink Few Liquids at Mealtime

Sip just 1/2 cup of hot water with a meal to add a little moisture to food but not more. If eating liquid foods like dahls and soups, limit your serving size to 1/2 cup. Avoid alcohol with your meal as alcohol interferes with proper and complete digestion. Consider a yogurt lassi drink {Aug 29} with your meal.

MARCH 22
KAPHA DINACHARYA—DAILY ROUTINE

All through the natural world we see creatures with daily routines. As humans, we have gotten away from this habit but benefit from it. Our physiology is adapted for routine and it is potent medicine for us. A daily routine or dinacharya is self-love. Ayurveda especially focuses on early morning routines. Let's keep in mind though that Kapha can get into a rut with too much routine and does need some excitement and variety as well. But that variety will be better received if there is a routine in place. Here is a typical healthy routine for Kaphas, and others during Kapha season.

IN THE MORNING

1. Choose a consistent time to awaken, even weekends preferably before 6 a.m.
2. Scrape tongue.
3. Empty bladder and bowels.
4. Brush teeth. Do oil pulling {Oct 23}.
5. Drink a large glass of warm water or hot water with lemon.
6. Move with morning kundalini yoga, a brisk walk, or other exercise.
7. Dry brush skin. Shower or bathe. Do a neti pot if mucus is excessive. Drop nasya oil into nostrils. Do an abhyanga self-massage if skin is not too oily.
8. Meditate.
9. Eat a Kapha-pacifying breakfast—fresh fruit or cooked grains {Mar 18}.

THROUGHOUT THE DAY

1. Keep a slow and steady work pace to honor your Kapha.
2. Eat lunch on time as your main meal.
3. Take a brisk walk.
4. Eat a light supper early in the evening.

AT BEDTIME

1. Turn off electronics at least 30 minutes before bedtime.
2. Brush and floss teeth.
3. Go to bed by 10 p.m. during Kapha time.
4. Take 1–2 triphala tablets or drink triphala tea.
5. Release tension with soft yogic breathing.

AYURVEDA ACTION
Ginger Up Your Daily Spice Water

Add a slice of ginger to your spice water. It is heating for Kapha and breaks up mucus.

MARCH 23
KAPHA SUPER HERBS

In Ayurveda, herbs are part of a comprehensive approach to balance and health. With this guidance in mind, let's look at herbs known to be particularly balancing for excessive Kapha.

Kapha is composed of earth and water and is responsible for structure and lubrication in our mind and body. When Kapha is vitiated, meaning impaired, conditions such as sinus problems, weight gain, diabetes, water retention, and excessive sleep can arise. Herbs that are light, heating, and stimulating balance Kapha's cool, heavy, and stuck qualities. Pungent herbs fill this bill.

TURMERIC—pungent, astringent, bitter and heating. Turmeric may be the most researched medicinal herb of all. (A great site to check this out is greenmedinfo.com.) Turmeric moves lymph, cleanses blood, lowers cholesterol, inhibits cancer cells, soothes the digestive system, and inhibits growth of bacteria, yeast, and viruses. A primary active ingredient in turmeric is curcumin. Some herbal companies have isolated curcumin and tout it as more effective than turmeric. Ayurveda does not support this thinking. An herb's power and influence is most noted when it is whole.

GINGER—pungent, heating. This versatile herb improves digestion and can alleviate nausea. Ginger contains powerful anti-inflammatory phytonutrients and is a strong antioxidant and antibacterial agent. Ginger is very heating, particularly in its intense powdered form, and is often used to treat typical Kapha conditions such as sinus congestion, sluggish digestion, and overweight issues. Ginger kindles agni.

CLOVE—pungent, heating. Cloves improve blood circulation, and we know Kaphas sometimes have trouble with that! These aromatic, dried-flower buds promote digestion by increasing hydrochloric acid production in the stomach, and are anti-inflammatory.

BLACK PEPPER—pungent, heating. Black pepper is warming and pacifying for Kapha and Vata. Use it freely to warm and stimulate your Kapha. Too much aggravates Pitta. Generally, use it as a powder, but peppercorns can be added to recipes and teas.

AYURVEDA ACTION
Add Ginger to Reduce Kapha Qualities

KEEP FRESH GINGER on hand and add it to meals. Sauté ginger in ghee, coconut oil, or avocado oil to release the herb's intelligence. Have a ginger pickle before your meal. {Mar 19} Add a slice of fresh ginger to your daily hot spice water.

MARCH 24
KAPHA WORK AND PLAY

The Kapha influence at work leads to slow and steady progress. Co-workers like Kaphas' sweet nature—for the most part. When in balance, Kaphas can listen intently, and are receptive to working together. They also are strong, with stamina. They may be slow to get started and rely on others for the spark of a fresh idea, but once going, they endure and get the job done. Loyalty is strong—perhaps too strong.

However, a Kapha stuck in a sedentary job can be sluggish, stuck in a rut, and exhibit withdrawn behavior. This could bring out possessiveness as well. Although routine may be comforting, the Kapha in everyone needs to beware of getting bored from repetitiveness or lack of physical movement. Seek ways to add variety and movement to your workday.

Kapha people make compassionate leaders and are good in helping professions. They can be great at manual labor. They are caring and patient. They are good at creating security, cohesion, and stability for themselves and others.

Kapha play comes down to one key quality—plays well with others. Kaphas enjoy people immensely, so when they play, they want to be with a group or a companion. While not crazy about lots of active play, which is what they need, they're more likely to "join in." Kaphas generally prefer slow and steady activities, like cross-country skiing. Kaphas left alone too long can slip into sadness.

Even if your dosha doesn't have a strong Kapha influence, you almost surely work or socialize with Kaphas. Even if you work from home you are likely to have opportunities to engage with others by phone or online. This knowledge can help you appreciate Kapha style and contributions.

AYURVEDA ACTION
Seek Out Challenges that Move You

Find motivations in your work or with co-workers. For example, allow yourself to feel and act on healthy competition. Find ways to move at work. Park your car far away from the entrance to your job, take the stairs, walk at lunch hour. Watch your tendency to snack on sweets. When you want something sweet, drink a cup of warm tea first to circumvent the desire and habit. Time to play? Find a buddy—you are more likely to follow through.

MARCH 25
KAPHA SKIN

A core Ayurvedic philosophy is that beauty radiates from within and is an essential aspect of your being. Skin is an outer shell that reflects the inner workings of your body. Healthy, radiant skin begins with diet and lifestyle choices. Eating in ways that balance your dosha(s) and making good daily lifestyle decisions give you the best shot at awesome health, which shines through your radiant skin.

Kapha skin type tends to have the qualities of water and earth—it can be oily, thick, pale, soft, cool, and more tolerant of the sun. It tends to age more slowly and form fewer wrinkles. What a blessing! However, Kaphas may also struggle with dull complexion, enlarged pores, excessive oil, blackheads, pimples, moist types of eczema, and water retention/puffiness.

Since Kapha skin is often moist, brushing it with a natural bristle skin brush or with Ayurvedic silk garshana gloves is highly recommended. This keeps the lymph system moving, which is critical for Kapha health. Abhyanga self-massage {Dec 6} is generally advised, unless there are skin issues. Doing abhyanga with 1/2 cup or less of warm sesame oil supports the movement of toxins to the lymph system for removal and brings toxins to the skin's surface to be rinsed away.

AYURVEDA SKIN CLEANSER-TONER-EXFOLIATOR FOR KAPHA

- 1 Tbsp organic cornmeal, chickpea, or oat flour
- 1/4 teaspoon triphala, triphala guggulu, or almond powder
- Rosewater or 1/2 tsp fresh lemon juice

First, rinse your face with warm water. Mix powders and dab dry powders on moist face. Next, spritz your face with rosewater until you make a paste. Massage in powders/rosewater to cleanse and exfoliate. Rinse. Or—mix dry powders and add lemon juice for a paste to put on your face.

Experiment with this treatment to determine whether it is okay to use on your skin daily. If redness or dryness occur, reduce the times per week or eliminate.

AYURVEDA ACTION
Cleanse and Tone Skin Each Night

Develop a nighttime ritual of using the cleanser-toner-exfoliator above. After cleansing, massage a small amount of light warming oil, such as jojoba or sesame, on the face to tone it. If your skin is oily, apply oil sparingly—just enough to replenish the skin and see a balanced glow.

MARCH 26
KAPHA SPIRITUALITY

MEDITATION IS ONE of the most basic practices to support spirituality for any dosha. The practice involves sitting quietly without movement. Kaphas are good at this because they are devotional by nature and can find bliss in daily spiritual practice.

Kapha types also will benefit from active, engaging meditation that helps release emotional attachments and counters lethargy. They might also find it helpful to do active yoga (such as kundalini) or to exercise before meditation to avoid falling asleep.

Walking meditations are particularly good for Kapha. Stay warm and take a short walk in nature, away from public sensory stimulation, if possible, in a place where you feel safe. Breathe deeply. Notice your breath. Notice your experience.

Pranayama, or controlled breathing, is good to stir up the sticky Kapha in any of us. Mantra meditations also are good for Kapha. Sit upright and avoid slouching. A stimulating mantra meditation is chanting OM. For visualization meditations, focus on fire and sun elements, or on moving wind. Meditate with a candle to engage fire, or with a fire-colored golden or orange shawl. Kirtan—group chanting—can be beneficial for Kaphas, as they express spirituality best in communities of like-minded others.

Kundalini yoga, combined with mantra chanting and meditation, can be particularly stimulating for a Kapha. It serves spiritual advancement by moving energy. Pranayama can also be stimulating and thus serving to Kapha.

AYURVEDA ACTION
Practice to Move Prana and Cleanse

PRANAYAMA MEANS CONTROL of the prana or life energy. Pranayama can be practiced on its own or combined with meditation. Many forms of pranayama exist, but one that benefits Kapha is "breath of fire" or "kapalabhati" because of its cleansing, energizing nature.

Sit quietly in a chair or cross-legged on the floor. Relax and breathe evenly. Begin kapalabhati by inhaling then exhaling forcibly through the nose while simultaneously pulling in your diaphragm/abdomen toward your spine. After a brisk, forceful exhale, the inhale happens naturally as the lungs open and act as a vacuum. Begin slowly. Over time, increase the speed and length of practice. Contraindications are cardiac condition or illness. Practice on an empty stomach.

MARCH 27
KAPHA LOVE

Healthy Kaphas are sweet, sweet, sweet. They are teddy bears, sharing their love and offering hugs. Kaphas are calming for the fire of Pitta and grounding for Vata. They are devoted, but can get too attached if out of balance.

Kaphas often have the big, round cow eyes that are easy to fall into. They're good listeners, but need to feel safe and invited to open up. Kaphas are sincere and mean what they say. If you are thinking of traveling with a Kapha, they prefer warm climates.

Want to honor the Kapha in your life? Here are things you can do, or let others know if these would be well received:

- Cook a meal for a Kapha. You can reach their heart through their tummy.
- Snuggle up to watch a movie together, or be okay if they are doing that while you work on a project around the house.
- Kaphas are slow to build their fire. Be patient with passion.
- Give space. Kaphas need time to consider what you have shared and like to make sure their response is not edgy or harmful. Even when they are angry, they know they still love you.
- Move with your Kapha person, especially around water. They may not be fond of too much action, but if it is gentle and encouraging, they will appreciate how they feel afterward. Time in nature is good for all doshas but is especially healing for Kaphas.
- Routine generally pleases Kaphas, but try gentle encouragement for something new, maybe just one thing in one day. They don't naturally gravitate toward the novel, but generally feel better after stimulation.
- Want to really make a Kapha swoon? Write them a poem.
- For more romance, try stimulating the sense of smell. A nice perfume, essential oil, or an aromatic food might provide the right stimulation. Just a little food, or your Kapha might focus on eating and forget about romance.

AYURVEDA ACTION
Communicate Your Love Needs

Remember, we all have Kapha qualities. The Kapha in you reveres love relationships. Communicate to a loved one what makes you come alive in relationship. Try to share your need or preference as a request and not a demand. Explore resources on Compassionate Communication, also known as Non-Violent Communication, for principles and practices. An example of what you might express is, "I feel loved, appreciated, and safe when you prepare a meal for me."

MARCH 28
KAPHA CHILDREN

KAPHA CHILDREN GENERALLY have larger frames with heavier, stockier builds. A Kapha child can be prone to excess weight. They love sweets and may need discipline to keep this tendency in check. They are likely to have a stable, tranquil personality. Although their Nature is to harmonize with other children, they can dip into sadness if they have too much time alone, or if they are not getting along with their peers.

Their natural hunger is mild, and digestion is slow. Kapha children shouldn't eat beyond satiation, as they develop the wrong habit. Kapha children might be slow to grasp learning but they generally retain what they have learned longer. They have good long-term memory. According to Dr. John Douillard, Kapha children prefer to learn kinesthetically.[13] Good gifts are things they can build or assemble.

Kapha children make more mucus than the other two types. Excess mucus traps bacteria and viruses in the sinuses, leading to colds and other conditions. Kapha children should avoid mucus-producing foods like cheese, even though they love gooey foods. A cooked-grain cereal makes a much better breakfast than cold cereal with milk for a Kapha child.

Kapha children are not naturally inclined toward exercise. Encourage them by making it fun and social. Team sports are ideal. A balanced Kapha child will be strong, affectionate, gregarious, and pleasant, with strong immunity. If imbalanced, you will find too much mucus, weight gain, asthma, excessive attachment, and low mood.

AYURVEDA ACTION
Reduce Excess Mucus Before It Causes Problems

DO YOU OR a child you care for have too much mucus? Reduce raw, cold foods, especially cheeses, ice cream, cold cereal, milk, and iced/cold drinks. Increase warm, cooked foods, steamed or lightly sautéed but not deep-fried. If the mucous membranes are irritated, consider taking turmeric to repair them.

Sitopladi is an herbal formula often used to mitigate excess mucus. It contains bamboo manna, long pepper, cardamom, cinnamon, and rock sugar, which combine lubricating and mucus-liquefying properties, without drying out the sinuses.

Turmeric and sitopladi can be mixed in equal amounts with raw honey. Typically children can take up to ½ to 1 teaspoon of the paste 1-3 times daily. Some children take as much as twice this amount, but test first for adverse reactions. You can make enough to last for a few days. The herbs can be taken in boiled water that is cooled to drink. Add a tad of raw honey or grade B (unrefined) maple syrup.

Raw honey should not be given to a child under two years old.

MARCH 29
KAPHA AROMAS

Kaphas are stimulated by the sense of smell. The wafting aroma of food cooking is gratifying, and a home-oriented Kapha will enjoy a home-cooked meal much more than eating out.

Walking in nature with the fragrance of trees, fresh-cut grass, and flowers—or receiving a fragrant bouquet—may be of special interest to Kaphas.

Essential oils, extracted directly from the root, seed, bark, flower, fruit, or leaf of a plant, are also great for balancing Kapha. These oils are nature's way of protecting plants from insects and a harsh environment. By using these concentrated essential oils, we humans can protect ourselves.

Never apply essential oils directly to skin and never take them internally. Add a few drops into a mild carrier, such as almond or jojoba oil, or in water, before dabbing on pulse points or using in massage. Emit essential oils from an oil diffuser or in sprays of oil and water. Always first test a small amount of oil for allergies or reactions. Essential oils to reduce excessive heaviness and coolness of Kapha include these wonderful choices, each with a special benefit.

To lift mood

   eucalyptus, orange, bergamot, lavender, ylang ylang

To relieve attachment and greed

   tulsi, basil, rosemary

To engage confidence

   jasmine, ginger, clove, cinnamon

To support weight loss

   grapefruit, peppermint, ginger, cinnamon

AYURVEDA ACTION
Consciously Take in Pleasing Aromas

Please your Kapha nature by taking in aromas as you prepare a meal or, if you are lucky, having one prepared for you. Wave the aroma toward you with your hand, take a deep breath and pause for a moment as you experience the aroma's flavors. Kaphas like to invoke memories. When have you enjoyed similar aromas?

MARCH 30
COMMON CONDITIONS ARISING FROM IMBALANCED KAPHA

Ayurveda treatments focus on balancing people's particular imbalances. Some conditions are more common to Kapha imbalances. Since Kapha qualities are heavy, slow, dull, cool, oily, liquid, slimy, smooth, dense, stable, and sticky, health concerns that tend to arise when these qualities are imbalanced include:

- Wet coughs with mucus
- Colds
- Allergies
- Asthma
- Shortness of breath
- Excessive weight/obesity
- Diabetes
- Edema/swelling
- Sinus and lymph node congestion
- Skin issues such as acne
- Digestive issues from sluggishness
- Toxicity
- Excessive sleep
- Depression
- Tumors

In addition to balancing Kapha imbalance, research Ayurveda strategies for healing these conditions. The three biggest strategies for Kapha-related conditions are to cleanse, move, and eat a heating and drying Kapha balancing diet.

AYURVEDA ACTION
Make Warming & Cleansing Kapha Tea

This tasty tea supports Kapha balancing to boost fat digestion, detox, release mucus, and promote weight loss.

- 1/16 tsp cayenne pepper
- 1/4 of whole lemon
- 1/8 tsp raw apple cider vinegar
- 1 cup boiled water
- 1 tsp raw honey or grade B maple syrup

Combine pepper, lemon, vinegar, and water. When cool enough to drink, add honey or syrup.

MARCH 31
RECAP AND WHAT'S AHEAD

KAPHA IS COMPOSED of earth and water elements. When balanced, they combine those two for strength and structure. When Kapha is imbalanced, you have mud and slime. Kapha qualities are heavy, slow, dull, cool, oily, wet, smooth, dense, stable, and sticky.

Balance Kapha by introducing opposite qualities—light, quick, sharp, hot, brittle, dry, rough, subtle, mobile, and clear.

Kapha often shows up as excess—too much weight, too much mucus, too much sleep, and too much lethargy.

The most effective strategies for balancing Kapha are daily movement, regular cleansing, and warm, cooked food. Heating, pungent spices like pepper, cinnamon, ginger, and cumin are good in food and drink. Sweeteners should be limited to modest amounts of raw honey.

WHAT'S AHEAD?

IN APRIL WE will focus on cleansing, an essential strategy to keeping Kapha in balance. Slow-moving Kapha can lead to toxin accumulation, so cleansing is a must.

MONTHLY REFLECTION TIME

WHAT ACTIONS DID you try and what was your experience? Did the new action feel worthwhile? Did you like it? Did you have adverse reactions? Put a check in the third column for actions you plan to incorporate daily, weekly, monthly, seasonally, or on occasion.

What New Actions This Month?	*Your Experience?*	*Habit Worthy?*
		☐
		☐
		☐

APRIL 1
SPRING CLEANSE FOR HIGH IMPACT RESULTS

Ayurveda suggests a cleanse at the transition between each doshic season, but spring—the transition from Vata season to Kapha season—is the most important and March through April is a good time to cleanse. Here's why.

- More than any other Ayurveda season, Vata winter (November through February; adjust time frame for your climate) invites toxin accumulation. Body systems become drier in winter, so toxins get stuck and stored, primarily in winter fat reserves. To manage Vata's qualities—dry, windy, light (weight), dark (visual), and cold—people often consume sugar and fats and just plain overeat. Major holidays in the winter invite travel, rich foods, and alcoholic drink. The season often also means more time indoors doing low-key activities.
- Nature returns moisture—like sap returns to trees—in late winter and early spring. So Kapha moisture begins moving into the dry area of stored toxins to loosen them for removal. Kapha season brings spring rains—March through June in many parts of the U.S. (Adjust time frame for your climate.)
- If all goes well, winter toxins move into your elimination systems and out. But with too many accumulated toxins, or if you have a dry system, or you lack strength or sufficient agni (digestive fire), then toxins, or ama, might not be efficiently eliminated. Instead, ama loosens and moves sluggishly until it hits a vulnerable spot and deposits. Consequences such as swollen glands, headaches, allergic reactions, muscle aches, weight gain, or depression could result.

The release of toxins and the blockages they create, restores the flow of energy and information throughout your body, bringing light to every cell and every thought. Rejuvenate and welcome spring with renewal by doing a little extra to detox.

AYURVEDA ACTION
Drink Ayurveda Hot Spice Water Tea...with a Punch

Continue or renew your commitment to drinking hot spice water. This is a daily detox, but give it a boost this month! Simply add thinly sliced fresh ginger root and/or fresh turmeric to the original hot spice water recipe. If you do not have the fresh roots, add a small amount of organic ginger powder and/or turmeric powder.

APRIL 2
LEVEL 1 CLEANSE (DAILY)

April often alternates between cold temperatures and warm days. We listen expectantly for the soft sounds of spring. We feel moisture return after a dry winter. Depending on your locale, you may see the ground swell with melting snow, early rains to bless us, the sap in the maple trees begin to flow, the lakes and rivers rise. And just as in nature, our own moisture returns.

Ayurveda cleansing is a healthy, everyday ritual for the transition of seasons. Two easy ways to detox every day are sipping hot spice water every 15 minutes or so and allowing 3–6 hours between meals (no snacking) to allow complete digestion.

- **Drink Hot Spice Water:** Always the best tip.
- **Avoid snacking:** If you constantly feed your body, it's constantly burning whatever you eat. That negates the need to burn stored fat, which contains much of the ama you host. Unless you are hypoglycemic or have other conditions that could be exacerbated, non-snacking is a good approach for regular detox. Be hungry at mealtime. If you are salivating with anticipation, the digestive juices are ready to do their job.

AYURVEDA ACTION
Try Sugary-Snack Alternatives

Are you challenged to make it through a day without snacks? Try flavorful teas with a dab of raw honey. Honey is "predigested" by bees, so it does not engage the physiology like other sugars. Remember, add honey only when the tea is cool enough to drink, or it could have a negative effect on health.

If you need something more substantial, eat a juicy piece of fruit. The liquid nature of fruit, like a soft pear or grapes, makes it easier to digest. Consider a brief walk instead of a snack. Do what you can. If you want to do more, check out Level 2 and 3 cleanses coming up.

APRIL 3
LEVEL 2 CLEANSE— DETOX DIET (1-2 WEEKS)

In addition to Level 1 cleansing described yesterday, a detoxing diet for one or two weeks clears out toxins and reboots your energy. Do Level 1 {Apr 2} along with these additional Level 2 recommendations.

1. Avoid ama-producing foods. These include GMO and non-organic foods, leftovers, and processed foods (packaged, canned, and frozen). Avoid heavy and aged cheese, butter and yogurt, although yogurt lassi {Aug 29} is fine. No fried or oily foods, raw foods of any kind, yeasted breads and crackers. Stay away from refined sugar. Avoid heavy fruits, such as mangoes and bananas.
2. Eat ama-reducing foods. Favor warm, fresh cooked, vegetarian foods, especially watery foods like brothy soups and dahls. Cook vegetables like leafy greens, asparagus, zucchini, carrots, Brussels sprouts and cabbage. Choose light lentils and beans such as yellow mung beans, red lentils, and puy lentils. Light grains offer fiber—choose quinoa, barley, amaranth, white basmati rice, and couscous. Cook fruits such as prunes, apple, pears, and pineapple. Raisins or dried cherries are okay if soaked and then chewed well.

    Be liberal with warming and detoxing spices like ginger, pepper, turmeric, coriander, fennel, and fenugreek. These spices support the flow of toxins from the skin, urinary tract, colon, and liver. Do not use salt. Use oils such as ghee, avocado, and olive in small amounts. Raw honey is the only detox sweetener recommended, in small amounts and never heated.
3. Use ginger to stimulate agni (digestive fire). Try a ginger pickle {Mar 19} 15 minutes before a meal—slice ginger the size of a quarter or smaller and sprinkle with lime juice and salt. Cook with ginger. Add fresh ginger to spice water.
4. Prepare foods with love. Eat in a peaceful, blissful environment.

AYURVEDA ACTION
Review Your Shopping List/Try Triphala

Look at the food recommendations above. Make a list of ama-reducing foods to buy. Add ginger and other heating spices to your shopping list. Consider taking 1 or 2 triphala {May 8} or triphala guggulu tablets (or 1/2 tsp powder in warm water as tea) at bedtime to support overnight digestion and elimination.

APRIL 4
LEVEL 3 CLEANSE (3 WEEKS)

INTENSE CLEANSES ARE recommended if you can complete them without compromising health. They are not recommended for those who are ill, frail, pregnant, or nursing. A level-3 cleanse is best done with the support of an Ayurvedic practitioner or in an Ayurvedic cleanse class. The details are provided here so you know what to expect.

1. Preparation: For the first three days, follow Level 1 and Level 2 strategies, including triphala or triphala guggulu at bedtime.
2. On days 4 through 7, eat ghee first thing in the morning in increasing amounts daily. Melting the ghee and drinking it while holding the nose helps some people get it down. Start with four teaspoons on day 4 and work up to 12 on day 7 if possible. Eat an easily digestible mono-diet of rice porridge for breakfast, kitchari {Mar 19} for lunch, and mung bean soup for supper {Mar 20}.
3. On day 8, drink 1 1/2 cups organic prune juice, do a warm oil abhyanga {Dec 6}, and take a warm bath or shower. This needs to be a day when you can be at home, as you will likely have a soft to watery stool that may come on quickly.
4. On days 9, 10, and 11, eat a simple light, vegetarian diet without fats and oils—soup or sautéed vegetables and rice.
5. On day 12, take a strength-building rasayana (longevity-promoting herbal remedy), such as chyawanprash, or herbs, such as ashwagandha. After a cleanse they reach deeper into physiology.
6. Continue with an ama-reducing diet for another week. You'll likely be tempted by sugary treats to restore energy, but energy should be built with very healthy foods. Many people fail at this step because they rush back into old habits or introduce bad ones. Prepare menus ahead of time.

To re-emphasize, please seek out resources for support if you choose to do this type of cleanse. Working with an experienced Ayurveda professional is recommended.

AYURVEDA ACTION
Gather & Use Support Resources

- Look for Ayurveda cleanse classes or support groups in your community.
- Check out free information from Dr. John Douillard on his cleanse at lifespa.com.
- Banyan Botanicals provides free info plus herbal and food supplies for cleanses at banyanbotanicals.com.
- VPK by Maharishi Ayurveda has cleanse resources in the "Explore Ayurveda" tab at mapi.com.

APRIL 5
DETOX LIFESTYLE PRACTICES

The way you conduct yourself during detox is as important as the foods you eat. Try on healthy behaviors. By reflecting on regular habits and choosing actions consciously, you can enter an attentive, sacred space. Can you commit to trying at least three or more practices during detox from the following list?

1. Include activities like yoga, meditation, and time in Nature in your dinacharya (daily routine).
2. Drink hot spice water or plain hot water throughout the day. No liquids immediately before or after a meal. Limit liquids with your meal to 1/2 cup of hot water.
3. Eat in a settled, quiet atmosphere with reverence for your food.
4. Do not work, read, do email, or watch TV while eating.
5. Rest for 15 minutes after a meal and then take a leisurely walk.
6. Have routine times for eating and bedtime.
7. Eat supper before 6 p.m.
8. Create beauty in the food you make and the table you set.
9. Prepare food with love and know that you are nourishing yourself with light and intelligence with every scrumptious, aromatic, flavorful bite.
10. Enjoy. Detox is like a lever that gives you larger effects than the effort. Be sweet with yourself.

AYURVEDA ACTION
Eat in Bliss

Start with one special, freshly cooked meal a week, or if you are already eating some fresh cooked meals, add at least one more per week. Focus on a freshly prepared breakfast or lunch. Play relaxing music, perhaps new age or classical. Use real plates and a cloth napkin, with fresh flowers or a plant on the table. Take a moment to appreciate the colors and aromas of your food. Notice your emotions during the meal. How satiated are you at meal's end? How does your digestive process feel? If you feel good, try eating at least two meals a week like this.

APRIL 6
HERBS—AMBASSADORS OF CONSCIOUSNESS!

The coherence and energy of herbs make them Nature's wise and compassionate sages. Herbs' intelligence resonates within like a tuning fork, bringing vibration and balance. Herbs are used to rejuvenate and treat disease, but beyond these correcting and strengthening qualities, herbs also awaken higher consciousness. They stimulate vital energies (prana) and higher mind.

According to Vedic knowledge, the sap of an herb contains a life essence called "soma," the home of the herb's inner intelligence. The whole herb is superior to the "active ingredient." For example, turmeric as a fresh root or powder is more effective than supplements that pull out its active ingredient, curcumin. Soma nourishes, sustains, and offers comfort and enjoyment at all levels. The amount and quality of soma depend on the conditions in which the herb grew and was harvested. For instance, plants grown in the mountains and near streams and lakes are purported to have more soma. Organically grown is always best.

The soma, or life-essence, of an herb combines with ojas (essential life energy or vigor) to boost activity. When you produce ojas, the vital nectar of life, you feel blissful. A good diet and lifestyle support the creation of ojas, and herbs stimulate and expand that process.

Herbs' effects manifest over time. They are not drugs—they work in concert with diet and lifestyle. Herbs operate on a more subtle level than food and can stimulate prana flow through nadis, the energy channels that carry prana to every cell.

The daily use of herbs offers great benefits. Herbs catalyze processes that clear ama (toxins), strengthen muscles and organs, deeply nourish, stimulate prana, and awaken potential for bliss. Plant the seeds that nourish you.

AYURVEDA ACTION
Nutrient Dense Foods Require Spicing

Proper nourishment starts with wholesome food (organic, whole foods freshly prepared) that is properly and fully digested. For this we need healthy, strong agni (digestive fire). Spices are the key to the strong agni that transforms food into healthy tissue. You are better off eating lightly this time of year, but when you eat heavier foods they especially need proper spicing. Nutrient-dense foods (fats, sweets, meat, desserts) require spicing or they will quickly lead to excess heaviness, incomplete digestion, and clogging of the physiology.

APRIL 7
HERBS & THEIR INTELLIGENCE TO SERVE

Below are herbs to consider in food preparation, teas, or as supplements. You likely recognize the Western herbs listed. Ayurvedic herbs might be less familiar. As supplements, powders are generally the best form—tasting the herbs has a healing benefit and stimulates internal effects. However, if powders seem too inconvenient for you, try tablets or elixirs. Better to get them in you, even if not in the most optimal way.

- Basil, pippali, sage—stimulate senses, improve perception, open your energy channels and remove mucus
- Ashwagandha, shatavari—increase awareness and intelligence, strengthen mind and body
- Valerian, nutmeg, skullcap, hops, chamomile, spearmint, red clover – calm the mind, emotional release
- Black pepper, cardamom, coriander, fennel, ginger, peppermint, turmeric, neem (not if pregnant), cinnamon, cloves, hing (also known as asofoetida)—stimulate digestion
- Cinnamon, clove—improve circulation
- Bay leaves, hing, cinnamon, coriander, mint, dill, ginger, basil – relieve intestinal gas, bloating
- Cayenne, ginger, triphala, and triphala guggulu—invite weight loss (with proper diet)
- Sarsaparilla, goldenseal, aloe vera, cayenne pepper, licorice, sage, cinnamon, cloves, cumin, ginger, turmeric—cleanse and purify

AYURVEDA ACTION
Drink Pungent Teas

Upgrade your daily spice water in Kapha season by adding fresh or dried ginger. Or make a simple tea with any of the pungent spices. Try cinnamon with a few peppercorns and a dab of honey. When your Kapha is craving something, this might satisfy.

APRIL 8
HERBS—HOW MUCH & HOW TO CARRY

Proper dosage of any herb should be done in consultation with an Ayurveda practitioner. However, for those who want to take herbs on their own, here is information on dosage to help you make a good decision. The most important advice is to start with one herb, in a small amount. Make sure you are not having adverse reactions, and if you have negative effects, reduce or stop taking the herb. If you are taking medications, check with your doctor or a pharmacist for contraindications. In the U.S., herbs are not recommended if you are pregnant or nursing and dosages should be reduced for children.

With those cautions, here are guidelines to consider:

- Start with a small dose—one tablet once a day or 1/4 tsp powder. A large dose would be 1 to 3 tablets up to 3 times a day or 1 tsp of powder daily. Standard dosage should appear on the pouch or bottle. If you have sensitivities, start with less.
- If you experience discomfort, dial down or stop dosage. If you take an herb with a cleansing action, for example, perhaps too many toxins are being removed too quickly. Try a smaller dosage.
- If taking powder, place it right on your tongue and perhaps follow with water. You can also choose a carrier, called an "anupan" in Ayurveda. The most common carrier is heated water as a tea, but warmed raw milk and alternative milks work as well. Sometimes cleansing herbs are taken with water plus lemon juice or vinegar. Sometimes herbs are mixed with an anupan of ghee or raw honey.

Focus on balancing just one condition at a time, and select one or two herbs/formulas to support that condition. Physiology can get confused, as some herbs work counter to others. Plus, sometimes clearing one condition will address other issues as well.

AYURVEDA ACTION
Cook with Spices

The term "Ayurveda herbs" refers to all Ayurveda medicines. Ayurveda medicines can be roots, resins, barks, oils, spices, and other natural sources. Add these herbs to your recipes to reduce Kapha: fresh ginger, chilies, black pepper, cumin, clove, and turmeric.

APRIL 9
HERBS—WHEN TO TAKE & FOR HOW LONG

Herbs are food and need time to show their effect. Give the herb at least a few weeks before expecting results. The best time to take Ayurveda herbs can vary. If you have sensitivities or are just starting a protocol, taking with food can buffer strong effects. Taking herbs on an empty stomach can increase the effect but might also increase side effects, such as nausea. In general, taking about 30 minutes after you begin eating is a safe approach. The exception would be herbs that fire up digestion, like ginger and cinnamon. Those should be taken about 15 to 30 minutes before a meal.

HERBS ARE USED TO RESET FUNCTION, NOT FOR LIFE-LONG DEPENDENCE.

Some herbs take effect quickly; most others need time for the effect to build. This can be tricky. When balance seems to have been achieved, the condition might return because it didn't rebalance down into all the layers of tissue. On the other hand, continuing an herb too long can mean passing through a state of balance into imbalance. Become sensitive to what is working for you.

No hard-and-fast rules govern when it is best to continue or suspend. An Ayurvedic practitioner can help you to navigate this terrain. If you are taking an herb to correct an imbalance or heal a condition, Ayurveda generally recommends taking an herb for 6–8 weeks. Then stop. Has the reset taken hold? Do you feel any difference? If you feel worse, the reset function might need to continue, or maybe it's the wrong herb. If you feel good, perhaps the herb has done its work. Take a break for 2–3 weeks to allow your system to adapt and rise up to restore functioning on its own.

Triphala is the one herb that does not generally fall into a time limitation. Triphala is tri-doshic and aids digestion in a gentle way. Many people take triphala for years, with occasional breaks. Triphala is usually taken at bedtime to aid overnight digestion. It can also be taken in the morning as well, especially if there is constipation, as triphala has a slight laxative effect.

Brahmi and ashwagandha can also be taken at bedtime to induce sleep or used at other times for its benefits. Chyawanprash is an Ayurveda jam that is a tri-doshic rasayana {Oct 18} and can be used as a daily regimen.

AYURVEDA ACTION
Take Herbs Seasonally

Some herbs are best taken seasonally. Cleansing herbs might be used in the spring {Apr 7}, and cooling and Pitta-pacifying herbs in the summer {July 23}. In the winter, immune-building and strengthening herbs/formulas {Feb 4} like ashwagandha and chyawanprash are worth considering.

APRIL 10
AYURVEDA ALL-STARS

Ayurveda is not about simply adding years to your life but adding quality and supporting spiritual evolution. According to Maharishi Ayurveda, "Advances in medical sciences will add about two years to your life, but changes in your personal behavior—read lifestyle—can add 15-plus years."[14] We keep coming back to some of these to reinforce them as sustained habits that need to develop over time.

Healthy Ayurveda Lifestyle Habits:

- Meditate.
- Drink herbal, nourishing teas with herbs that support health.
- Get to bed by 10 p.m. and rise before dawn.
- Eat in a settled environment.
- Cook with herbs and spices—fennel, cumin, cinnamon, and cardamom are good for digestion.
- Avoid foods with toxins or preservatives and avoid leftovers.
- Add more cooked greens to your diet—turnip and mustard greens, spinach, Swiss chard.
- Eat your biggest meal at noon—a warm cooked, freshly prepared meal.
- Sip hot spice water throughout the day—1/2 tsp of fennel, 1/4 tsp of cumin, 1/4 tsp of coriander (all seeds) in a quart thermos of boiled water. Add a slice of fresh ginger for more pizzazz.
- Attune to the joy in life and other people.
- Keep a regular routine—meals, bedtime, etc.
- Do yoga or gentle exercise, or walk daily.

AYURVEDA ACTION
Sauté Your Herbs First

Some herbs are fat (oil) soluble and some are water soluble, meaning that when heated in these environments they release intelligence and render their qualities available. Rather than be concerned with which herbs are which, sauté all herbs and seeds for 1–2 minutes in oil that is good for high temperatures: ghee, coconut, or avocado. Then add the herbs to your dishes, which will contain moisture from vegetables or water you have added.

This is an essential knowledge bit and you will see this tip reinforced at various points in this book.

APRIL 11
PAYING ATTENTION TO BALANCE/IMBALANCE

For good health, balance is key in Ayurveda. And awareness of balance may be cultivated. Think about your day so far.

1. Select one thing you did or thought or experienced today that disturbed your balance.
2. What one thing today reinforced your health or connected you to Nature or your nature and helped you rebalance?
3. Were you aware of the effect of either balance or imbalance at the time? Did the balancing and imbalancing events feel like choices, habits, or something else?

Start your journey with mindfulness. Take stock of your sense of life balance or imbalance overall. Do you know when you are out of balance? Do you feel it when you have done something good for yourself?

For example, on more than one occasion I have checked my email and social media first thing in the morning, while still in bed. This delayed my arising—and I felt my balance disturbed. My meditation was delayed and sometimes shortened, but even some meditation felt restorative. I am not always aware of what is disturbing or restorative to my balance, but I know the benefits when I am in a state of awareness.

We are always negotiating balance. My friend wrote a poem that speaks of falling as the first act of walking. To walk, we fall forward, then we adjust to regain footing. A healthy Ayurveda lifestyle is like this. It is impossible to always be in balance. If you do not move (walk), then you stagnate, and the forces of Nature throw you out of balance. But you can gently, frequently rebalance when you have gone too far in one direction. No guilt necessary here—just notice. This is the key to internal wisdom.

> *"Self-reflection without judgment is the highest form of spiritual practice."*
>
> —Swami Kripalu

AYURVEDA ACTION
Pick a Simple Rebalance

Pick one simple thing that you can do to rebalance. Maybe you have been working or playing too hard or you have been on a sugar binge. Set one change in motion to serve as an exemplar for good things to come. Set an achievable goal so you feel successful. One of my favorites is to return to drinking hot spice water daily. Perhaps do a daily meditation, even if it's only 5 or 10 minutes. Maybe an Epsom salt bath at night will help. Just do one simple thing to get back in the groove.

APRIL 12
DISEASE PROCESS AND PREVENTION

Disease is the end result of a long process of imbalance. With Ayurveda, imbalance can be determined early and corrected before disease manifests. Ayurveda is known to prevent disease but also has capacity for correction after disease has occurred. Let's look at what we can do to intercept the disease process through prevention.

The six stages of the disease process are:

1. ACCUMULATION – Doshas in their own place; see "governs" row in the Three Doshas At-A-Glance {Appendix} to see the seat of each dosha. No symptoms.
2. AGGRAVATION – Dosha is provoked to leave its seat. No symptoms.
3. MIGRATION – Aggravated dosha moves and preliminarily manifests as nonspecific symptoms.
4. RELOCATION – Doshas stick to ama in a particular organ or tissue type where srotas (physical and energetic channels in the human system) are disturbed. Symptoms of disease begin to develop.
5. MANIFESTATION – Symptoms appear in specific, related locations, such as joint pain and stiffness, skin eruptions, labored breathing.
6. CHRONICITY – Disease becomes chronic or complications manifest such as a heart attack, arthritis, eczema.

To interrupt the disease process, intercept after accumulation or aggravation stages with balancing actions. Accumulations and aggravations are natural—this is the way of the world as you engage with daily and seasonal stressors. It is not an Ayurveda goal to stay in perfect health—that does not happen. Awareness of your current state and introducing balances when you are off-center is what you're aiming for. These stages will be reviewed in more detail. {Oct 1}

AYURVEDA ACTION
Recheck Your Doshic Imbalance

LOOK AGAIN AT your Vikruti, or current dosha imbalance {Assessment 1} and observe present health issues. If you think the imbalances are in stage 1 or 2, adjust your diet or seasonal and daily routines to prevent disease manifestation. If issues are into stage 3 or 4, purge toxins from your system with a focused cleanse or daily moderate cleansing strategies. Stages 5 and 6 require myriad strategies including panchakarma (five actions of deep cleansing), herbal therapy, aromatherapy, spiritual deepening, and the benefits of conventional medicine.

APRIL 13
THREE PILLARS OF GOOD HEALTH

Wholesome well-being is built on the three pillars of good health: proper digestion (ahara); proper sleep (nidra); and regulated lifestyle/sexual drive (brahmacharya). These three are referred to as Eat, Sleep, Love. When one of these is not strong, the whole construction falls over like a three-legged stool with a leg missing.

Improper eating, or living out of sync with the laws of Nature or your own nature, causes imbalance that, left uncorrected, leads to discomfort and possibly disease. Ayurveda cures by removing or correcting the cause of the imbalance and by emphasizing positive choices, such as eating sattvic (pure, natural, energy-containing, clean) foods.

Ayurveda balance is more than treatment; it is a way of life. Balance brings you into harmony with the nature of your environment and your personal nature. The greatest balance of all is awareness of true self, the consciousness of our unification with the Nature of the absolute. A healthy and balanced body, mind, and life force energy form conditions to know your true Self or Soul.

You can learn a lot about Ayurveda this year; however, the most important learning is about who you are. You are the wise one in this adventure. The knowledge in this book is intended to help you remember that internal wisdom. Increased clarity about the effect of thoughts and actions upon your life is key. It's easy to ramble along in the dull fog of busyness and to operate by rote, according to our habits. But as you develop awareness, you will naturally be drawn to activities in every one of the Three-Pillar areas that feel good. The reward comes little by little, day by day. A virtuous cycle builds good upon good, one step at a time.

AYURVEDA ACTION
Invite Good Sleep

The Ayurvedic term for sleep is nidra. The term for "without sleep" is anidra. Any of the three doshas can be involved in restful or unrestful sleeping. Try this: At bedtime, heat a cup of raw cow's milk or alternative milks like coconut, almond, or hemp. Add 1/4 to 1/2 tsp ashwagandha powder to soothe Vata sleep imbalances. Ashwagandha is revered for calming the nervous system. Or drink a relaxing tea made with brahmi leaves.

APRIL 14
SPRING CLEANING WITH NATURAL PRODUCTS

One form of ama is called garavisha, or the bioaccumulation of environmental toxins. Environmental toxins assault our minds and bodies daily. The U.S. Environmental Protection Agency ranks indoor air pollution among the top environmental dangers, yet does not regulate common cleaning products, which are a primary cause. Exposure to indoor pollutants can cause headaches, fatigue, and respiratory illness. Babies and children are particularly susceptible to the effects of pollutants in enclosed spaces.

A healthy Ayurvedic lifestyle means avoiding exposure to toxins. One way to make your home less toxic is to use natural cleaning products. The star players? BAKING SODA has proven virus-killing abilities and cuts through grease. CASTILE SOAP is made from 100% plant oils. WHITE VINEGAR's acidity cuts grease and scum. ESSENTIAL OILS help your DIY cleaners smell better, and many have antibacterial, antifungal, and antimicrobial qualities. Test natural ingredients, especially essential oils, to make sure they are okay for you and any others sharing your home.

Borax is listed in many DIY cleaning products; however, research shows it can irritate skin and eyes and disrupt hormones.

AYURVEDA ACTION
Make DIY Cleaning Products

MAKE ONE PRODUCT, such as glass cleaner or a general-surface cleaner. Store DIY products in glass jars rather than plastic. Add a new product each month. Before you know it, your home is cleaner and you are also helping the environment, as these cleaning products go into the air, down drains, and into septic or sewer systems. Here is another version of an all-purpose cleaner for you.

All-Purpose Cleaner:

- 2 Tbsp baking soda
- 1/2 cup white vinegar
- 10 drops tea tree or lemon essential oil (for disinfectant properties)

Put the baking soda in a 12 oz glass spray bottle. Add water to near full; then add essential oils and vinegar. Gently shake before each use. Wipe dry with a cloth.

APRIL 15
NONTOXIC CLEANING

Nontoxic cleaning products are worth additional discussion. Volatile Organic Compounds (VOCs) are included in many conventional cleaning products because they evaporate quickly. VOCs have been associated with health problems related to the liver, kidneys, and nervous system.

Moving to green cleaners gives you a healthier home and a cleaner environment, with less expense and a smaller impact on ozone depletion and global climate change. Government regulations do not require ingredients to be listed on cleaning products. There is no oversight on safety. You know the ingredients when you whip up your own cleaning products. Back to basics is a good thing.

AYURVEDA ACTION
Make Kitchen & Bathroom Cleaning Products

Surface & Glass Cleaner

- 1/2 cup white vinegar
- 2 cups water
- 1/4 cup rubbing alcohol
- 5 drops orange or lemon essential oil
- 1 Tbsp cornstarch—to reduce streaking

Mix all ingredients together in a glass spray bottle. Shake well before each use. Spritz on a rag or directly on glass; wipe dry.

Toilet Scrub

Pour 1/2 cup baking soda and 10 drops of tea tree or lemon essential oil into the toilet. Add 1/4 cup vinegar to the bowl. Scrub while the mixture fizzes. To clean toilet surfaces, fill a spray bottle with 1 cup vinegar and a few drops of essential oil. Spray and let it sit for a few minutes. Wipe clean.

Drain Cleaner

- 1/4 to 1/2 cup baking soda
- 1/4 cup white vinegar

Pour baking soda down a clogged or sluggish drain and follow with vinegar. The mixture will bubble. Let sit for an hour or so; then pour boiling-hot water down the drain to rinse. Repeat if necessary.

APRIL 16
HEALTHY WEIGHT, AYURVEDA STYLE

Your perfect weight, size, and shape are rooted in your constitutional make-up. Not everyone can be thin, nor should they be, no matter what messages advertisers and society send. Vatas by nature tend toward thinness. Kaphas tend to be solid and roundish, and Pittas are likely strong and medium-sized.

By understanding your true nature and living in balance with your natural rhythms, the perfect weight is revealed. When you panic or worry, or if your weight constantly fluctuates, the body reacts to an "emergency state." The result of this stress prompts the body to store fat or to short-circuit a healthy appetite.

Weight-loss strategies focused on deprivation or on specific nutrients—such as no carbs or only protein—are not advised in Ayurveda. Healthy weight might be slower to arrive, but it will last longer. Slow and steady is better.

If weight is a concern, what can you do? Slow down. Listen to your inner intelligence. Engage in mind-body-spirit practices that lead to a healthy weight. If you recognize and embrace your body constitution, eat consciously for the dosha you need to balance, maintain strong agni (digestive fire) and low ama (toxins in the body), then the body's support system finds its resting point in the correct weight.

Begin by adding a few new foods, spices, or behaviors. Check the Kapha tip below, or look at weight tips for Vata {Nov 15} and Pitta {Jul 15}. Employ the Ayurveda concept of "add and squeeze": As you take on healthy actions, you squeeze out what is no longer needed.

Kapha overweight imbalance is typically due to low digestive fire and slow metabolism. Even if you eat small meals, you may put on weight. In addition, digestive impurities from processed food deposit ama in fat tissue and accumulate over time. Even if Kapha is not predominant in your constitution, it's likely that your Kapha will become imbalanced/excessive in this season of Kapha.

AYURVEDA ACTION
Introduce Fire for Kapha Weight Imbalance

Introduce fire to your diet to balance Kapha. Eat freshly prepared foods with pungent spices like pepper, fresh ginger, and turmeric. Add green leafy vegetables, broccoli, cauliflower, and Brussels sprouts—all sautéed or steamed. Eat quinoa cooked with a little olive oil. Exercise is critical to balance Kapha. Add fire with hot spice water daily.

APRIL 17
STRENGTHEN YOUR AGNI

Strengthen your agni to burn stored fat and detox from a winter of improper eating.

WHEN YOU EAT

- Eat three meals a day at regular times and not later than 6 p.m.
- Eat the largest meal midday when digestive fire is naturally highest; supper should be the smallest meal.
- Eat only when hungry—skipping your regular breakfast or supper is fine—but don't snack to make up for it.

Note: When you snack, there is no call for the body to metabolize stored fat. Fat is burned in between meals. If you have hypoglycemia, do what is best to take care of that—perhaps eat small meals throughout the day. Otherwise, avoid snacking.

HOW YOU EAT

- Slow down, relax, enjoy your meal.
- Be at peace when you eat.
- Digestion functions better if you eat without engaging with media, or arguing.

Note: If you relax when you eat, you digest and utilize food energy without sending signals to store fat. You will feel full when you have eaten enough food to nourish.

WHAT TO EAT

- Eat more foods that are good for you.
- Ayurveda recommends enjoying seasonal foods. As soon as spring greens break forth, go for them! The same for foods such as berries and asparagus.
- Eat warm cooked foods that are freshly prepared.

Attend to when, how, and what you eat. Pace yourself. You don't want your body to see eating as a stressful emergency and store fat.

AYURVEDA ACTION
Spice Up Your Metabolism

Add metabolic boosters to your meal with hot peppers or a liberal sprinkling of black or cayenne pepper on your food. You burn more calories when meals are hot and spicy.

APRIL 18
RIGHT WEIGHT

Many people eat well generally, but on occasion good habits go out the window. Exhibiting abandon for the sake of joy and community is a good thing once in a while. Just remember to restore balance after you have gone too far in one direction.

Select, prepare (with spices), and consume natural (non-processed) foods that support your doshic balance to enjoy the Ayurveda goal of perfect digestion. Proper nourishment reduces cravings and improper assimilation of food.

Ayurvedic principles teach you to:

- optimize digestion
- eat to detox and balance your doshic type
- fire a healthy metabolism
- pay attention to *how* you eat

Weight change is not the goal of Ayurveda, but its approaches lead to a healthy, consistent size for your doshic type. The idea is to *lean into* an evolution of health, not to make radical changes that you won't sustain.

AYURVEDA ACTION
Exercise Properly to Burn Fat

If you want to be an efficient fat burner, choose a way to exercise that is slow and moderate, like walking and moderate forms of yoga, says Dr. John Douillard, a noted Ayurveda author and educator. You will burn more sugar at this pace. Maintain calm by breathing through your nose.[15]

Vigorous exercise, with gasping, open-mouth breath (as in some popular anaerobic-style classes), signals an emergency state to your body and triggers a response to store fat.

APRIL 19
AYURVEDA VIEW ON DIETING

Diets that focus on consuming or eliminating certain foods result in cravings. Ayurveda's basic foundation calls for a healthy, balanced diet and lifestyle. Perhaps the greatest dieting myth is the low-calorie and low-fat diet. Calorie restriction can signal the body that there is a food scarcity, which can slow metabolism and store fat.

With Ayurveda, you learn to increase metabolism, burn stored fat, and clear toxins. Detoxing is a core factor in finding and living with your right weight. Ama accumulation prevents proper digestion. Unprocessed or improperly processed food is stored as fat or as dried toxins in the colon. Keep the system clean by avoiding toxins and regular, mild daily cleansing.

Triphala, a premier Ayurveda rasayana, is an excellent daily cleanse. It promotes proper, complete digestion that can lead to weight loss. Rasayanas are highly refined herbal/fruit combinations that promote ojas {May 19}. Ojas leads to radiant health and long life. Triphala combines three herbs—amalaki, bibitaki, and haritaki—and has a slight laxative effect.

Mucus in the digestive tract helps lubricate the eating process. Over time, however, mucus can accumulate and clog the villi, millions of small projections in the small intestine. This inhibits the function of absorbing nutrients and removing toxins. Toned, healthy villi help with efficient food digestion and prevent partially digested food from remaining in the intestinal lining.

AYURVEDA ACTION
Partner with Triphala for Weight Loss

Taking triphala is often recommended as a bedtime practice to aid digestion during sleep and to support a morning bowel movement. For weight loss, take triphala after each meal as a tablet or as a tea: 1/4 tsp powder in 1/2 cup of warm water.

APRIL 20
TONGUE SCRAPING

Have you ever noticed the white film that accumulates overnight on your tongue? Once you start looking at your tongue in the morning, you will be amazed at the presence of this white coating. It is comprised of toxins that have been pulled out of your system during overnight digestion. The white gunk is ama.

You don't want to rinse that gunk back into your system or brush your tongue, which sends the ama back in. Scrape your tongue in the morning before drinking fluids or brushing teeth.

Scraping your tongue is an important part of daily oral health. It removes accumulated ama. You don't want to scrape your tongue in the evening or middle of the night, because that stimulates the organs that have receptacles on the tongue and could make it difficult to sleep.

Tongue scraping improves breath and your ability to taste. It also tones the associated organs and tissues represented on the tongue.

AYURVEDA ACTION
Scrape Your Tongue Each Morning

Use a tongue scraper or spoon. Hold the two ends of the tongue scraper and place the rounded part of the scraper as far back on the tongue as is comfortable. Gently pull the scraper forward while the coating accumulates. Rinse the scraper clean after each pull. You may need to scrape several times. A thin white coating always remains, so just scrape off most of the ama.

If using a spoon, tilt it to the side and pull the edge along your tongue until you reach the front. The spoon side will have accumulated the white ama. Rinse between scrapings as you would a tongue scraper.

Once you experience the incredibly clean mouth feeling, you will wonder how you ever got along without this healthful habit.

APRIL 21
SELECTING AND PREPARING LEAFY GREENS

Most of us just don't eat enough cooked greens—and they are incredible for longevity and radiant health. Leafy greens contain antioxidants that prevent aging and disease.

Buy greens that still have their bitter taste. Agribusiness has sweetened up greens to make them more palatable. Try a farmers' market, grow your own, or take just a little snip of the greens in the grocery store to test if they have the bitter taste.

- Select organic greens that are crisp, with a fresh, brilliant green color.
- Wash greens in a full sink of water several times to eliminate hidden sand and dirt embedded between leaves.
- Keep the leaf part whole when cooking.
- Remove tough stalks or slice into bite-sized slices and cook longer than the leaves. Tender stalks can be cut into small pieces and cooked just before adding leaves.
- Cook in ghee with spices suited to the dosha you wish to pacify.
- Do not cook greens in aluminum or copper pans, as sulfur in greens can interact with these metals.

Some Ayurveds recommend eating leafy greens every day for great skin and good health.

AYURVEDA ACTION
Try Dandelions!

Nutrient-dense dandelions arrive in spring when they're most needed. Use all parts of the plant—leaves, roots, blossoms—to cleanse the liver and gallbladder. For a tasty side dish, steam the leaves lightly with mint to improve digestibility. Or, make a tea from the leaves. Boil roots lightly to allow removing their peels; then cook and season as you would parsnips or carrots. You can even eat the yellow flower or buds (info online).

Buy dandelions organically or forage from areas that have not been treated with fertilizers, herbicides, or pesticides.

APRIL 22
DIABETES EVERYWHERE

We are in the midst of a diabetes epidemic. About one-third of the U.S. population is diabetic or prediabetic, and the numbers are quickly rising in the rest of the world as well. Bad as it is, diabetes can also lead to heart/coronary disease, high blood pressure, stroke, fatty liver disease, cancer, and other chronic conditions.

What can be done? You can start right now to prevent diabetes or reverse its effects. Diabetes is often associated with Kapha imbalance, so now is a good time to act.

THE SCIENCE OF THE GLUCOSE AND INSULIN DYNAMIC

The body uses glucose, sugar from the foods you eat, for energy. In the small intestine, glucose is released from food and in turn causes the glucose level in the blood to rise. For its part, your pancreas continually produces and directs insulin to the blood to match up with the glucose level.

Tiny blood vessels take glucose and insulin close to each cell in the body. Insulin acts like a key, which unlocks the door to each cell. When the cell door is open, glucose can enter. Glucose provides energy to recharge the cell's battery and allow it to work. With diabetes, either the pancreas does not produce sufficient insulin or cells do not receive the insulin, leading to high blood-sugar levels.

AYURVEDA ACTION
Add Cinnamon for Diabetes Issues

Cinnamon contains large amounts of antioxidants which protect against the development of nearly every chronic disease, including diabetes. Cinnamon may help lower blood sugar and fight diabetes by:

- imitating insulin's effects
- increasing glucose transport into cells
- increasing insulin sensitivity, making it more efficient at moving glucose

Ceylon cinnamon is called "true cinnamon." Ceylon is typically more expensive, and most effective for health. Cassia cinnamon is common and has a stronger flavor but is less effective and is not advised for people on blood thinners. There are other types of cinnamon as well. Get more cinnamon in your diet by adding it to coffee (perhaps a cup daily) or tea, or including it in rice dishes or soups. Desserts usually spike blood sugar, but adding cinnamon might mitigate that, according to recent research.

APRIL 23
DIABETES DEFINED AND CAUSES

TYPE 1 DIABETES

The pancreas is unable to make insulin. Only 5 percent of diabetes diagnoses are for Type 1, and onset is usually in childhood and your genes likely play at least some role.

TYPE 2 DIABETES

The pancreas can make insulin, but cannot unlock the cell door, resulting in glucose and respondent insulin levels rising. Eventually the pancreas becomes dysfunctional from working so hard. Fatigue and a host of other health issues can emerge because cells are not getting needed energy.

PREDIABETES

A state of progressing insulin resistance, which leads to higher-than-normal blood glucose levels but is not yet at the marker for diabetes. Prediabetes is easier to reverse than a diabetes diagnosis. Prediabetes is easier to reverse than a diabetes diagnosis.

WHAT CAUSES DIABETES?

Diabetes has increased 300 percent in the U.S. in the past 15 years.[16] What is happening? For starters, diets have become metabolically deranged with processed foods, in particular through the use of high-fructose corn syrup (HFCS). HFCS is particularly hard on the hormone leptin, which regulates appetite, satiety response, and body weight. When leptin is disrupted, the body craves food and loses the ability to feel "full," which results in overeating.

Eating large volumes of food regularly, especially processed carbs and sugary foods—burdens the pancreas and its ability to produce sufficient insulin. Leptin and insulin disruption go hand-in-hand. Over time, the disruption leads to unbalanced blood sugar levels, which is diabetes.

AYURVEDA ACTION
Bottom Line—Eat Real Food

Processed foods—with sugars such as HFCS, hidden fillers, and various other toxins—are a primary culprit of bad health. They certainly aggravate the conditions that contribute to diabetes. It's this simple: Eat real food, preferably organic and freshly prepared. Take a look in your kitchen today for processed foods; then read the ingredient lists. Wow, huh?!

APRIL 24
DIABETES—PREVENTION AND TREATMENT

Here's your smack-down-diabetes checklist:

- Limit processed foods and eat more real foods (whole, organic, local, vegetables).
- Exercise regularly—even 20 minutes three times weekly helps immensely.
- Get at least 20 minutes daily of outdoor sunshine, or if you cannot, consider a quality liquid Vitamin D3 supplement.
- Reduce food intake; maintain a healthy body weight.
- Add blood sugar-regulating herb intelligence to your diet.

HERBS TO SUPPORT HEALTHY BLOOD SUGAR

- Turmeric
- Cinnamon
- Tulsi
- Fenugreek seed
- Triphala
- Triphala guggulu

More research has been done on turmeric and its healing qualities than any other herb. Turmeric is especially helpful for regulating blood sugar and preventing and treating diabetes. Systemic inflammation, which impacts insulin secretion and function, is emerging as a root cause of diabetes. Turmeric's antidiabetic properties are related to its well-known anti-inflammatory properties.[17] Note: Visit greenmedinfo.com for research on natural approaches to healing, including turmeric.

AYURVEDA ACTION
Consume Turmeric Daily

Here are five easy ways to get the benefits of turmeric every day:

1. Add it to scrambled eggs or tofu, or to oatmeal.
2. Add to rice.
3. Use in soups.
4. Add to most freshly cooked foods.
5. Make a tea by adding 1/4 to 1/2 tsp turmeric powder to 1 cup boiled water. Simmer 10 minutes, strain, and drink. Skip the draining if you don't mind drinking the powder slurry. When cool enough to drink, you can add raw honey.

APRIL 25
WOMEN'S HEALTH

Rather than managing a woman's life changes with an isolated element, such as hormone replacement or antidepressants, Ayurveda instead looks at underlying imbalances in lifestyle, diet, and beliefs. Corrections are made with natural practices. For you or for the woman in your life, here are general tips for common concerns.

- MENSTRUAL CRAMPS—Drink aloe vera juice, 2 to 4 Tbsp daily in juice (such as organic pomegranate). Cooking with ghee throughout the month can ease menstrual cramps.
- OVERWEIGHT—Avoid sugar. Use moderate amounts of good fats in cooking, like ghee and avocado oil. Drink warm tea with honey to fight hunger cravings.
- SADNESS/DEPRESSION—Soothe with meditation, time in Nature, mild exercise like yin yoga, or massage. Sweeten your heart with roses. Read spiritual literature. Turn on the lights literally and figuratively. Eat quinoa, couscous, and amaranth.
- PREGNANCY—Everything you taste, touch, smell, see or feel should nourish. Eat warm, cooked, organic foods that easily digest like raw cow's milk, ghee, fresh vegetables.
- MENOPAUSE—Symptoms can result from any dosha imbalance, and treatment is based on that assessment. Drinking 1/4 cup of aloe juice daily helps with hot flashes.
- OSTEOPOROSIS—Avoid caffeine. Get 15 minutes of sunshine daily. Exercise. Get calcium from sources like organic milk, sesame seeds, almonds, broccoli, and greens.
- URINARY TRACT INFECTIONS—Drink 100% organic cranberry juice; its D-mannose is effective at attaching to the bacteria of many UTIs and flushing them from the body.

AYURVEDA ACTION
Cultivate the Divine Feminine (Regardless of Gender)

- CULTIVATE COMMUNITY. Allow love to be part of your beloved community. Love is healing for you and others. Healing, inclusion, and love are the essence of the divine feminine. Invest time and celebrate the facets of your community.
- RECOGNIZE AND PURSUE DESIRES. Feel your passion and act on it in ways that respect others. Feel your sensuality. Take time to express it with yourself and others.
- FLOW WITH EMERGING REALITY. Divine feminine does not try to control; it is confident in its ability to flow with what emerges. The divine feminine is observant and adaptable.

APRIL 26
HEALTHY WEIGHT BY DOSHA

Kapha Weight Imbalance

KAPHA OVERWEIGHT IMBALANCE is due to low digestive fire and slow metabolism resulting from Kapha ama. Kapha ama is thick, sticky, and foul-smelling and tends to accumulate in the stomach, lungs, and sinuses. It often leads to congestion, colds, and coughs. You might put on weight even if you eat small meals. Digestive impurities from processed and junk food deposit as ama in fat tissue, accumulating over time.

AYURVEDA ACTION
Balance Kapha

INTRODUCE FIRE INTO your diet. Eat freshly prepared foods with pungent spices like pepper, fresh ginger, and turmeric. Enjoy mung dahl soup, broccoli, green leafy vegetables, cauliflower, Brussels sprouts—all cooked—and quinoa cooked with a little olive oil. Exercise is essential to balance Kapha. Add fire daily with hot spice water.

Pitta Weight Imbalance

PITTAS COULD HAVE long-term ama build-up that clogs srotas (energy channels), especially around the stomach, creating too much heat in the body. Pittas are usually fiery—you would think that comes with great digestion. However, without regular meals to feed that fire, ama will coat the digestive system and lower metabolism, resulting in weight gain. Appetite might be high, along with excessive thirst.

AYURVEDA ACTION
Balance Pitta

EAT THREE MEALS a day at regular times. A stewed apple or oatmeal is a good start for breakfast. Try drinking a tea of ¼ tsp each of coriander (detox), licorice (cooling), and fennel (digestion). Eat lots of sweet, juicy fruits. Zucchini, asparagus, and yellow mung dahl are cooling and detoxing for Pitta. Quinoa and basmati rice are also good. Cooling spices like fennel and small amounts of cumin and turmeric balance Pitta.

Vata Weight Imbalance

VATAS ARE OFTEN thin, but not always. Sometimes Vatas can be too thin and require more nourishment. They are susceptible to mental stress and emotional eating of sweet, sugary foods. When ama accumulates, even Vatas can become overweight.

AYURVEDA ACTION
Balance Vata

IF UNDERWEIGHT, BE sure to nourish and fortify Vata. Eating warm, cooked, grounding foods such as winter squashes and practicing a daily rasayana such as chyawanprash help nourish and fortify. If you are overweight with a Vata imbalance, continue to nourish as well and really focus on grounding your energy. When Vatas overdo—which can easily happen—they burn up their energy reserves and might just start grabbing sugary treats to get through. If you focus on stable nourishment, you can avoid the energy depletion that leads to unhealthy cravings.

APRIL 27
WHAT ABOUT KETO, PALEO & OTHER DIETS?

The research on diet effectiveness for weight loss is mixed. The customized principles of Ayurveda apply here: What one person needs for weight loss could be very different from what another needs.

Finding and maintaining your right weight is a customized path of lifestyle choices over time. Ayurveda does not generally recommend diets that isolate out real foods long term. You need a broad range of nutrients and operational information from the underlying field. Missing something important in your diet invites unhealthy cravings.

Keto and Paleo diets both recommend moderate to high fat and low carbohydrates. Protein recommendations vary. I did once try the keto diet for a few months and found it helpful for weight loss. But the real benefit of strict keto for me was complete elimination of added sugar. I had been inattentive to my afternoon sugary-snack habit. This diet helped me treat my sugar attraction as an addiction. By also adding more fat, I felt satiated and energetic, which allowed me to get off the sugar train.

Historically, late winter and spring were natural times for ketogenic cleansing because food was hard to come by. The body was forced to burn its own fat, which is the goal of a ketogenic diet. This scarcity provided a natural cleansing reset each year.

Dr. John Douillard advises that the "ketogenic diet can be a great way to reset fat-burning for two-week, maybe three-week stints," but is not a continuous way of life. Once fat burning has been reestablished, return to a dosha-balancing diet and focus on food that is seasonally available. Paleo may offer the same short-term benefits.

AYURVEDA ACTION
Become a Better Fat Burner

- Avoid sugar.
- Avoid bad fats found in processed foods, especially cooked oils in processed foods—even bread.
- Enjoy moderate exercise, which is more fat-burning than endurance walking, swimming, or biking.
- Eat balanced meals with real food and use moderate amounts of good fats. I only use ghee, coconut oil, or avocado oil for cooking.
- Do not snack between meals so you can metabolize stored fats.

APRIL 28
CLEARING MENTAL CLUTTER WITH MEDITATION

MEDITATION IS AMONG the best practices for our overall health and well-being. Choose a meditation practice for your purpose. Here are five to consider.

Mindfulness Meditation—Open your awareness to sounds and activity around you. Allow your mind to be fluid, flow from one thought or one sound to the next. The idea is not to get involved with thoughts, simply to be aware of what arises and let it pass. Notice what patterns you see. Be the observer.

Prayer or Spiritual Meditation—Commune with God or the Underlying Field in a calm, quiet space. Offer up a prayer of gratitude or listen for guidance.

Mantra Meditation—Mantras are words/sounds that resonate with higher consciousness. This meditation purifies through inviting the presence of the mantra, which "bumps into" thoughts and beliefs and releases them on the journey to pure consciousness. This is the meditation that I teach.

Concentration Meditation—Focus on a single point such as a sound, a candle, or the breath. This practice leads to a refined sense of concentration and clarity. It can be challenging for beginners. Start with a few minutes and slowly add time.

Movement/Breathing Meditation—Focus on the slow, mindful movement of the body when walking for instance or if a breathing meditation, focus on inhalation and exhalation.

AYURVEDA ACTION
Practice Breath Awareness

1. Find a comfortable position in a firm chair or on the floor and let hands rest.
2. Notice the shape and weight of your body. Be aware of—and curious about—body sensations as you relax.
3. Tune into your breath. Feel the natural flow, in and out. Notice where you feel your breath—in your abdomen, or in your upper or lower chest. Be gently aware.
4. Having thoughts is completely natural. As you become aware of thoughts, return to breath awareness. If it helps, you can say "thinking" or "wandering" softly in your head.
5. Continue with breath awareness for 5 or 10 minutes.
6. Check in with body sensations once more before completing the meditation.

APRIL 29
CLEARING YOUR ENVIRONMENT OF CLUTTER

I AM WORKING on removing clutter from my home, so hopefully by the time you read this, I will have made great gains. I have done well with restricting clutter to my office, the basement, and my closets. I can tell you from experience that clutter comes at a cost.

One day I was going through my books, culling those I have never read and never will. I found two copies of *The Feng Shui of Clutter*. It made me laugh, and helped me lighten up about releasing—no, pushing out the clutter.

Drowning in clutter? Feeling overwhelmed? Here are four strategies I found helpful.

1. Gretchen Rubin from "The Happiness Project" suggests employing the 1-minute rule. If you can do a task in less than 1 minute, do it—don't procrastinate. It takes less than a minute to decide on a piece of mail, put a dish in the dishwasher instead of the sink, or place clothing in the hamper instead of on the floor. Just Do It!
2. I set my oven timer for 15 or 30 minutes and commit to cleaning and clearing until the buzzer sounds. The time limit motivates me to be productive.
3. The third strategy, which I use in my "walk-in closet" office, is to envision the end result. For example, I clear everything from one area, such my file cabinet or desktop. I put back only those things that I really want or need in that area. Everything else gets tossed or given away.
4. Clearing clutter can be spiritual, a practice at releasing attachments. Look at an item and avoid thinking about how it was once meaningful or might still useful. Instead ask, "Does it excite me with meaning today? Is it highly useful to me right now? Will I actually use this item, or wear this clothing, or hang this art?" If the connection is nostalgic, or you think it only has potential use, peel away the attachment. Let it go.

The internet has a plethora of sites with more ideas to support you in clearing clutter.

AYURVEDA ACTION
Try the Timer Trick

SET A TIMER for 15 minutes and see how much clutter you can eliminate. Short, clutter-clearing sprints are better than marathons. Next time, maybe try 20 minutes or even 30. Once you make a good start (or two), you will feel how nice it is to have the space. Let that motivate you to keep going.

APRIL 30
RECAP AND WHAT'S AHEAD

April is a great time to cleanse and to clear your body, your mind, and your environment. Intense cleansing can help you adapt to seasonal changes. Daily cleansing of body, mind, and environment is the way to go over time.

Spring is the best time to cleanse your body and digestive system, allowing you to eliminate winter's accumulated toxins. If you are only going to do one cleanse a year, now is the time.

Daily cleansing is also important to sustain a healthy mind, body, and spirit. This means:

1. Eat freshly prepared, organic foods whenever possible.
2. Use cleansing herbs like triphala, black pepper, cinnamon, cloves, coriander, cumin, and turmeric.
3. Meditate daily to keep the mind clear.
4. Keep up with clutter around your home and/or place of work.

WHAT'S NEXT?

May continues the cleanse trend and begins restoration through light eating. After cleansing, you might be ravenous. However, it's advisable to restore gently with fresh foods and not overeat. Metabolism slows in spring and summer, so plan on eating for low volume and high nutrition. This month we gave you a taste of greens, and now spring greens are on their way. Go for them!

MONTHLY REFLECTION TIME

What actions did you try and what was your experience? Did a new action feel worthwhile? Did you like it? Did you have adverse reactions? Put a check in the third column for actions you plan to incorporate, whether daily, weekly, monthly, seasonally, or on occasion.

What New Actions This Month?	*Your Experience?*	*Habit Worthy?*
....	....	☐
....	....	☐
....	....	☐

MAY 1
ALL LIFE FORMS EXIST TO NOURISH AND BE NOURISHED

Every form of life both receives and transmits energy to all other forms of life. Even "things" like trees and rocks are not as solid as we think. Everything has energy and vibrates in a range of frequencies and exchanges this energy with every other form of life in a tapestry of influence and engagement. As humans, in reality we are in constant connection with every bit of this vibratory life, although often we have no awareness of it and therefore do not act in ways that acknowledge this connection.

Let's take an example. Think about your diet for a moment. Plants serve up not only nutrition to fortify us, they also supply us with energy from the sun through light that they transmute into their composition, which we ingest. The sun animates the life of the plant and then the plant carries the light and animates our human experience.

Humans then transmute light into consciousness, or love, through perception. This is our special calling as humans. Think of images you see of awakened persons. They are radiant with light. Through plants and experiences in Nature, you commune with the outer sun and receive light. When you meditate, live with mindfulness in the moment, and ingest food and experiences with reverence, you commune with and fortify your inner sun. The alchemy of outer and inner sun is our true Self-awakening.

You may eat the same foods at a meal as does another person, but when your system is fairly clean because of your Ayurveda practices and you eat with reverence for the food and those who toiled to bring it to you, then you experience the true intelligence and radiant power of the food on your plate. Take a moment to experience communion and gratitude for the food you eat.

AYURVEDA ACTION
Plant Ayurveda Herbs

What better way to revere your relationship with the plant world than to grow and enjoy your own fresh herbs? These are easy to grow yourself:

CILANTRO/CORIANDER
  Pitta digestive stimulant, heals Kapha upper respiratory

GINGER
  Digestive stimulant, breaks up agni, grounding

HOLY BASIL
  Also known as tulsi; opens heart and mind, bestowing love

LEMON BALM
  Treats headaches, relieves anxiety, pacifies Vata

MINT
  Helps digestion, lowers high blood pressure, calms mind, detoxifies

SAGE
  Treats swelling, infection, and pain; eases digestion

MAY 2
HOW DOES FOOD NOURISH FROM THE UNDERLYING FIELD?

Food carries more than calories for energy and nutrients for building and sustaining cells and tissues. It carries intelligent information about Nature and its composition received from the underlying field of consciousness. Nature designed a way for carrots to be in this world. Carrots have a unique structure and a dynamic.

Eating and digesting real food carries Nature's intelligence into our bodies. That intelligence becomes part of us. Elements in food stimulate actions and nourish you on all levels. Food is filled with code which looks for receptors in the body to unleash processes that lead to well-being.

With good food and practices to promote perfect digestion, you receive and transform Nature's intelligence, which is transformed into radiant health. For instance, a carrot has information at an energetic and cellular level. It sends signals to body organisms to turn on or off certain proteins, which then signals hormonal and other processes to engage or to shut down.

With genetically modified and processed food, your body still gets operating signals, but they don't support proper digestion or transmission of Nature's intelligence. Junk signals deplete, and they can result in disease.

This integrated, sophisticated system of intelligence connects you to everything. A goal of Ayurveda is to live closer to Nature and your own nature. Being healthy and vibrant allows you to receive the vibrations of higher consciousness and live with more bliss. Ahhhh...beautiful.

AYURVEDA ACTION
Try One Day with No Processed Food

Try going an entire day without eating processed food. Eat only real food, brimming with intelligence from the underlying field. Bless the food as you prepare it. Play or chant soothing music during meal preparation. Be grateful for the many hands involved in getting food to your plate.

No TV or cell phones or computers during dinner. Chew until your food is gone from your mouth—do not rush. Sometimes I set my fork down between each bite instead of getting the next one ready, an easy and effective practice.

Imagine your food coming from the underlying field, connecting you with the cosmos. Imagine food coming from that source, because it does!

MAY 3
IMMUNE SYSTEM BALA

Maintaining a healthy immune system is key to staying healthy, especially during outbreaks of the flu or during "cold season." In Ayurveda, this is called bala. All people are exposed to germs continually. Some will become ill and others won't. A big factor is the strength and response-ability of your immune system.

If you do become ill, do your best to rest, drink fluids, and eat for health. Remember, illness can be a way to keep the immune system at peak condition and boost intelligence in the fight against invaders. A strong immune system can get you through illness more quickly and with less severity.

STAYING HEALTHY WHILE TRAVELING

Travel, especially air travel, puts you into tight quarters with people who might be ill. Whether you get sick depends more on susceptibility than on exposure.

Airplanes are filled with dry air. When sinuses become dry, they produce more mucus. Mucus can be a breeding ground for bacteria or viruses. Keep nostrils lubricated with sesame oil (massage variety, not the cooking oil) or an Ayurveda mixture called nasya oil. {Sep 28} Dab oil inside nostrils regularly before, during, and after a plane trip.

AYURVEDA ACTION
Take a Thermos with You—Everywhere

Carry an empty thermos with herbs for hot spice water or immunity tea on the plane. When you get past security or find your seat on board, fill the thermos with hot water. It's a great way to hydrate and protect your immunity while traveling.

I take a thermos of hot spice water with me nearly everywhere—traveling in the car, going to a meeting, or taking my dog to the park. Daily hot spice water is a good way to flush toxins and build bala.

MAY 4
BITTER TASTE FOR SPRING

DESIRE FOR GREEN! We want to see it, we want to walk in it, we want to honor the earth by being "green," and if we want radiant health, we should eat green!

The green that greets us in the spring grasses, flower stems, and early garden treats is vibrant, luxurious, radiant. Do your eyes just dance like mine when you see grass bounce to new life with the unbelievably attracting shade of spring green? With the sometimes brutal or drab winters in many parts of the world, we are probably extremely hungry for green. And green is just right for us at this Kapha time of year (generally March–June). Kapha Nature is cool and wet—just right for producing spring greens.

As a reminder, the six tastes of Ayurveda are sweet, sour, salty, pungent, astringent, and bitter. We need to eat foods that have all six tastes for balanced daily nutrition. However, we should favor the tastes that will balance our imbalanced dosha and support the influences of the dosha season we are in. We left the Vata season of the three S's—sweet, sour, and salty—a few months ago and now it is time to continue to restore balance by focusing more on PAB: pungent, astringent, and bitter. Check in. How are you doing with that transition?

The bitter taste is especially healing and is often missing from our typical diet. The bitter taste is available to us in all sorts of greens—turnip, collard, swiss chard, and spinach for example. Cultivate greens in your diet this spring. Bonus: it's part of an earth-friendly lifestyle to find balance with Nature, leading to personal health and the health of our dear planet.

AYURVEDA ACTION
Eat Bitter Herbs/Foods Daily

TRY WORKING THE bitter taste into your diet with these:

- Arugula
- Broccoli rabe
- Collard greens
- Dandelion greens
- Dark chocolate
- Dill
- Fenugreek seeds
- Kale
- Mustard greens
- Sesame seeds
- Turmeric

MAY 5
GO LEAFY GREENS!

Leafy greens are rich in antioxidants, calcium, magnesium, iron, potassium, vitamin A, vitamin K, and vitamins B1 and B2. They contain nutritious juices to hydrate your system and purify the subtle srota channels. Leafy greens are rich in prana.

These dynamo greens help balance Pitta and Kapha. Vata, however, can be aggravated by the bitter and astringent qualities of greens. If you need to balance Vata, eat greens sautéed in oil or ghee and add digestive spices like cardamom, cumin, fennel, ginger powder, turmeric, and hing (aka asafoetida). To get the nutritional advantages of greens while not aggravating Vata, add them to brothy vegetable soups or other watery dishes.

Bitter foods activate taste buds, which stimulate enzyme production and the flow of bile that leads to better digestion. (Even a nutrient-rich food won't provide benefits if it can't be absorbed.) Greens' high-fiber content also helps with smooth elimination.

Bitter greens naturally detoxify the liver too. Leafy greens contain antioxidants to prevent aging and disease. It is best to keep the leaf part whole when cooking. Tough stems should be sliced into bite-sized slices and cooked longer. {Apr 21} Some Ayurveds recommend eating cooked leafy greens every day for great skin and good health—just do so moderately if you have a Vata imbalance.

AYURVEDA ACTION
Eat Leafy Greens for Super Nutrition

Leafy greens are super food. Get them in your diet. In addition to being abundant in nutrients, they're low in calories so you can eat enough to get full. Greens contain unique enzymes that support the immune system like no other food. They are good for your skin and hair and remove ama from the body. They purify the subtle channel srotas of the body as they hydrate. If you don't already eat greens regularly, consider a goal of preparing cooked greens for one meal a week. Experiment with different ways to prepare them and keep them on your go-to shopping list.

MAY 6
NOT SO FAST ON THE GREEN SMOOTHIES

With the need to get more bitter greens into your diet, green smoothies might sound like a perfect solution. Maybe not. Green smoothies are aggravating for Vatas, and many people have Vata imbalances. Vata is affected by stress, so Vata is the dosha most out of balance about half the time.

While greens are exceptional to represent the bitter taste and therefore pacify Kapha and Pitta, eaten in excess or over a long time, greens can aggravate Vata. In addition, green smoothie drinks are typically cold. Vata does better with warm, cooked food. So Vatas, beware of green smoothies. Kaphas are pacified by the bitter, but they are aggravated by cold, so Kaphas should drink their green smoothies room temperature. Pittas? Green smoothies are great for you, especially as warmer weather arrives.

What's more, smoothies often mix vegetables with fruits, which are digested differently. Ayurveda recommends eating fruits and veggies at different times to support proper digestion. Food remains in the stomach until the most difficult ingredient is digested. If it stays too long, it can ferment rather than digest. That results in ama accumulation.

Vata imbalances over the long term break down tissues. You might initially feel energy from the catabolic release of tissue breakdown, but this is short-lived and leads to depletion over time.

AYURVEDA ACTION
Adapt Smoothies to Be More Ayurvedic

So Vatas and Kaphas, if you love a smoothie, adapt it to make it Ayurvedically sound. Add fresh or powdered ginger and turmeric to your smoothie to turn up the heat. Drink at room temperature rather than cold—no ice! Experiment with recipes. You can add greens of your choice, water, and perhaps flax seed. Keep it simple.

Ayurveda would also recommend using fewer ingredients in your smoothie (3 or 4). And separate fruits and veggies: choose a green veggie blend with water or a fruit smoothie. Do not use yogurt—dairy products have a faster rate of digestion, so Ayurveda says to eat them separately.

Protein powders are highly processed and thus not recommended. Get your protein from real food. See {May 23} for ideas on getting more protein in your diet.

Of course—it's always more nourishing and better for digestion to eat greens warm and lightly cooked.

MAY 7
YOUR SATTVIC LIFE

Sattva is one of the three gunas, or qualities, of Nature. It is positive qualities of spiritual goodness and equanimity, or translated simply, means "pure." Sattva is the observer and harmonizer of positive and negative forces. In your natural state of awareness, virtue, and joy, you are of sattvic mind. The other gunas are tamas, meaning inertia and stability, and rajas, meaning movement {Jan 20}.

Your daily choices can build ojas, the juice of a sattvic life. Sattva Vijaya is a Vedic term that means "winning over the sattva." Success is based on engaging daily dietary, behavioral, and environmental strategies to form sattvic habits. The Ayurveda information and actions in this book will help you to lean in to sattvic life, day by day.

Eating sattvic foods is a good way to build a sattvic life. They are soothing and nurturing, and promote purity of body and mind. Cooked with love, they nourish us deeply and create positive spiritual qualities. Sattvic foods both quiet the mind and sharpen it. Naturally grown, vegetarian foods are sattvic. They contain no preservatives, artificial flavors, or other unnatural additives.

Intelligent, sattvic foods include:

- Fresh organic fruits and vegetables
- Whole grains, nuts
- Dairy such as raw milk and ghee
- Beans and lentils
- Natural, unrefined sugars like raw honey and pure maple syrup
- Spices such as cinnamon, basil, coriander, ginger, and turmeric
- Herbs blends, such as ashwagandha, shatavari, and brahmi

Doshic diets are used to balance, and sattvic diets are followed to improve the mind. Consider doing a cleanse before getting deeply into sattvic foods, and introduce more sattvic foods after a time of cleansing.

AYURVEDA ACTION
Add Sattvic Foods to Your Diet Now

Consider a few of these for your shopping list: almonds, raw honey (never use for cooking or baking), the freshest/most colorful organic vegetables at your market, plus juicy fruits like grapes, pears, and mangoes.

MAY 8
TRIPHALA—A POWERFUL TRIO

Triphala is a perhaps the most popular herbal formula in all of Ayurveda. In India, there is a saying that any condition can be healed by a vaidya (Ayurveda physician) who knows how to use triphala properly. The formula is cleansing and a rasayana, which is an herbal combination that offers rejuvenation, long life, and promotes ojas, the material equivalent of bliss.

During each meal, the intestinal tract produces mucus to lubricate the digestive tract. Over time, digestive mucus builds up, clogging the little hair-like villi in the small intestine that help the body absorb nutrients and remove toxins.

Triphala, an Ayurvedic rasayana formula, helps cleanse the mucus from digestive villi, making for more efficient food processing and absorption of nutrients. This formula is comprised of three fruits that support the eliminative process:

1. Amalaki supports the health of intestinal tissue and villi and is loaded with vitamin C.
2. Bibhitaki pulls old mucus and toxins off the wall of the gut.
3. Haritaki strengthens and tones intestinal muscles to contract more efficiently when the bowels need to move.

Thus, triphala scrubs the intestinal tract in three important ways. I use triphala daily, as do many people. Others use it occasionally for cleansing or when traveling. It is typically taken at bedtime to support overnight digestion and morning elimination. That is when I take mine. Research suggests that triphala after a meal can help with weight loss. Find more information at Dr. John Douillard's website lifespa.com.[18]

Although some people do take triphala continuously, Dr. Douillard recommends stopping once digestion is stabilized—meaning you are having a bowel movement within an hour of awakening or you have lost weight. There are mixed views on whether to take triphala continuously or to take for a while and then break. Personally, I choose to take triphala continuously as it is tri-doshic and supports regular digestion. If stools are loose, stop taking triphala. A registered Ayurvedic practitioner can help you decide what is best for you.

AYURVEDA ACTION
How to Take Triphala

Triphala is best taken in hot water as a tea. Typical dosage is to add 1/4 to 1/2 tsp of triphala powder to a cup of boiled water. Allow to cool and drink on an empty stomach or, for weight loss, take after completing a meal. You may also use triphala tablets; 1–2 at bedtime is typical. These are not as effective but are certainly more convenient. Or you can drink about 30 drops of triphala liquid extract in a small amount of water up to 3 times daily.

MAY 9
AMA DETOXING TIME!

We are in the middle of Kapha season, the time where ama accumulation can be high. Everyone has ama. Stressful demands, fast food, rushed meals, and lots of change all invite ama to stick around. It's a good time to encourage ama to *leave*.

Ama busters:

1. Use ginger—in all forms. Cook with minced fresh ginger or powdered versions. Add fresh ginger to boiled water for tea.
2. Sip hot spice water throughout the day—my go-to strategy for daily radiant health. Add 1/2 tsp fennel, 1/4 tsp cumin and 1/4 tsp coriander seeds to a quart of hot water in a thermos. Add a slice of ginger as well.
3. Spend time in Nature.
4. Practice meditation and deep breathing.
5. Chew fennel seeds after a meal to improve digestion.
6. Soak in a hot Epsom salt bath—put one quart of salt in your tub and enjoy for 20 minutes.
7. Good sleep is important: Be restful in late evening, turn off electronic stimuli with screens, and go to bed by 10 p.m.

Even though it is Kapha season and you want to balance the Kapha influences this time of year, also be mindful to balance the dosha that is out of balance for you.

AYURVEDA ACTION
Add Detoxing Spices to Everything

Ginger, turmeric, coriander, cumin, fennel and fenugreek help open the srotas, the body's energy channels, to support flushing of toxins via the skin, liver, urinary tract, and colon.

Sauté spices in ghee, coconut oil, or avocado oil to release their intelligence.

MAY 10
PURE IN → PURE WITHIN → PURE EXPRESSION

"Pure in" is pureness experienced, followed by pure out. What you take in becomes part of you and forms the essence of your expression in the world. Small changes can be levers for large change. Increasing purity increases sattvic life.

Take a scan of yourself right now. Are there aches anywhere? Do you feel heavy or airy in your digestive system? Are your thoughts or emotions unsettled or aggressive?

11 IDEAS TO INCREASE PURE INTAKE:

1. Do not eat leftovers.
2. Do not eat GMO (genetically modified organism) foods.
3. Do not drink ice water, especially not with a meal.
4. Do not read or watch TV when eating.
5. Do not microwave food.
6. Do not eat when you are upset.
7. Eat mostly vegetarian.
8. Eat the freshest food you can find.
9. Eat organic—especially thin-skinned fruits and vegetables.
10. Eat food that is colorful and healthy looking.
11. Eat food that is prepared by a loving, settled cook.

Food provides the intelligence and operational codes for your biochemical system. When we scramble the code of foods, as we have with GMOs in the past few decades, the signals that our human systems have been built upon are scrambled. Eat real, clean, and fresh whenever possible.

AYURVEDA ACTION
Avoid the Most Damaging Foods

If you are not eating totally organic, start by avoiding foods known to be damaging to your health because they are GMOs or are treated with toxic pesticides. Food will retain pesticide residue even after scrubbing.

Genetically modified foods to avoid include corn, soy, sugar, aspartame, papayas, canola oil, dairy, zucchini, and yellow squash.

According to the evidence-based EWG (Environmental Working Group), these are some of the worst potentially toxic foods and organic is strongly recommended: strawberries, spinach, nectarines, apples, peaches, pears, cherries, grapes, celery, tomatoes, sweet bell peppers, and potatoes.

MAY 11
GHEE IS GREAT

GHEE, PURE CLARIFIED butter, carries nutrients and lubricates the intestinal tract and tissues. Ghee is a concentrated form of butyric acid, the primary fatty acid in butter. Butyric acid is also found naturally in the intestinal tract along the gut wall. The cells of the colon use butyric acid as the preferred source of energy securing gut wall integrity and health.

Ghee is loaded with a full spectrum of short-, medium-, and long-chain fatty acids, as well as omega-3 and omega-9 fatty acids. It also boasts vitamins A-D-E and K, plus other beneficial elements and minerals. Even lactose-intolerant people are often able to eat ghee because the milk solids have been separated and removed. In Ayurveda, ghee is revered as the most ojas-producing food.

Get ghee in your diet, but as with all Ayurveda tips, use it moderately. A tablespoon a day is advised. Ghee is wonderful and healing. Enjoy.

AYURVEDA ACTION
Make Your Own Ghee

MANY PEOPLE PREPARE ghee in a pot on the stove. You can find instructions online. Heating to the correct point is critical. I have found a simple and foolproof way to make ghee.

- Put two pounds of unsalted, organic butter in a crockpot. If you have warm-low-high settings, leave overnight on warm. If you only have low-high settings, put on low for about 4 hours. When the ghee has properly separated, water will have cooked off and milk solids will rise to the surface, making a popcorn-looking coating with golden highlights. Creamy milk solids will fall to the bottom. About 95 percent of the clear golden liquid in between is your ghee.

Crockpots differ so use your skills of observation to determine the timing.

- Scrape off the top layer of milk solids.
- Pour from crockpot through a sieve or colander lined with cheesecloth into a mixing bowl. (One with a pour spout is preferred.) Stop pouring when you get to the milk solids on the bottom. The cheesecloth captures the popcorn milk bits.
- Pour from the mixing bowl into small jars. Cover with lids. Store in a cool, dark place—never in the refrigerator. Always use a clean spoon when handling ghee. Untainted ghee can last for years on the shelf. Some people eat the popcorn milk solids, but most discard the top and bottom milk solids. This is the part of butter that goes rancid with time.

MAY 12
DEVASTATING EFFECTS OF HIGH-FRUCTOSE CORN SYRUP

Processed foods with high-fructose corn syrup (HFCS) are among the unhealthiest foods you can consume. This highly unnatural sweetener creates ama and is a major contributor to Type 2 diabetes.

HFCS and other non-real food ingredients disrupt leptin, the hormone that regulates appetite, satiety response, and body weight. Disrupted leptin initiates food cravings, and because you lose the ability to feel full, it's easy to overeat.

When you eat large quantities of food, you often choose unhealthy kinds, too—like processed carbs with high sugar content. This burdens the pancreas's ability to produce sufficient insulin. Leptin and insulin disruption go hand in hand. Over time, this leads to unbalanced blood-sugar levels, which is the hallmark of diabetes.

HFCS is cheap to make, and because it makes foods addictive, it is added to many processed foods. Check labels but be aware that food manufacturers have started using different names for HFCS. The safe bet is to eat real, unprocessed food.

AYURVEDA ACTION
Eat Real Food with Ease

Enjoy real foods for one breakfast and one lunch or supper meal at least once a week for the next three weeks. If you already have this habit increase the number of real-food meals you eat for the next three weeks. Real food is the key to radiant health. For convenience, consider purchasing a rice cooker—avoid buying Teflon versions. The better stainless-steel pot rice cookers are a little pricier but worth it.

While rice is cooking, lightly sauté some veggies. You can also use a rice cooker to prepare hot cooked cereal. Set it up the night before with your grain, water, and spices and turn it on in the morning. Easy!

MAY 13
HOW SKIN WORKS

The skin has three layers—epidermis, dermis, and subcutaneous (sometimes called hypodermis). The epidermis is the surface. New skin cells are made at the bottom of that layer and move their way to the top. Teenagers produce a new skin surface every two to four weeks, but by age 60 or so, this process takes 12–13 weeks.

The next layer down is the dermis. It is full of tiny blood vessels that deliver oxygen and nutrients to skin cells and take away waste. The dermis contains the sebaceous glands that produce sebum oil to keep your skin lubricated and protected. Third is the subcutaneous layer, made mostly of fat to keep our bodies warm and to absorb shocks when we bump into something.

A primary purpose of skin, besides holding us all together, is to regulate body temperature. Exertion, especially in summer, prompts the brain's thermometer, called the hypothalamus, to move blood vessels closer to the skin's surface to release heat. This is why you get red-faced when you're overheated. Sweat glands also release sweat, which evaporates and cools.

Skin processes work miraculously to keep you warm, moist, and protected. In hot weather, those processes can get taxed. Ayurveda offers refreshment for all the skin layer processes, including sloughing old skin, opening the blood vessels, and eliminating ama from fat cells.

AYURVEDA ACTION
Make Ayurveda Cleanser–Toner–Exfoliator

Exfoliate 1–3 times a week. Determine how often is best for your skin. Recipe:

- 1 Tbsp chickpea flour—exfoliates and moisturizes naturally
- 1/4 tsp triphala or triphala guggulu powder—provides vitamin C to support collagen and skin elasticity while pulling toxins from deep tissue layers
- Mix into a paste with rosewater

If you like, add a dosha-specific option.

Vata skin	Pitta skin	Kapha skin
1 tsp raw honey and/or sandalwood powder	1/4 tsp powdered neem (not if pregnant) or mint leaves	1 tsp raw honey and 1/2 tsp lemon juice and/or 1 tsp turmeric

Wet your face and rub on paste. Allow to set for a few minutes. Wipe off with a wet washcloth. Moisturize with an appropriate oil for your skin type. Some preferred oils are sesame oil for Vata and Kapha and coconut oil or sunflower oil for Pitta.

MAY 14
DEPRESSION AND SADNESS

Everyone feels sadness and depressed moods from time to time. Clinical depression and grief are something else. While Ayurveda provides strategies and support for fleeting sadness, clinical depression should be accompanied by other treatments as well.

Three types of sadness arise from doshic imbalances. Vata anxious depression arises from the colon, Pitta agitated depression from the small intestine, and Kapha sluggish depression from the stomach. These dosha imbalances enter general circulation and lodge in the nervous system.

Vata depression could be triggered by loss of a loved one, a job, or a relationship. These losses create emptiness, the air/space nature of Vata. Balancing Vata with more water and earth elements can restore a sense of cohesion (water attribute) and enduring stability (earth attribute).

Pitta sadness might be triggered by burnout or perceptions of not living up to expectations. Getting fired from a job or failing at a task or relationship leaves Pittas irritated in their depression experience. Cooling foods and time with Nature can help Pittas relax their need to be in control. Time in Nature gives Pittas a sense of being held in something larger and gentler than their own ego.

Kapha depression shows up as sluggishness. It's a can't-get-out-of-bed sadness and could be triggered by resisting a change in work or relationships. Kaphas have excessive desire for solitude when not in balance. Some solitude is good of course, but to avoid Kapha depression, it's best to move physical energy with exercise and activity and animate emotional energy by spending time with others, especially fun and/or spiritual groups.

AYURVEDA ACTION
Lift Dosha Sadness with Herbs

The bedrock for balancing emotional imbalance is nourishing foods and lifestyle actions. Also consider these herbs known in Ayurveda for lifting mood:

Vata anxiety and sadness

brahmi, shankhpushpi, jatamansi, ashwagandha, kappikachu

Pitta anguish and sadness

brahmi, gingko biloba, arjuna

Kapha sluggishness and sadness

ginger, punarva, kappikachu, arjuna

MAY 15
THE JOY OF EMOTIONAL BALANCE

After lifting yourself from ongoing sadness or depression, support a sense of daily joy in one or all of these ways:

- Meditate—daily practice is the greatest key to a blissful, joyful life.
- Get good sleep—go to bed before 10 p.m. and rise early by 6 a.m..
- Wake up with the rising sun—or before. Sleeping past 6 a.m. can clog the srotas (energy channels), leading to dullness in your day.
- Spend time in nature. Take a walk every day. Exercise moves ama and blocked emotions out of the body. It increases agni and releases positive neurohormones that elevate mood and spark positive thinking. Early morning sun is the most sattvic (pure).
- Eat real food—a major way that intelligence from the underlying field engages physiology and leads to health. Ojas is the product of real food and experiences. Ojas nourishes a blissful life.
- Have real experiences—time in Nature is real, authentic conversations are real, loving without expectations is real.
- Don't suppress natural urges and don't force them—this includes everything from flatulence to sex to sharing your voice.
- Enjoy daily abhyanga massage to clear toxins from the body, calm the mind, and soothe emotions.
- Surround yourself with love and beauty.

AYURVEDA ACTION
Choose Herbs for Joy

The deep source of joy is a healthy diet and lifestyle. However, herbs can lift moods.

- Ashwagandha—tones the nervous system, increases energy and vitality, calms the mind
- Kapikacchu—soothes nervous system, natural source of levodopa
- Arjuna—soothes the heart and emotions (sadhaka Pitta), especially grief and sadness
- Cardamom—strengthens heart-mind connection and clears the lungs for deep breathing

MAY 16
CANCER—
AN AYURVEDIC PERSPECTIVE

Healing involves your spiritual, emotional, and intellectual nature, as well as the physical. Healing is always possible, whether or not cure is the outcome. Cures in mainstream, Western medicine are often turned over to physicians, their treatments, and drugs. Ayurveda puts each person at the center of his or her healing process. This goes beyond cure, and healing is a long-term lifestyle.

Cancer is the second leading cause of death in the U.S., following heart disease. The true causes of cancer need to be understood to make changes where we have influence. New evidence-based knowledge is emerging about natural approaches to prevent and heal cancer. Alignment with Nature in every way is key.

In its origin, Ayurveda did not speak of cancer by that term. Ayurveda does, however, offer time-tested knowledge for the two primary strategies for preventing and healing from cancer—reduce inflammation and improve the immune system.

Please be clear: I am not suggesting that you forego treatments by mainstream medicine. I have friends and clients who have had cancer. That gets your attention. I know people who have chosen a completely natural approach; I know those who have used natural/Ayurveda strategies in combination with chemo and other treatments, and those who have stayed with mainstream medicine. Some have survived cancer, others have not. Dealing with cancer is a personal journey, without one right answer. I feel great respect for those who have gone through, and are going through, this life experience.

AYURVEDA ACTION
Benefit from Daily Turmeric

Turmeric is the most researched herb in terms of its efficacy for healing. Turmeric has been shown in many studies to prevent and treat inflammation and strengthen the immune system.[19] Both of these are at the root of creating a body environment that will not be a good host for cancer. Get more turmeric by adding it to meals or taking it in tinctures or tablets. Of course, it's good as turmeric tea; recipe here.

Add to one cup boiling water:

- 1/4 tsp turmeric powder
- 1/4 tsp ground cinnamon
- 1/4 tsp ground ginger

Add a bit of lemon and raw honey (when cool enough to drink) to taste. Strain out the powders if you want; I like to drink them in the tea.

MAY 17
KEY TO UNDERSTANDING CANCER

Everyone has cancer cells. How do you prevent them from multiplying and causing problems? Or if cancer cells have taken hold, how do you combat their progress and reverse effects?

I have taken an interest in natural approaches to preventing or dealing with cancer. Research is being conducted by natural health leaders, and new perspectives on cancer are emerging. They combine well with the ancient wisdom of Ayurveda.

Cancer may be a body's predictable response to innumerable attacks from cancer-causing toxins in the air, water, and food system: these include GMO foods introduced in the past couple of decades, with more on the way every day, it seems. Cancer cells are caused and aggravated by inflammation, and an overwhelmed immune system is unable to rid the body of these cells. Cancer cells are tricky—they have a positively charged energy coating covering a negatively charged cell. White blood cells do not recognize or perceive the threat of the positively charged coating.

The immune system, and only the immune system, rids us of cancer effects. Simply put, treatments such as surgery, radiation, and chemotherapy attempt to reduce the number of cancer cells to give our own immune system a fighting chance.

Mainstream medicine's typical approach is to "fight the cancer." Ayurveda and other Natural healing methodologies seek to understand causes and work to shift those so that your miraculous body can heal itself.

This information above was gleaned from the video series *The Truth about Cancer*.[20] It features many doctors who have rejected what their medical training offered in favor of natural approaches, which they say are more effective in treating and curing cancer.

AYURVEDA ACTION
Reduce Sugar & Use Raw Honey Instead

It's thought that sugar fuels cancer cells. Read more in the next entry {May 18}. So, everyone should reduce intake of added sugars found in processed foods and even the "healthy" raw sugars added to recipes. Because raw honey is predigested by bees, it operates differently in our body than other sugars. To sweeten a recipe, look for ways to use raw honey and local honey if you can find it. (Beware of pseudo-honeys, meaning most of the honey on grocery store shelves.) Don't cook or bake with honey, as that changes its composition and becomes a negative for health. When tea or any other item is cool enough to eat or drink, then add the honey.

MAY 18
NATURAL APPROACHES TO PREVENT & TREAT CANCER

- **EAT AN ALKALINE DIET.** Whole vegetables and fruits are generally more alkaline. Beets, broccoli, cauliflower, kale, spinach, sea vegetables, berries, grapes, and lemons are especially good. Almonds, Brazil nuts, cinnamon, and ginger are also recommended.
- **ELIMINATE PROCESSED SUGARS.** We know cancer feeds on sugar. To detect cancer in a PET scan, D-glucose is injected because it is quickly taken up by cancer cells. New research gets more specific about sugar and right- and left-spinning molecules. Have you noticed the "L" in front of amino acids like L-lysine? The L stands for left-spinning, and that is good. Unnatural, processed sugar is right-spinning, and should be avoided.

    Natural, unprocessed sugars like honey, molasses, maple syrup, sugar cane, and natural sugars in fruits are left-spinning. New research is proposing these do not feed cancer. Blueberries spin left and are often promoted as cancer preventing.
- **ELIMINATE HIGH-GLUTEN GRAINS** like wheat, rye, and spelt—even if they are whole grain. Enjoy non-gluten grains such as rice, buckwheat, quinoa, millet, and amaranth.
- **REDUCE DAIRY.** Dairy is high in casein protein, which has been found to be cancer promoting. Dairy can be acidifying and cause inflammation. Exception: raw cow's milk.
- **USE ORGANIC OLIVE, COCONUT, AND AVOCADO OIL.** Coconut oil has a mild antibacterial and antifungal effect, so is helpful if the immune system is compromised. It is cooling, which helps to balance inflammation. Avoid GMO oils, processed oils, and hydrogenated (hard) oils. Do not heat olive oil.
- **DRINK FRESHLY MADE VEGETABLE JUICE, CLEAN WATER, HERBAL TEA, AND LEMON WATER.** Avoid processed drinks of any sort. Helpful herbal teas include green, sage, mint, or ginger. Carrot or carrot-beet juice strengthens the immune system. When juicing, keep it simple—using just a few vegetables in one drink makes them easier to digest.

AYURVEDA ACTION
Explore the Alkaline Diet

YOU MIGHT BE doing many of the strategies noted above. To prevent cancer, do more. To deal with cancer, become even more vigilant. Explore a more alkaline diet—good for everyone, but especially if you are trying to treat or prevent cancer.[21] The pH number tells you how acidic (0) to alkaline (14) a food is. Seven is neutral. Meats, grains, dairy, and alcohol are more acidic. Natural fats, starches, and sugars are neutral. Fruits, legumes, and vegetables are more alkaline. A good vegetarian diet aligns with the alkaline diet to prevent and treat cancer.

MAY 19
OJAS—THE JUICE OF LIFE

OJAS IS THE byproduct of perfect digestion. Ojas is life's vital energy and exists on the physical level, at least in the ancient texts, if not yet discovered by modern science. The functions of ojas are nonphysical.

Think of ojas as similar to a crystal that takes energy waves and transforms them. Ojas transduces the "waves of consciousness" into the life force that animates us. It's a beautiful, virtuous cycle. More consciousness means more ojas; more ojas means more consciousness. Ojas is responsible for contact with the underlying field and is responsible for bala—strength and immunity–that maintains the integrity of our body.

Signs of high ojas include:

- Glowing complexion and eyes
- Abundant strength and energy
- Heightened senses
- No aches and pains
- Ease of body movement
- Robust immunity
- Mental clarity
- Joy and happiness
- Overall sense of well-being

Freshly preparing foods (and spices) with love, cultivating bliss, and being grateful for your abundant blessings—all of these nourish the gift of ojas.

If you have issues with ama, you need to cleanse first before building deep nourishment. Perhaps try an intense cleanse or a regular habit of daily cleansing. If you try to engage more ojas-producing foods while you have a lot of ama, you will overwhelm your system. When you are on a good path of reduced ama and have good, not perfect, daily health habits, it is time to build ojas.

AYURVEDA ACTION
Boost Your Ojas Today

GOOD FOODS TO promote ojas are raw milk if you can get it, whole grains, fresh organic fruits and vegetables (especially leafy greens and avocados), dates, and nuts (especially almonds). Avoid leftovers, processed foods, dense foods like meat, dry and raw foods, and stimulants like caffeine. What can you eat or avoid today?

MAY 20
OIL PULLING

People are buzzing about oil pulling, also known as "kaval" or "gundusha." It is a simple practice of swishing about one tablespoon of oil in your mouth for 10–20 minutes and then spitting it out.

Oil pulling helps maintain a neutral pH and keeps particles from building up in the mouth. If food particles are left to settle in the mouth, decay and gum infection can occur. Tongue scraping {Apr 20} and teeth brushing help, but oil pulling added makes a complete strategy. Oil swishing pulls fat-soluble toxins out of tissues. Be sure not to swallow the oil, because it has accumulated toxins. Always spit it out.

Benefits of oil pulling include toning the sinuses, keeping mouth joints flexible, relaxing the neck and jaw, and moistening the skin inside and around the mouth. Oil pulling brings nutrients right to the mouth to build strong bones and teeth.

Typically, sesame massage oil is recommended for oil pulling, although coconut oil also can be used, especially for Pittas.

In the morning, I generally brush my teeth, take the tablespoon of oil into my mouth, then swish while in the shower, and spit it out after.

AYURVEDA ACTION
Add Oil Pulling to Your Daily Routine

---

1. Swish the oil in the mouth from one side to the other.
2. Bring the oil to the front of the mouth, and ooze it between the teeth.
3. Spit out in the toilet or trash. Spitting oil in a drain could clog it.
4. Rinse the mouth with warm water.

MAY 21
THE TONGUE MAPS YOUR INNER WORKINGS

WHAT CAN YOUR tongue tell you? Your tongue's coating and characteristics reveal the state of your health. You can study your own tongue for clues about what is going on.

Look at size/shape, color, coating, and terrain of the tongue. The Vata constitution tongue is thinnest—small and a bit dry and rough—the qualities of Vata. A Pitta tongue is redder and medium sized. A Kapha tongue is large, light pink, and moist.

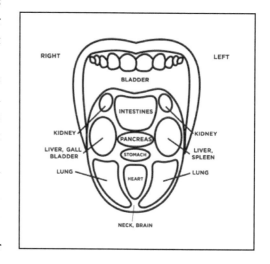

A healthy tongue has uniform color and is sufficiently moist, with no cracks, no shininess, and no tooth marks on the side. If you notice cracks in a particular area, see which organ on the tongue is affected. Excessive Vata might be in that organ. Teeth marks on the side of the tongue are a sign of malabsorption. Glassy shininess on the side indicates liver concerns. A shaky tongue is another sign of Vata imbalance.

If the tongue is red and too moist, excess acid is in the stomach. Too smooth and buff—as though the taste buds are hiding—indicates excess mucus in the stomach and small intestines.

Other qualities to look for:

- Slimy tongue/thick white coating—mucus accumulation, Kapha imbalance, ama
- Dry tongue or cracks or brownish color—Vata imbalance of digestive organs or nervous-system
- Swollen tongue—low digestive fire, lymph congestion
- Yellow-green tongue—Pitta derangement
- Pale tongue—undernourished rakta dhatu (blood cells)
- Depression in the heart area—can indicate grief
- Pimples—possible signs of toxins and Pitta pushing them out
- Crack down the middle—spinal cord or Vata emotional or digestive issues

AYURVEDA ACTION
Examine Your Tongue

LOOK AT YOUR tongue a few times throughout the day to notice changes in the coating. A thin white coating is good, but if the coating is thick and gooey, or dry, you have signs of ama. Always start your morning with tongue scraping {Apr 20}, and if your tongue is showing ama, engage ama-reducing strategies. Pay attention to small signs and make minor corrections to prevent problems.

MAY 22
REALIZATION AND FIRST BREATH

Let's take a fresher perspective on "morning breath." Before getting out of bed, look around at positive things to set your perspective for the day. Be open and inspired.

- Upon awakening, dedicate your first breath of the day to Spirit.
- Sense the energy of the day.
- Notice how the sun lights up your bedroom or honor the dark if you awake in the wee hours.
- Connect with the cosmos by opening your arms wide.
- Connect to earth by feeling energy gathering in your feet.
- Breathe into your heart space.
- Sing a few lines from a song like "Oh, what a beautiful morning" or ask Alexa or Google to play it for you. The Mormon Tabernacle Choir has an inspiring version.
- Imagine a luminous stream of golden love, compassion, and understanding coming from realized beings and all of your teachers—past, present, and future.
- Gently rub your palms together briskly to generate warmth; then gently massage your entire body.
- Sit on the edge of your bed and say a prayer or an affirmation.

AYURVEDA ACTION
Breathe Deeply Throughout the Day

According to Ayurveda author and educator Dr. John Douillard, deep breathing calms nerve receptors. It also helps you stay calm yet alert. Shallow breathing triggers upper-chest receptors, where most of the fight-or-flight receptors are located.

Put your hand on your belly. Are you breathing down to your deep calming receptors? If not, try to do so. Then during your day, when you are in your car or in a meeting, or watching TV, do a check-in. About to give a speech or ask for a raise? Breeeeathe. It's one thing to be able to breathe deeply when getting ready to meditate, but we want to extend the habit to the activities of our everyday life.

MAY 23
SOURCES OF COMPLETE PROTEIN

Protein sources are considered complete when they contain the eight essential amino acids the body cannot make. Ingested and—most importantly—properly digested protein maintains, replaces, and builds body tissues.

Animal sources of complete protein include:

- Fish
- Seafood/shellfish
- Poultry
- Milk
- Eggs
- Cheese
- Meat

Vegetarians need to be thoughtful about eating a wide variety of protein-rich vegetables and grains to get their essential amino acids. All essential amino acids aren't necessary at each meal; just get them some time during the day. Only a few plant-sources of protein provide all eight amino acids in the necessary proportions to qualify as a "complete protein." They are: quinoa, buckwheat, hempseed, and soybean. Asparagus and lentils are also big winners, with a whopping 27 percent of their calories supplying protein. Conventional wisdom for vegetarians suggests combining foods to meet complete protein needs—rice and beans, for example. However, recent research suggests these combinations don't have to be in the same meal. Some amino acids are "pooled" in the body. For most moderately active people, a vegetarian diet of varied and mostly freshly-prepared foods will suffice. For active athletes or women who are pregnant, protein combining could be important.

AYURVEDA ACTION
Add Vegetarian Protein to Your Diet

Soybeans are a great source of protein. Soy powder is generally not recommended because of its affect on hormones. Cook soybeans in the pod with a little salt for part of a meal or as a nice snack alternative to popcorn, which is drying to your system. Add beans to your diet, along with the spice mixture hingvastak (main ingredient hing, or asafoetida) to balance their air quality. Quinoa is a great source of protein, with about 8–9 grams per cooked cup.

MAY 24
PROTEIN—GETTING ENOUGH? TOO MUCH?

Most Americans get enough protein. In fact, meat eaters often get too much. To gain sufficient protein from a vegetarian diet, one needs to commit to preparing fresh, nutritious foods. Dr. John Douillard identifies four signs of protein deficiency:

1. Constant craving—you may especially crave carbs, because of blood-sugar instability.
2. Muscle and/or joint pain—protein stored in synovial fluid around joints is the first to be depleted.
3. Can't sleep well—if you are protein deficient, it can cause sugar craving.
4. Low energy, moodiness – protein stabilizes blood sugar and evens moods.

The recommended serving of protein is up to 55–60 grams/day for men and 45–50 grams/day for women. That level of protein is achieved by eating yogurt and 4 oz of meat daily. If you don't eat meat, be conscientious about getting protein through meals with other foods. Good protein sources are:

- 1 egg 7g
- 1 oz beef 7g
- 1 oz almonds 6g
- Avocado 4g
- Cooked peas 8.5g
- 1/2 cup tofu 10g
- 1 cup quinoa 8g
- Oatmeal 6g
- Basmati rice 4.4g

Excessive protein can cause intestinal discomfort, indigestion, exhaustion, nausea, irritability, and headache. Chronic protein overconsumption overworks the organs, which can lead to cardiovascular disease, and liver and kidney issues. Too much protein acidifies the body, which can leach calcium from the bone marrow to neutralize acid. This weakening of the marrow increases risk of osteoporosis. Protein from fatty meat sources also can add excess weight. As always, the key in Ayurveda is balance.

AYURVEDA ACTION
Analyze Your Protein Balance

If you experience the signs from too little or too much protein, analyze food intake, starting with the most recent 3-day period. Find a reliable chart on protein in foods. Analyze how much protein you are getting—don't just guess. Get the facts to decide if you need more or less protein.

MAY 25
DIGESTING NATURE'S INTELLIGENCE

Herbs and spices are powerhouse messengers of Nature's wisdom. They contain minerals, vitamins, enzymes, and proteins. Herbs support healthy circulation, digestion, respiration, elimination, and physical/emotional balance. They strengthen from within, not by addressing symptoms.

Spices, often used in seed form, contain concentrated forms of Nature's intelligence rising up from the underlying field of consciousness, also known as the quantum field. While most foods begin to deteriorate as soon as they are picked, seeds hold potency and a productive blueprint for more than a year to enable planting.

AYURVEDA ACTION
Add These Top 7 Hero Spices to Your Shopping List

To activate the intelligence of spices, lightly sauté in ghee or avocado or coconut oil.

- Cinnamon is a rich source of antioxidants, has anti-inflammatory properties, eases digestion, promotes weight loss, and may reduce blood sugar and cholesterol.
- Cloves are antibacterial, anti-inflammatory, and antifungal. They have been studied for use in aiding detoxification from environmental pollutants.
- Coriander seeds (from the cilantro plant) have antioxidant, anti-inflammatory, and antibacterial qualities. Coriander soothes the stomach and relieves bloating.
- Cumin is a traditional herbal diuretic (helps the body shed water), relieves diarrhea and bowel spasms, relieves morning sickness, and eases carpal tunnel syndrome.
- Fennel seed is a powerful antioxidant and contains fiber, folate, potassium, and vitamin C. It is believed to boost the immune system, reduce blood pressure, and aid in detoxification. Fennel is also a mild appetite suppressant.
- Ginger treats nausea from morning or motion sickness. Ginger also has anti-inflammatory properties for muscle and joint pain. It is good to cleanse and detoxify the body, stimulate circulation, and ease bronchitis and congestion.
- Turmeric, the queen of medicinal herbs, promotes healthy cell replication. It contains the flavonoid curcumin, which is known for its anti-inflammatory properties and may relieve the effects of chemotherapy, improve cognitive function, detoxify the liver, and boost immunity.

MAY 26
ARE YOU BUGGED?

BUGS, OR MORE inclusively, insects, are an important, contributing part of our ecosystem that support the balance of Nature. Then again...ouch.

Bugs benefit the ecosystem through pollination by bees, moths, flies, beetles, and butterflies, which is essential for our food supply. We often don't think about this benefit, but bugs also are responsible for decomposing old life—plant and animal—to nourish and aerate the soil, providing the base for new life to form.

But some insects just "bug" people, and a few can even be dangerous. Once in a while, you want or need to keep certain bugs away. You can do this in a natural, nontoxic way.

AYURVEDA ACTION
Make Natural & Effective Insect Repellents

Lemon Eucalyptus Insect Repellent

- 1 part lemon eucalyptus oil
- 10 parts sunflower oil or carrier oil of your choice. Spritz or rub it on skin.

Lemon eucalyptus oil has been touted as a natural insect repellent for decades. It even has the backing of the U.S. Centers for Disease Control (CDC) as an effective ingredient in insect repellents.[22]

Lavender Essential Oil Repellent

- Drop lavender essential oil on a clean cloth and rub it on your skin. Lavender is one of the few essential oils that can be applied directly to skin. Always check a small area first.
- Try growing lavender around your home to keep mosquitoes away. Grab a few sprigs of lavender and crush/rub them on your skin to keep the "skeeters" away and to smell good.

Citronella Mosquito Repellent

- 2 Tbsp neem seed oil
- 1 Tbsp carrier oil, such as almond
- 1 tsp melted coconut oil
- 10–15 drops citronella essential oil

Rub sparingly onto exposed skin. CAUTION: *Do not use neem seed oil if you are pregnant or trying to get pregnant, as it is an abortifacient.*

MAY 27
PREVENT THE OUCH!

A CORE PRINCIPLE of Ayurveda is to live as close to Nature, including your own nature, as you can. So, get out there and enjoy the outdoors. That means being with bugs, so take care that your preparation includes healthy strategies. Homemade products are not only healthier for your body, they often are less expensive to make. Here's to a healthy summer!

NATURAL BUG REPELLENT FOR OUTDOOR LIVING

READY FOR RELAXING alone time or a get-together in the great outdoors, but "bugged" by pesky mosquitoes? Here is another recipe to keep them away.

Put these items in a mason jar, set on your picnic table, and light the candle: 1–2 lemon wedges - 1–2 lime wedges - 2 sprigs rosemary - Active Ingredient: 7–10 drops lemon eucalyptus oil or citronella oil - Water (fill remainder of jar with water) - Floating tea candle

AYURVEDA ACTION
Treat Mosquito Bites

DID YOU ALREADY get bitten?

- Put ice cubes or a cold pack on the bite, wrap with towels, and hold in place 10 minutes. The ice numbs and controls swelling.
- Press a used tea bag on your bite until itching subsides. Tea tannins are astringent, drawing toxins out of the body.
- Make a paste of baking soda and water. Apply to the bite. The paste pulls toxins from the body, and baking soda's alkalinity helps neutralize the pH of the affected area and reduce swelling.

MAY 28
USING A NETI POT

Kaphas tend to accumulate mucus, and Kapha season can bring on the mucus, too. Using a neti pot—similar to a small teapot with a long spout—helps keep sinuses clear.

INSTRUCTIONS:

1. **CLEAN YOUR NETI POT.** Clean before each use with natural soap and rinse.
2. **MAKE A SALINE SOLUTION.** Mix 1/4 tsp finely ground, non-iodized salt with 8 oz warm distilled, boiled, or filtered water. Do not use tap water. Use finely ground mineral, sea, or kosher salt, not table salt. Stir until dissolved.
3. **GET INTO POSITION.** Tilt your head over a sink so that one ear is parallel to the sink. Breathe through your mouth.
4. **INSERT THE SPOUT IN THE UPPER NOSTRIL.** Lift the neti pot to the upper nostril and slowly pour in half the solution, letting it run out of the lower nostril. Reverse the head position and pour the remaining solution.
5. **REMOVE EXCESS WATER FROM NOSTRILS AND SINUSES.** With your face over the sink, gently blow through your nose until dripping has subsided.
6. **RINSE YOUR NETI POT WITH SOAP AND WATER.** Dry it and wrap it in a cloth to store.
7. **RUB OIL INSIDE BOTH NOSTRILS.** Put a drop of sesame, almond, olive, or coconut oil on your finger and wipe the inside of each nostril. Select an oil that is pacifying for the dosha you are balancing. Vata-sesame or almond; Pitta-coconut, Kapha-small amounts of sesame.

Using a neti pot can be drying. I recommend only doing neti when you have excess mucus in the sinuses. Always use oil in the nostrils afterward to keep them toned. (search for instructional videos online.

AYURVEDA ACTION
Clear Chest Congestion

IT IS NORMAL and protective to have mucus in your nasal passages and chest. Mucus keeps bacteria and viruses from entering the sinuses and lungs. However, thick mucus build-up is not good. When the mucus cannot eliminate trapped intruders, infections can result. Coughing and sneezing are functions of clearing mucus. Try these:

- Inhale steam.
- Diffuse peppermint or eucalyptus oil.
- Drink more tea—ginger, lemon, green—add raw honey.
- Gargle with warm water; add salt or turmeric.
- Drink more fluids.
- Eat hot, spicy foods if your throat is not sore.

MAY 29
LIVING AN AWAKENED LIFE

Ayurveda is commonly known for its capacity to support healing of many conditions and to extend life itself. But Ayurveda is more than a science of picking the right foods and choosing balancing lifestyle practices. At its very core, Ayurveda is a psycho-spiritual, energy science of consciousness. Ayurveda science is based on the idea that we are, in our essence, souls on a path of evolution to enlightenment or unification with God, the Infinite, or Source, or as you prefer to think about it.

Along this journey there are challenges to inspire us to go deeper within, to know and return home to our true, unchanging soul identity as we loosen the grip of our conditioned up-down ego identity. Challenges may come in the form of health, work, relationships, or societal pressures. These challenges are just what we need; they are our grit and gift. Without them, we would not be motivated to become the spiritual adventurer that is our deepest, truest, healthiest nature.

Being in harmony with this deep inner nature leads to radiant health. And radiant health prepares our physiology and energy body to recognize, call in, and hold the higher energies of this deep inner nature of pure consciousness. This is a mutually beneficial two-way relationship. They go hand-in-hand.

Sattva { Jan 20} is the radiant guna of clarity and purity. When our minds are pure we are connected to God or pure consciousness. Sattva is the sole cause of health. Sattvic actions include eating real, pesticide-free food in a peaceful environment, meditating, spending time in Nature, going to bed and arising early, and loving. All 3 Gunas show up in our lives, but when we increasingly lead a sattvic life, we are able to enter the state of Sattva where we are awakened to the light within.

Why is it so difficult to lead a Sattvic life? Because we are not yet fully awakened to our deepest spiritual nature. Our human nature desires what gives us pleasure and the highs, even though those moments are fleeting. Even with occasional highs, we wind up not very satisfied and desiring more. We reject the lows, although often not very easily. Ayurveda and the Sattvic life bring us peace that sustains us and brings blissful joy. Be sweet and patient with yourself as you do your best in a formidable world. Enjoy that pizza with friends and an occasional glass of wine. In my view, there is nothing more Sattvic than to enjoy your life and the people in it.

AYURVEDA ACTION
Live a Sattvic Life

---

1. Meditate
2. Go Within
3. Cook with Love
4. Eat in Bliss

MAY 30
MAKING VIGOR!

OJAS IS VIGOR. Vigor is not magically bestowed by a fairy godmother—you make or diminish your own vigor for life. When you consume fresh, ripe, pure fruits and vegetables, you are taking in the nutrients and absorbing the energetic ojas of those foods. A walk in the sunshine gives you vitamin D as well as an appreciation of Nature, boosting your ojas reception. When ojas is maximized, all with whom you come in contact benefit. People in your life are lifted, your plants are healthier, your pets are shiny, your children glow.

Abundant ojas helps you connect to your divine wholeness. Vigor is evident in radiant skin, shining eyes, strong body, good digestion, and bliss. Ways to build ojas:

- Eat a sattvic (pure, clean, wholesome) diet—ghee, fruits, rice, almonds, mung beans, dates, honey, and pure oils like olive, avocado, and coconut.
- Eat locally and seasonally and to balance imbalanced doshas.
- Attend to what brings you bliss and joy. Do not repress worrisome thoughts, but do not entertain them. Catch and release.
- Avoid drugs, alcohol, processed foods.
- Stay active daily with 30 minutes of walking, yoga, or other exercise.
- Get adequate sleep.
- Meditate.
- Eat in a peaceful environment, honoring your food and those around you.
- Eat with consciousness by noticing smells, tastes, and colors.
- Avoid iced drinks. Ice slows digestion and can cause indigestion or weight gain.
- Eat mostly cooked food, which is easier to digest. Eat local.

Don't get overwhelmed. Choose a few things, try them out, notice the difference, and watch as you are naturally drawn to more healthy choices.

AYURVEDA ACTION
Enjoy a Nightly Ojas Drink

START WITH RAW local milk or use non-homogenized vat pasteurized (low temp) organic milk available in health stores. If you don't drink dairy, substitute with drinks made from coconut, almond, rice, or hemp. Add a small amount of any or all of these to a cup of heated milk:

- 1 Tbsp chopped skinned/pitted dates
- 1 Tbsp chopped skinned almonds
- 1 Tbsp coconut flakes
- Up to 1/4 tsp each saffron, nutmeg, and/or cardamom
- 1–2 tsp ghee
- 1/4 tsp shatavari and/or ashwagandha powder

MAY 31
RECAP AND WHAT'S AHEAD

In many climates, life returns in May. Green appears, bringing purity and crispness to the environment and to our bodies. Eat lightly with what is in season, such as early greens. Emphasize the bitter taste. Bitter helps complete the detoxing process that started with cleansing in March or April. Eating greens is a gentle cleanse.

Enjoy lots of greens, even dandelion greens. Microgreens, which are nutritionally dense, are a great option. Be cautious with green smoothies. They might seem healthy, but cold drinks aggravate Vata, an imbalance that affects many. Greens, yes, and some raw is okay, but mostly consume lightly cooked foods that are easier to digest. Perfect digestion is the No. 1 goal of Ayurveda.

You also learned about the miracle three-herb formula called triphala often taken at bedtime. It can be taken as a tea or as tablets. Triphala scrubs the intestinal tract, which gets lined with excess mucus, to aid the digestive process.

Tongue scraping and oil pulling were other cleansing strategies discussed. I hope you have included both of those in your dinacharya, or daily routine. You also learned about using the neti pot when sinus mucus needs to be cleared.

Last but not least, you learned about natural approaches to health—from DIY bug repellents to serious issues like depression and cancer.

WHAT'S NEXT?

In June we will get into happiness, joy, getting your vitamin D, and the benefits of raw honey. You also will learn about the Ayurveda perspective on cholesterol and why it is often vilified. The end of the month will feature summer slumber, which can be challenging with such long days.

MONTHLY REFLECTION TIME

What actions did you try and what was your experience? Did the new action feel worthwhile? Did you like it? Did you have any adverse reactions? Put a check in the third column for actions you plan to incorporate daily, weekly, monthly, seasonally, or on occasion.

What New Actions This Month?	Your Experience?	Habit Worthy?
		☐
		☐
		☐

June 1
Research on Happiness

The Framingham Heart Study, published in the British Medical Journal, collected data over 20 years from a network of 4739 individuals.[2,3] The findings? Happiness spreads through social networks of family members, friends, and neighbors.

According to the study, you are 15% more likely to be happy if someone you directly know is happy, 10% if a friend of a friend is happy, and 6% if a friend of a friend of a friend is happy.

Basically, happiness is contagious! It spreads quickly like a chain reaction and is self-sustaining.

Ayurveda Action
Embrace Gratitude

Conventional wisdom suggests that if you are happy, then you will feel grateful. Well, that idea should be turned on its head. Intentionally cultivating a state of gratitude leads to feelings of happiness. Some people use gratitude journals, although that practice didn't work for me. However, when I lie down to sleep most nights, this very genuine phrase comes into my mind: "Thank you," for the many blessings of the day. I do not make myself say it out loud; but the statement is just an honest reflection on the day.

Happiness

> *"Happiness is a continuation of happenings which are not resisted."*
>
> —Deepak Chopra

JUNE 2
INCREASING JOY!

What does how and what you eat have to do with joy? Sluggish digestion and poor assimilation profoundly affect your emotional and mental experiences and the perceptions that filter experience. When digestion is not optimal, physical and emotional toxins clog the body's energy channels and block its vital life flow. Here are tips from Maharishi Ayurveda to support healthful physical and emotional digestion:[24]

- Eat easily digestible foods. Watery vegetable soups and vegetable rice dishes are good this time of year.
- Eat foods spiced according to the dosha you need to balance.
- Eat the biggest meal at midday when the digestive fire is at its peak.
- Prepare meals with love, and eat in a pleasant atmosphere.
- Avoid overeating, which can be a major cause of feeling low.
- Stimulate digestion by eating a little fresh ginger before or with meals.
- Avoid eating dead, unintelligent foods—leftovers, processed foods, sweets.
- Do a daily abhyanga (warm oil massage) to ease emotions and release toxins.
- Raw honey, in moderation, enhances digestion and helps with Kapha.
- Seek the stimulation of new sights, sounds, and people.
- Meditate daily.

Ayurveda beautifully describes the Nature of a happy and unhappy life:

> *Sukhayu* (Happy) *is mental and physical satisfaction, good thinking, physical strength, healthy body, life satisfaction, energy.*
>
> *Dukhayu* (Unhappy) *is full of tension, a diseased body, and dissatisfaction.*

According to Ayurveda, happiness comes from feeding your body and mind with good food and knowing the ease of good digestion. Cultivate healthy relationships with friends and family. Most importantly, nourish your soul. Ayurveda summons you to better living and a long life.

AYURVEDA ACTION
Make a Spice Mixture for Emotional Balance

- 3 parts cumin
- 2 parts turmeric
- 2 parts coriander
- 1 part black pepper
- 1 part black cumin
- 1 part cardamom
- 1 part ashwagandha root pieces

Grind spices together and store in an airtight container. Sauté small amounts in ghee to spice vegetables and grains. You can also leave seeds and roots whole to make tea.

JUNE 3
GET VITAMIN D

When I was young, sunbathers would slather on baby oil and sit directly in the sun, working to get maximum skin color. That color often wound up being red. Strong skin color was equated with health. Today it is understood that is not a healthy practice.

Now people avoid midday sun, slather on high-intensity sunblock, and purchase clothes made to block UV rays. Our work worlds often keep us out of the sun during daylight hours. Is that going too far? Many scientists and spiritualists believe so.

Sunlight is an important catalyst for life. Sunlight synthesizes vitamin D in the body, which is necessary for strong bones. Digesting sunlight has many benefits, including regulating your hormones for physical and emotional health.

Sunburn is not healthy, but you want to strike a healthy balance that offers a life in harmony with the sun's catalytic energy.

Although it's called vitamin D, it is actually a hormone, and in a class by itself. In fact, vitamin D in the active form, known as D3 or calcitriol, is understood to be the most potent steroid hormone in the human body.

AYURVEDA ACTION
Get High-Impact Sources of Vitamin D

---

1. Humans get 90% of vitamin D naturally, from sunlight exposure.
2. Oily, cold-water fish—tuna, sardines, mackerel, salmon—are sources of vitamin D.
3. A good quality supplement also provides D3, as well as tanning booths (although it is unclear if the latter are healthy—your call).

Note: While sun overexposure carries risks, that idea is mostly promoted by the cosmetic industry. No research has shown harmful effects from regular, nonburning exposure to UV light. In contrast, the tally of ill health effects—such as chronic fatigue, bone pain, and muscle weakness—from insufficient vitamin D is growing daily.

Sunshine is your best bet. Full-body exposure to sun for 15 minutes produces 3,000–20,000 IU (international units) compared to eating fish: fresh wild salmon 600–1000 IU and farmed salmon 100–250 IU.

JUNE 4
MAL-ILLUMINATION

In 1932, Dr. Wendell Krieg, professor of anatomy at Northwestern University (Chicago, U.S.), concluded that lack of specific light wavelengths causes a biochemical or a hormonal deficiency in plants and animal cells. He referred to that as "a condition of mal-illumination similar to malnutrition."[25]

THE SKIN ALPHABET: UVA, UVB

UVA are the sun's long-wave ultraviolet rays (type A) that penetrate the skin deeply and cause skin cells to age. They are considered the more harmful primarily because of their abundance.

UVB are short-wave ultraviolet rays (type B) that convert cholesterol on the skin's surface into vitamin D3 and result in tanning and sunburns if you get too much. UVB rays have been linked to skin cancer. Sunscreens block UVB, which is being discovered as essential for vitamin D and good health. The jury is still out on danger vs. benefits of UVB rays; however, there is a movement afoot suggesting we are blocking too much sun and getting insufficient vitamin D. Watch the emerging research on this as you make your personal decision.

The healthy balance may be to get sun exposure in the early-morning hours and use a good, natural sunscreen or block when the sun is directly overhead during peak sun hours.

AYURVEDA ACTION
Make Your Own Natural Sunblock

- 1/2 cup coconut oil
- 1/4 cup almond oil
- About 10 drops essential oil of your choice (add sandalwood, frankincense, or grapefruit essential oil if you also wish to repel mosquitoes)
- 2 Tbsp non-nano zinc oxide powder

Melt oils in a double boiler. Remove from heat and add zinc oxide. Stir and do a skin test. Use as needed, reapplying about every 2 hours. You can store this mixture at room temperature in a dark place.

JUNE 5
VITAMIN D'S EMERGING ROLE

For the past 80 years, the common belief was that vitamin D was important for regulating calcium and building bones. That seems to be its first duty when low levels of vitamin D exist. However, the natural health community is excited about a broader range of benefits that is emerging when vitamin D levels are higher, as reported by the Vitamin D Council:

- Vitamin D protects more than 2000 genes (about 10% of the total) from expressing negative traits.
- Vitamin D defends the body against microbes (bacteria, viruses, etc.).
- Vitamin D acts as a hormone, regulating calcium and phosphate concentration in the blood. This helps promote bone formation and growth and assists in preventing osteoporosis (porous and weak, degraded bones).
- Vitamin D looks after nerve-muscle coordinate functioning, reduces inflammation, and influences gene action.

As expanded contributions come to light, vitamin-D deficiency is implicated as a major factor in the pathology of cancers, stroke, heart disease, hypertension, diabetes, autoimmune diseases, and more. We really need to get out more!

AYURVEDA ACTION
Optimize Sun Exposure, But Don't Overdo

During the summer, UVB rays are strongest between 10 a.m. and 2 p.m. For most people, 15 minutes of direct sunlight on unprotected skin will be enough to manufacture about 3,000–20,000 IU of vitamin D3. Consider your skin type. People with pale skin should get just enough sun to turn skin slightly pink. Darker-skinned people should increase sun exposure to optimize vitamin D levels.

JUNE 6
GET SUN NOW TO STORE FOR WINTER MONTHS

CAN YOU REALLY do that? According to the U.S. News and World Report, the UVB rays necessary for vitamin D production are available only when the UV Index is at 3 or above.[26] For most of the U.S., this doesn't happen in the winter. UVB rays convert cholesterol in the skin to vitamin D3, superior in many ways to the popular vitamin supplement D2.

You need healthy fat cells to store vitamin D3 longer and to help you endure a UVB-deficient winter. If you are obese, though, your fat cells are reluctant to give up the stored vitamin D. The vitamin D stays stored for only about two to three months. This may be why so many northern-climate people need to get into the sun around December through February.

Don't be quick to shower after being in the sun—you might wash off the good effects. It takes about an hour for the cholesterol on the skin to convert and absorb beneficial D3. Many animals get vitamin D by licking their oily fur, which has absorbed the UVB rays to make vitamin D3.

AYURVEDA ACTION
Use Healthy Sunscreens

DAILY EXPOSURE TO sun is a good thing, but if you're going to be outdoors a long time, consider a sunscreen or sunblock. The Environmental Working Group tests and reviews sunscreens, which is what the FDA requires them to be called, even if they work to block sun's rays (e.g., zinc oxide) rather than absorb them (chemicals). Most are ranked inferior. A few recommended "safer and effective" brands include:[27]

- Aveeno Baby SPF 50
- Badger SPF 35
- Dr. Mercola SPF 15-30-50
- Kiss My Face Natural Mineral Sunscreen SPF 30
- Raw Elements USA SPF 30

JUNE 7
WHAT ARE PREBIOTICS?

PREBIOTIC SUBSTANCES PROVIDE food for the bacteria living in your gut in the form of high fiber and natural sugars. Prebiotics encourage beneficial species of gut flora to grow. They are a type of non-digestible fiber, meaning they pass through the upper part of the gastrointestinal tract undigested and get fermented by gut microflora when they reach the colon. This fiber scrapes and cleans the intestinal tract and supports the growth of good bacteria.

There are two types of prebiotic fiber:

- SOLUBLE PREBIOTIC FIBER attracts water and then dissolves, turning into a gel that supports and slows digestion and blood-glucose balance. It can be found in oat bran, barley, nuts, seeds, beans, lentils, peas, and some fruits and vegetables. Psyllium, a fiber supplement, also contains soluble fiber.
- INSOLUBLE PREBIOTIC FIBER does not dissolve in water. It adds bulk to the stool, and helps food pass through the stomach and intestines more quickly. Insoluble fiber is found in foods such as wheat bran, some vegetables such as beans and broccoli, and whole grains. Psyllium husk is known as one of the most effective fibers for maintaining regular digestive health. It comes from the seeds of the plantago ovato plant and is a source of both soluble and insoluble fiber.

PREBIOTIC FOODS YOU MAY ALREADY LOVE

- Asparagus
- Bananas
- Onions
- Garlic
- Cabbage
- Beans/legumes
- Bran
- Artichokes
- Leeks
- Root vegetables
- Apples

AYURVEDA ACTION
Balance Gut Flora with a Prebiotic

FIRST, DRASTICALLY DECREASE or eliminate sugar intake, especially from processed foods. Increase consumption of fermented foods such as kefir, kimchi, and sauerkraut. Fermented foods are nutrient rich, especially in vitamin K2, which is known to counteract hardening of the arteries and osteoporosis. Sauerkraut is easy to make and lasts a long time. Eat a small portion of prebiotics with one of your meals today, and strive to include some with each meal. Apple cider vinegar is also a prebiotic. I frequently drink detox tea made with apple cider vinegar in the morning {Jan 27}.

JUNE 8
PROBIOTICS

Probiotics are showing up everywhere in natural health circles, and thank goodness, because they are essential for well-being. I mean really essential! But knowing how and why they work and knowing what to eat can be puzzling.

Basically, your body is loaded with good and bad bacteria. Ideally, the ratio is 85% good bacteria and 15% bad, but for most people, that is not the case. Probiotics are the good bacteria naturally found in your body, and also can be found in foods. Good bacteria drive your immune processes. Daily diet practices are essential to keep the good bacteria stronger than the bad and effectively replenish and build your immune system.

Strengthen your internal probiotic environment by eating high-probiotic foods or taking refrigerated supplements daily, although it is tricky to keep probiotics active in supplements. Ayurveda offers natural approaches that will restore resiliency to your probiotic environment and build your immune system.

GOOD POPULATION EXPLOSION—PROBIOTIC/GOOD BACTERIA

- Eat a diet of whole, unprocessed foods.
- Increase intake of probiotic/fermented foods daily {Jun 9}.
- Take high-quality probiotic supplements if you just can't get from foods—must be refrigerated to maintain live probiotics.
- Eat antioxidant green foods.
- Avoid toxins in foods, cleaning products, and the environment when possible.
- Make your own pre- and probiotics—always better than store bought.

AYURVEDA ACTION
Eat Pre/Probiotics When Taking Antibiotics

Antibiotics are just that—ANTI. When absolutely necessary, they can aid healing. However, they indiscriminately kill intestinal bacteria—good and bad. After a round of antibiotics, you need to restore healthy gut flora by consciously increasing your intake of pre- and probiotics. Identify your go-to prebiotic and probiotic favorites like homemade yogurt or sauerkraut. Make some every once-in-a-while so that when you need them post antibiotics, you are ready to go and experienced at making them.

JUNE 9
WHY FERMENTED FOODS?

Fermented foods are chock-full of probiotics, or good bacteria. Myriad research has demonstrated how the ideal balance of good and bad bacteria in your gut forms the foundation for physical, mental, and emotional well-being.

Consuming traditionally fermented foods provides a number of benefits, including:

- OFFERS IMPORTANT NUTRIENTS. Some fermented foods such as cheese curds and natto (fermented soybeans) are high in vitamin K2 and many B vitamins, which help prevent arterial plaque buildup.
- BUILDS YOUR IMMUNE SYSTEM. About 80% of your immune system is in your gut. Probiotics help build the mucosal immune system in the digestive tract and support antibody production.
- DETOXES. Fermented foods have beneficial bacteria that act as excellent chelators, which can draw out a range of deep-set toxins and heavy metals.
- HAS A BIG EFFECT. Add a small amount of a variety of fermented food to each meal. They are inexpensive and more effective than processed supplements.

AYURVEDA ACTION
Eat More Pre- & Probiotic Foods

YOGURT OR KEFIR
from raw-cow or goat milk

SAUERKRAUT
made from scratch or non-pasteurized

DARK CHOCOLATE
raw organic dark cacao; add your own natural sweetener

MICROALGAE
ocean-based plants such as spirulina, chlorella

MISO SOUP
with miso made from fermented rye, beans, rice, or barley

SOUR CUCUMBER PICKLES
and other pickled vegetables/fruits

TEMPEH
fermented soybean product

KIMCHI
fermented vegetables

KOMBUCHA TEA
fermented, effervescent, lightly sweetened green or black tea

SOURDOUGH BREAD
fermentation of dough uses naturally occurring lactobacilli

OLIVES
in brine to retain probiotic cultures

JUNE 10
FINDING EMOTIONAL BALANCE

When emotions are out of balance, such as when you are sad or perhaps fearful, Ayurveda says it is because of pragya aparadh, or mistake of the intellect. That means you have lost access to your primary identification with higher Self or divine soul. How did you get here?

Children learn early to recognize that the world is not completely safe. They can learn this at home, or at school. People learn to employ their minds, the manomaya kosha {Sep 8} to protect themselves with stories about what is safe and what is not. Some projections are accurate, and many others are exaggerated or even fabricated.

The mind does a great job at protecting the delicate heart space from insults and intruders. The mind's reactive impulses, like anger, shame, and insecurity, keep attention away from the deep hurt of separation from Self. Money, achievement, fashion, stuff—all are seen as a way to fill the void.

What started as a structure to protect turns into an impenetrable barrier that overlays a veil of self-protection. Our protector constructions now keep us from knowing and living as we truly are. The good news? This spiritual journey is filled with joy and delightful collaborators along the way.

For a particularly intuitive and spiritually identified person, the distance from true Self can create a sense of anguish. You can either let this take you down or use the discomfort as inspiration to dig deep and get under your levels of protection. You can find kind, respectful ways to see who you are in your state of innocence and pure consciousness.

AYURVEDA ACTION
Find Your Self/Your Soul

Notice today—as the day goes along—those moments when you feel more truly yourself. Are you alone, or with others? Whatever you notice, resolve to do more of that. Maybe it means spending more time in Nature, or with family and friends, or meditating. Pay attention and do more of what makes you feel true and real.

JUNE 11
EXERCISE—MUST WE?

Ayurveda's recommendation for daily exercise has myriad benefits, including increasing the efficiency of your digestive system with a balanced appetite and metabolism. Exercise also improves circulation, flexibility, ability to breathe deeply, posture, mental alertness, strength, vitality, and energy. All of these benefits are directly related to healthy digestion.

Many of us probably do not exercise vigorously enough, but it is not good to push too hard. As always, balance is key. Do not exercise to the state of discomfort. Do not exhaust yourself or strain muscles. When you push to the point of needing a day of rest after exercise, you create free radicals, the culprits of cell breakdown, early aging, and disease.

Ayurveda texts refer to the concept of balaardh—using half your strength or capacity when you exercise. Figure out what that 50% strength is for you. This principle isn't an excuse to be lackluster in your movement. Exercise will bring you brilliance and radiance if you push some, but not too much. Find your Zen with this.

Enjoy the exercise for itself, without focusing on how it might make you stronger or leaner. Just allow yourself to experience the activity. Focusing on your breathing will help.

AYURVEDA ACTION
Move Daily

- Exercise daily—If it is not a workout day, take the stairs or go for a walk. Move until you sweat, which is detoxifying.
- Develop a daily yoga practice—yoga is a perfect example of balaardh. Of course, even yoga can be done too little or too much.
- Consider doing tai chi daily.
- Strength training—helps with muscle tone and has also been shown to have more cognitive benefits than cardio workouts.
- Focus on breathing—no matter how you exercise, breathe deeply. Dr. John Douillard suggests using deep nasal breathing to avoid a fight-or-flight response. Deep breathing helps you remain calm and centered while exercising.[28] If you are unable to breathe through your nose, you may be exercising too hard.
- Abhyanga—do a warm oil self-abhyanga massage {Dec 6} as often as you can. Daily is great, but try for at least 1 day a week. This is a soft, nourishing way to move your muscles gently and keep them toned.

JUNE 12
LIVING IN NATURE'S WISDOM

Ayurveda calls for a strong, passionate relationship with Nature. Ayurveda is the pure knowledge of Nature's intelligence. Living with Nature in all aspects helps you be healthy in mind, body, and spirit. It's not just a "you have passed your annual physical" health, but a radiant glow that emanates from blissful experience. If you yearn for this kind of life, you can have it.

I have a lovely butternut squash growing in my garden. It knows exactly what to be. I use organic gardening methods. When the week is dry, I give the squash extra water. That's it. A good start in organic soil and balancing if the week has been dry—the result is a perfect butternut squash. That squash, raised in natural conditions, is full of natural intelligence. When I eat the squash, I am not just getting calories, I'm drawing that intelligence into my being. I am reminded of Nature's vibrations as butternut energy mixes with mine, especially if I eat with reverence for my dining companions as well as what I am eating.

A vegetable raised in harsh conditions with chemicals that defy Nature—well, Mother is not happy. Indeed, the old adage is true, "We are what we eat." When you live with the vibrations of Nature, you entrain to her intelligence with every cell and energy pulse.

AYURVEDA ACTION
Make Your Own Natural Deodorant

Harsh chemicals in commercial deodorants and antiperspirants are not in tune with Nature—and neither are their packaging and aerosol propellants. It's simple to combine the following ingredients (choose organic).

- 4 Tbsp baking soda
- 4 Tbsp arrowroot powder
- 4 Tbsp unrefined coconut oil
- 10 drops essential oil of your choice (consider lemon, lavender, tea tree, or lemongrass if you also want to repel mosquitoes)

Mix dry ingredients in a tin or dark jar (or purchase a roll-on deodorant container). Slowly add in oils until there is a smooth consistency. Store at room temperature with a lid. If deodorant becomes too soft from warming, store in the refrigerator for a bit. Scoop up with your fingers or the back of your fingernail and rub into your skin.

JUNE 13
CHOLESTEROL—DOES IT DESERVE VILIFICATION?

Short answer: No!

Cholesterol is essential to good health in so many ways. This soft, waxy substance is found in almost every cell of your body. Cholesterol is needed to make hormones, convert sunshine to vitamin D, digest food, protect nerve membranes, and repair and produce new cells. Cholesterol is essential for brain health, a growing concern as we live longer. Cholesterol numbers are a poor predictor of heart disease and can be a distraction from the real causes of heart disease, especially INFLAMMATION. Yet the myth persists that high cholesterol causes heart disease and should be reduced with medication.

Cholesterol shows up when there is inflammation, but it is an innocent bystander. Think of it as the calcification that shows up around a fractured water pipe. The calcification might clog the weakened area of pipe, or even seal the fracture, but it did not cause it. Same with cholesterol. When a blood vessel is injured through the inflammatory process, cholesterol shows up to help heal the inflammation. If a lesion occurs, more cholesterol is sent to cover the area like a scab and prevent further damage.

In keeping with Ayurveda, we need to uncover the true source of the problem rather than treat symptoms and after-effects. Reducing inflammation does more to keep the heart healthy. A low fat/high sugar diet is the opposite of what is needed to reduce inflammation.

In our culture, getting off of sugar is challenging. The food industry's hard marketing has led to a sugar addiction epidemic. Sugar addiction creates frequent food cravings, and this path will destroy health. Knowledge makes it easier to make dietary changes. The Ayurvedic primary strategy is to enjoy real food and avoid processed foods.

AYURVEDA ACTION
Avoid These to Reduce Reparative Cholesterol

SUGAR AND REFINED carbohydrates are the culprits for necessitating the formation of cholesterol. Especially avoid these:

- Candies, cakes, and cookies
- Jelly and jam
- Sodas and fruit drinks
- Sweets made with sugar
- Processed, refined grains
- Bread and pasta made with refined flour

JUNE 14
MORE ON CHOLESTEROL

Some cholesterol comes to us through food, but the liver manufactures 75% of the body's cholesterol. If you take in less, the body manufactures more to accomplish the job that we need it to do, which is often to heal inflammation. A low-cholesterol diet will not significantly affect cholesterol levels and keeps you from getting the healthy fats that you need.

Temporary inflammation from injury is a natural part of healing. But many people suffer from chronic inflammation due to an unnatural diet that includes lots of sugar and carbohydrates that convert to sugar. Persistent inflammation makes cholesterol numbers high. They will remain there, unless you understand what to do.

AYURVEDA ACTION
Reduce Chronic Inflammation for Healthy Cholesterol

The "what to do" is reduce inflammation, the source of the problems, which is caused by an unnatural diet and sedentary lifestyle. In his free e-book, Dr. Mercola recommends these high-impact strategies:[29]

1. Reduce sugars, grains, and carbohydrates.
2. Eat high-quality animal-based omega-3 fats found in ghee and fish like salmon, and tuna. Spirulina and algae are also good vegetarian sources.
3. Significantly reduce processed foods that contain high-fructose corn syrup. HFCS is seriously damaging and is common in processed foods.
4. Eat foods with good fats such as extra virgin olive oil, coconut oil, organic raw butter and other dairy, raw nuts, cheese in moderation, eggs cooked with yolks intact, and organic, grass-fed meat.
5. Include fermented foods in your diet such as sauerkraut, kimchi, kefir, and homemade yogurt without added sugars.
6. Eliminate high temperature frying, which can cause healthy fats and foods to oxidize within the body. Oxidized cholesterol can cause blood clotting.
7. Get the right amount of exercise for you.
8. Don't smoke, of course, and consume only moderate amounts of alcohol—no more than two alcohol drinks a day for men and one for women.
9. Optimize vitamin D with appropriate daily sun exposure.
10. Address emotional issues.

JUNE 15
WHY SO MANY ON CHOLESTEROL DRUGS?

Today, nearly one-third of Americans over age 40 take cholesterol-lowering drugs, such as statins, and nearly half of people over 75 take them for lowering the risk of heart disease. Though the research connecting cholesterol to heart disease has been debunked in the past decade, the myth continues. In 2015, the US Dietary Guideline Advisory Committee announced that "dietary cholesterol is no longer a concern of over consumption,"[30] yet physicians commonly prescribe drugs to lower cholesterol.

How did this happen? The original premise was faulty as well as some of the research methods. More than 100 years ago, German pathologist Rudolph Virchow studied arterial plaques from corpses. Because those with heart disease had cholesterol plaques, he assumed cholesterol caused heart disease. As noted, cholesterol is an innocent bystander that tries to remedy damage done by inflammation.

Dr. Ancel Keys conducted a seminal study on this, known as the Seven Countries Study, which linked dietary fats and coronary heart disease. This became the base for the feverish introduction of cholesterol as culprit. Although Keys had data from 22 countries, he only included the seven countries that supported his hypothesis. If all 22 had been included, he would have found no correlation.[31]

Since 1958, when this study was published, Americans were encouraged to cut out butter, red meat, animal fats, eggs, and dairy. Low fat/high sugar processed foods were introduced to the market based on this flawed research. It changed the course of the country's nutritional foundation, and health declined. Cholesterol-lowering drugs are among the most widely prescribed and are a multi-billion dollar industry.

Statins can lower total cholesterol but do not reduce injuries from inflammation to your arteries. Ultimately, statins do not reduce risk of cardiac disease and they can have harmful side effects. The first approach to lowering cholesterol is to reduce the body's need for so much reparative cholesterol. Insulin sensitivity is the primary culprit in heart disease. High triglycerides are a number you can pay attention to, because it means you are eating too many carbohydrates that convert to sugar.

AYURVEDA ACTION
Investigate Cholesterol Lowering Drugs—Now or Later?

If you are not facing this question yet, you likely will someday. It's good to think about this in advance. Investigate recent research about cholesterol, as well as the side effects of statins and other cholesterol-lowering drugs. Base your decision on good information. If you are taking drugs and wish to continue, a healthier lifestyle could help you reduce the dosage.

JUNE 16
HONEY—THE SWEET, SWEET HEALER

Honey is considered medicine in Ayurveda wisdom. The bees have had your back for a long time. Now modern science concurs. Scientists have found that the pollen in honey contains all 22 amino acids, 28 minerals, 11 enzymes, 14 fatty acids, and 11 carbohydrates.

Consuming small amounts of honey each day, one or two teaspoons, is an Ayurveda treat with a healing benefit. I have seen recommendations for up to 4 teaspoons daily, but only if you don't have blood-sugar issues or eat other forms of sugar. To be safe, keep intake low.

Because bees "predigest" honey, we can easily assimilate it. Honey enters the bloodstream directly, offering instant energy. Honey is a great anupana, which means "carrier," to transport Ayurveda herbal powders into the bloodstream. This knowledge puts new zing in the idea that a spoonful of "honey" helps the medicine go down.

Other anupanas are warm water or milk, alcohol, aloe vera juice, and ghee. An anupana can enhance an herb's medicinal effects and direct it to specific tissues. Honey especially directs healing to muscles.

Madhu, the Sanskrit derived word for honey, means "perfection of sweet." In Ayurveda terms, honey is heating and warms the cold qualities of Kapha and Vata. It could be too heating for Pitta.

AYURVEDA ACTION
Eat Honey—But Not Heated

The nutritive benefits and healing qualities of honey are destroyed when it is heated to pasteurize, which many shelf-stable honey suppliers do. Some say never heat honey above 104 degrees F. Ayurveda wisdom: when heated, honey becomes like glue and digests slowly, with a negative impact.

- Use raw honey and never cook with it or heat it in any way.
- Add honey to tea only when it is cool enough to drink.
- For a tasty dessert, drizzle a couple of teaspoons of raw honey on unsweetened yogurt or cooked barley; sprinkle with walnuts.

JUNE 17
OH, HONEY!—FAST FACTS

Here are some of honey's remarkable healing capacities:

- **Feeds good bacteria**: Bees add probiotic lactic acid bacteria to honey, which stimulates production of antibodies.
- **Fights "bad" bacteria** (i.e., MRSA [staph]): Honey breaks through the biofilm barrier that protects MRSA/staph, allowing the body's antimicrobial agents to get in and do their job.
- **Promotes digestion**: All digestive organs respond favorably to honey, which is heating and reduces bloating and gas. It is a mild laxative.
- **Reduces mucus in the lungs**: Eat some honey to cure a cough or excess mucus.
- **Can be used as ointment**: Honey is antibacterial, antiseptic, and antifungal. It can be used externally to treat skin conditions such as cold sores.
- **Builds blood**: Honey contains iron, copper, and manganese, which treat anemia.
- **Invites romance**: Because honey is sourced from flowers, the plant's reproductive organs, it is a natural aphrodisiac.
- **Protects against allergies**: Eating local, raw honey is known for preventing and treating allergies, hay fever, and asthma reactions to local pollen.
- **Offers antioxidants**: Honey is high in antioxidants that fight free radicals.
- **Contraindicated**: Children under age 2 should not be given honey.

AYURVEDA ACTION
Source Local, Raw, Real Honey

Artificial honey is abundant in the marketplace. A recent study by a Food Safety News group (foodsafetynews.com) found that three-fourths of honey on the market is not real. Water, sugar, and other unsavory ingredients may be added. Ultra-processing removes pollen, and the FDA has determined that honey without pollen is not considered honey.

Honey is such an awesome healer, it's worth the effort to find a source for the real thing! Buy local honey whenever possible and you will see how much thicker it is.

JUNE 18
HEALING HONEY FORMULAS

Use raw, local honey to create your own healing formulas for lots of uses.

Weight loss
A small dosage, 1 tsp daily, can reduce weight by reducing Kapha and increasing fat metabolism.

Coughs and colds
Mix 1/2 Tbsp each of ginger, black pepper, cardamom, clove, cinnamon, and turmeric (or as many of those as you have). Combine 1/2 or 1 teaspoon of this mixture with honey and take twice a day to clear mucus.

Eyesight improvement
Mix 2 tsp of honey with fresh carrot juice and consume before breakfast.

Skin treatment
Rub raw honey on minor wounds, burns, acne, and scars. Research shows that honey sterilizes wounds. Test in a small area first.

Energy boost
Take 1 tsp honey. This might be an alternative to morning coffee or an afternoon sweet.

Morning start/insomnia help
Take 1 tsp honey in warm milk or water. It is a healthy energy aid in the morning, and at night, allows restful sleep because it rejuvenates and is not a stimulant. If honey disturbs sleep, it is a stimulant in disguise and likely is not pure, raw honey.

Blood benefits
Just 1 tsp honey daily in tepid water raises blood's hemoglobin levels and increases iron, copper, and manganese absorption. Some evidence shows that honey can prevent low white-blood-cell count.

AYURVEDA ACTION
Mix Honey and Ghee Properly

Do not mix honey and ghee in equal proportions. This produces a chemical called hydroxymethyl furfuraldehyde (HMF), which has a negative effect on digestion. You can mix in unequal portions in food preparations.

JUNE 19
DISAPPEARING BEES...

HONEYBEE POPULATIONS HAVE plummeted in recent years—as much as 70%. This is called "colony collapse disorder" (CCD).[32] Some claim the cause is all the harmful pesticides used on crops, although agrichemical companies blame the problem on mite infestations in the beehives.

The U.S. Environmental Protection Agency (EPA) has been investigating CCD, yet it is unknown how political bias influences the EPA's research findings.

Five things you can do:

1. Check out actions you can take at savebees.org/petitions.
2. Grow dandelions and clover in your yard; plant flowers such as bee balm, echinacea, foxglove, and goldenrod.
3. Do not use toxic chemicals on your garden plants/lawn or in your home.
4. Eat raw honey from local beekeepers.
5. Buy organic, non-GMO fruits and vegetables

Let every wind that blows drop honey.
Let the rivers and streams re-create honey.
Let all our medicines turn into honey.
Let the dawn and evening turn into honey.
Let the darkness be converted to honey.
Let our nourisher, the sky above, be full of honey.
Let our trees be honey.
Let the sun be honey.

—RIG VEDA 1:90; 6-8

AYURVEDA ACTION
Create a Bee Bath

SUPPORT BEE POPULATIONS by buying local honey and plant flowers around your home, but remember that bees need water, too. Fill a shallow birdbath or a small dish with clean water that you change frequently. Arrange stones and pebbles to poke out of the water, so bees can land on these little islands to drink without risk of drowning.

JUNE 20
GLADDEN THE MIND

If you want positive experiences to take root in your sense of identity, purposely sustain attention on a positive experience. You do this by embodying the experience: feel, smell, touch. Enliven all the senses and thoroughly enjoy the pleasantness of experience for at least 15 seconds and try for 30 seconds. That is how long it takes for an experience to enter your implicit memory and become available for recall. You want joy and a sense of awe in life as well as preparedness for danger.

THREE WAYS TO GLADDEN THE MIND

Tara Brach, a psychologist, author, and teacher of emotional and spiritual healing, is a favorite of mine on this path of awakening.

Your mind rolls negative experiences over and over, which embeds them in your implicit memory. It is Nature's way. The brain isn't wired to embed positive experiences by default. By consciously cultivating positive experiences in an attentive, awakened way, you develop new cognitive capacities. But do not bemoan "negative" experiences. Accepting reality is important—don't bury difficult experiences. Acknowledge and process them. Stuffing them never helps. Tara Brach teaches three ways to "gladden the mind" and install positive experiences into memory to shape perception. [33]

GRATITUDE—Engage a sense of gratitude on purpose. Don't take life's goodness for granted. Find humor in your "inner grumbler," which might be active much of your day. Some people find a gratitude journal helpful, or a gratitude buddy.

SERVE—Being of benefit to others naturally engages the gladdening of our mind. Serving others frees you from the sadness that results from self-centeredness.

SAVOR—When something good is happening, savor the experience. Pause. Spend 15 to 30 seconds taking in the good. Use as many senses as you can. Appreciate the moment as meaningful as opposed to a neutral, unattended one. This is key to awakening to the delight of your life and inviting bliss.

AYURVEDA ACTION
Be Grateful, Serve, Savor

Be conscious of these three. You probably have thought about gratitude and serving. Enliven those. But really focus on savoring. Spend some time in Nature and I am sure you will come upon an experience worth savoring. Take a full 30 seconds of engaging as many senses as you can to really take It in. Higher levels of gratitude were found to be associated with better mood, better sleep, less fatigue and less inflammation. [34]

JUNE 21
SUMMER SKIN

Summer officially arrives June 21 in the U.S./North America. As days get longer and hotter, you often spend more active time outdoors, exposing skin to the elements. In Ayurveda, slathering products onto your skin is not where enhancement and protection start.

Ayurveda defines true beauty as an essential aspect of being that radiates from within. Skin is the outer shell that reflects the inner workings of your body and state of being. Dr. Manisha Kshirsagar, author of *Enchanting Beauty,* writes about three levels: 1) inner beauty, 2) outer beauty, and 3) lasting beauty.[35] According to Dr. Kshirsagar, inner beauty is a sense of self-love and value. Outer beauty is an expression of healthy, vibrant physiology. Lasting beauty comes from a healthy, balanced lifestyle and maintenance of inner and outer beauty. External and lasting beauty arises from inner beauty.

Beauty is more than skin-deep—it is consciousness-deep. According to revered Ayurveda author Atreya, physical beauty starts with connection to consciousness, and beauty forms from "your mental attitude, your capacity for strong digestion, your food choices, and your daily regime."[36]

Summer conditions can wreak havoc on skin. But it's the season of fresh fruits and vegetables, plus you can be more active around water and other soothing environments. Sunshine lifts the mood.

AYURVEDA ACTION
Make a Spice Blend for Healthy Skin

Ayurveda also provides special formulas for skin care! You eat this one.

- 5 tsp coriander powder
- 4 tsp fennel powder
- 3 tsp turmeric powder
- 1 tsp cinnamon powder
- 1/2 tsp black pepper powder

Mix spices together and store in a glass jar. Use when preparing cooked foods, or sprinkle on top. These spices work synergistically to cleanse lymph, blood, and fat tissues. Turmeric is an especially potent skin rejuvenator because of its antioxidant and anti-inflammatory properties.

Recipe reprinted with permission from *Enchanting Beauty* by Dr. Manisha Kshirsagar.[37]

JUNE 22
TICK...TICK...TICK...TICKED OFF!

Ticks are bothersome and can even be dangerous. Some carry a bacterium that can result in Lyme disease, which has flu-like symptoms and is difficult to treat and cure. It might show up anywhere from three to 30 days after being infected by a tick. At the site of the bite, you may see a circular red spot. Prevention is the way to go.

According to the U.S. Centers for Disease Control, black-legged ticks must be attached for 24 hours to transmit the disease. Check yourself and your pets regularly after being outside.

There are a lot of great recipes for tick preventatives online. Geranium oil is a common ingredient in DIY recipes to prevent tick bites.

TICK PREVENTATIVE RECIPE

- 4 Tbsp vegetable oil or almond oil
- 2 Tbsp aloe vera gel
- 30 to 40 drops geranium essential oil

Mix well. Use an eyedropper to apply the mixture to your skin and rub it in. Apply two to three drops to your dog's collar to repel ticks. Test first, of course, to assure you or your dog does not have an adverse reaction. Essential oils are not advised for cats; they can be life threatening.

If you find a tick on your body, use small tweezers and grab the tick as close to the mouth as you can. Do not grab the swollen belly. For detailed written instructions, search at: www.webmd.com.

AYURVEDA ACTION
Make & Use Natural Mosquito Spray

- 4 Tbsp distilled or boiled water
- 1 Tbsp witch hazel or vodka
- 1 Tbsp almond or jojoba oil
- Add 60 drops total of any of these essential oils: lemon eucalyptus, citronella, peppermint, lemongrass, clove

Place ingredients in a small blue or brown spray bottle. Shake before each use.

JUNE 23
MEN'S HEALTH

Ayurveda is customized to the person; however, there are some health concerns that may be particularly keen for you as a man or for the men in your life. These primary areas of concern are prostate issues, sexual function, and cardiovascular disease.

- The prostate naturally enlarges with age and can impinge on other tissues and organs in the genital area, leading to urinary-tract dysfunction that manifests as urinary hesitancy, urgency, or dribbling. Prostate inflammation can be painful. Prostate cancer has symptoms similar to an enlarged prostate, so it should be checked regularly.
- Good Ayurveda practices will help to prevent such issues as men age. Practices to prevent and treat prostate issues include Pitta pacifying foods to decrease heat and inflammation, such as coconut water, sweet juicy fruits, pomegranate juice, and asparagus. Barley soup is also identified as helpful.
- The most common herb suggested for men's virility along with muscle tone (men's and women's) is ashwagandha. Ashwagandha also tones the nervous system and combats stress, which supports a grounding that helps with the calmness of intimacy, tenderness, and conversations. Eating rice, dates, honey, ghee, and almonds also supports virility.
- Cardiovascular health in Ayurveda is not just about the physical heart, but also the emotional heart. Eating fresh food, enjoying moderate exercise, and using breath to reduce stress and lower the heart rate are good heart-honoring practices. The herb arjuna, named for the warrior who is guided by Krishna in the Bhagavad Gita, is touted for both physical and emotional benefits. In this epic tale, Arjuna represents the heart of humanity guided by the Divine. This hero herb strengthens the functions of the circulatory system, supports healthy blood pressure, and promotes emotional support for those experiencing grief. It is said to "mend a broken heart."

AYURVEDA ACTION
Take Care of Your Heart

The heart is not just a blood pumper—it is the fountainhead of all emotions. Seek experiences that promote well-being. Be with people who understand and support you and cultivate the positive in your thinking and habits. The heart is the seat of prana, your life force, and must maintain the delicate balance between agni (fire solar element) and soma (cooling lunar element). Stress eats away at soma. Find balance in your activity and rest today.

JUNE 24
RECOGNIZING GENETICALLY MODIFIED FRUIT

MANY COUNTRIES REQUIRE mandatory labeling of genetically modified ingredients in food, but so far, the United States has chosen not to.

However, checking the sticker on the fruit you buy is good way to determine if it's a GMO (genetically modified organism).

The number on the bar code tells you how the fruit was grown.

- 4 DIGITS means it was conventionally grown (using chemicals).
- 5-DIGIT NUMBER BEGINNING WITH 8 means it was genetically modified.
- 5-DIGIT NUMBER BEGINNING WITH 9 means it was grown organically.

Find organic produce by looking for stickers that begin with the number 9. If you are not buying organic, look for four digits. When there are five digits, here's your rhyme: Nine is fine—see eight? Not great.

AYURVEDA ACTION
Transition from Honey to Cane Sugar & Maple Syrup

RAW HONEY, IN moderation of course, is great for Kapha because it is heating. However, when hot weather arrives, avoid honey. Transition to less heating sweeteners such as raw cane sugar and maple syrup. Moderation in use of sweeteners is especially good in the heat. If you need a sweet summer drink, try coconut water, which is cooling, refreshing, and naturally sweet.

JUNE 25
COCONUT OIL FOR SKIN AND HAIR

Pitta season is associated with the fire element and is soon approaching around early July. Whenever it starts getting hot where you live, coconut is a great way to beat the heat. Use organic coconut oil daily to moisturize and nourish your skin. Your skin will drink it up, leaving it more supple and elastic. Coconut oil heals dry, damaged skin and cools excess body heat. It is soothing for eczema, psoriasis, and sunburn.

Using coconut in lots of ways can cool the Pitta imbalance by softening anger and lowering inflammation. You can drink it, slather it on your skin, cook with it and sprinkle coconut flakes on fresh fruit.

Some say plain coconut oil's cooling properties make for a good sunscreen with natural SPF properties. It also makes a good deodorant by itself or with supportive ingredients {June 13}. Put a little coconut oil on your hair before you wash {May 23} to protect it. Cooking with coconut oil is great, especially in the summer, because it can handle heat well and has a cooling effect. Even though it has a low smoke point, it does not oxidize easily when heated and thus is stable for high temperature cooking.

AYURVEDA ACTION
Use Coconut Oil + Shea Butter to Moisturize

These two make an outstanding combination for both skin and hair. Mix coconut oil and raw shea butter in approximately equal proportions. If needed, heat gently to soften. The concentration of natural vitamins and fatty acids in shea butter makes an incredible moisturizer that tones skin and conditions hair. And together with rich and fragrant coconut oil, you will love the results. The coconut oil by itself absorbs more easily if you are concerned with getting greasy.

JUNE 26
THE TRUTH OF LOVE

Dr. John Douillard speaks about radiant love as the awakening challenge of our times.[38] He is one of my teachers, and a warm, authentic, brilliant, and giving person.

Dr. Douillard encourages us to love like the sun—fully, without expectation. The sun does not decide if a flower is worthy of being shined upon. The sun does not say to the flower, "What have you done for me lately?" The sun shines on everything. That is the truth of the sun's nature, and Douillard says love is the deepest truth of our nature as well.

When you experience this truth, you cannot help but act upon it. Even the crankiest, most off-putting person is safe in this radiance and can let their own bud open. Certainly, make decisions about your boundaries with persons who are destructive to others. But you can still shine with love, even at a distance.

Dr. Douillard challenges us to be the source of love. It is a key to expanding consciousness. Prioritizing your physical and emotional well-being, spending time in Nature, staying committed to ongoing personal growth, sharing in a spiritual community, understanding the context of our evolutionary times—all of these support you in becoming more loving and practicing enlightened living.

AYURVEDA ACTION
Use Ayurveda Herbs for Love & Romance

Healthy habits and diet are the strategies for balanced life force. In Ayurveda, herbs are the powerhouses, used as remedies and for rejuvenation, but they're not a substitute for the basics.

Some of the herbs and foods recommended for love, romance, potency, sexual function, and vitality include:

- Dates—A well-known aphrodisiac in many cultures
- Ashwagandha—Especially vitalizing and warming for Vata weakness; tones muscles
- Shatavari—Moisturizing and cooling; supports healthy libido
- Raw milk and ghee—Vitalizing and rejuvenating; good carrier for other herbs
- Cinnamon—Increases circulation to genitals and supports erectile function
- Kappikachu—Natural source of L-dopa for elevating mood aspects associated with romance; promotes vitality and tones reproductive organs

JUNE 27
SLIPPING INTO SUMMER SLUMBER

Do you find it difficult to switch off mental chatter in the evening? As you lie down to sleep, your mind might become identified with the objects of your senses. That's because remembering the day's events reproduces the emotions and thoughts that accompanied those experiences. Unless you can detach, it might be difficult to fall deeply asleep. Do you grind your teeth during the night? It could mean you have emotions that have not sufficiently digested from the day or ongoing issues.

WHAT HAPPENS DURING SLEEP?

In sleep you reconnect with the underlying field, or source, to receive divine intelligence and energy for well-being. During sleep hours you process food, emotions, and experiences from the day. Properly processed food and experiences aid your concentration, emotional balance, zest for life, proper digestion and elimination, radiant skin, and energy. Restful sleep repairs and rejuvenates physiology for tissue growth and supports the immune system.

In the summer, the sun rises early and sets late. Often so do we, which results in insufficient sleep. Insufficient sleep affects physical, mental, and emotional health. Here are summer sleep tips:

- Go to bed by 10 p.m., while still in Kapha time.
- Eat an early, light dinner—lunch should be your large meal.
- Reduce evening stimulus: listen to soothing music, read a bedtime story to children, or do an easy breathing practice.
- Avoid alcohol and caffeine; drink soothing tea or warm milk with nutmeg in the evening.
- Apply coconut oil to scalp and feet to cool your system.

AYURVEDA ACTION
Drink Water from a Copper Cup

Ayurveds also recommend setting a copper cup of water next to your bed each night so you can drink from it in the morning (after you scrape your tongue), to prevent arteriosclerosis. Drinking therapeutic water from a copper cup is called tamra jal. The science is that water in contact with copper for more than 8 hours gets infused with small quantities of this essential metal. The process is called "oligodynamic effect," and enhances the water's capacity to destroy harmful microbes, molds, and fungi. Copper is a natural antioxidant that balances water's pH, making it "alive" again. Water can be stored for a long time in copper vessels without becoming stale.

JUNE 28
DIGESTIVE FIRE AND METABOLISM BY DOSHA

Agnis are the enzymes and endocrine factors governing digestive and metabolic functioning. Digestive activity is governed by the doshas and can become excessive or deficient, which is the basic imbalance that must be healed.

- Excess Vata in the body produces weak, irregular digestion and causes gas.
  - Solution: Eliminate cold drinks, which extinguish agni. Drink room-temp or hot drinks like hot spice water. Cook and make teas with fresh ginger.
- Excess Pitta is an out-of-control furnace, burning food quickly and maybe causing burning sensations, thirst, or acid indigestion.
  - Solution: Garnish your foods with cilantro chutney to cool overheated Pitta fire. A walk in the moonlight does wonders to cool Pitta.
- Excess Kapha in the digestive tract results in low digestive fire, making it difficult to digest food and causing nausea soon after eating. Symptoms are feeling dull and lethargic, and weight gain.
  - Solution: Try a tea with equal parts freshly ground black pepper and fresh ginger to trigger digestive enzymes. It is crucial to avoid cold drinks. Hot spice water is good for Kapha—it supports digestion for all three doshas.

AYURVEDA ACTION
Drink Detox Tea

Here is another option for a tea that will correct tri-doshic imbalances and promote digestion.

- 4 cups of water
- 1/2 tsp cumin seeds
- 1/2 tsp coriander seeds
- 1 tsp fennel seeds
- 1/2-inch slice ginger
- 5 black peppercorns
- 3 cloves
- 1 shard cinnamon

Steep ingredients in boiling water. Pour into a teapot or thermos flask. Strain out the spices before drinking. Drink throughout the day—but only 1/2 cup at mealtime, and stop in the evening after supper.

JUNE 29
SUMMER TIPS TO MAINTAIN METABOLISM

Keep yourself cool inside so that your metabolism does not need to slow down. Body heat can become so high that metabolism slows to lower your body temperature. If you eat harder-to-digest foods like burgers, pizza, French fries, and nachos, eat them at midday and eat less. Remember, your largest meal should always be midday according to Ayurveda, but especially in summer to allow a slower metabolism the time it needs. Here are cool tips:

- Alcohol increases heat, so easy does it.
- Eat less meat and more fruits and vegetables. Small amounts of raw food are okay, but lightly cooked is more digestible.
- Coconut oil and coconut water are cooling; ghee (clarified butter) is, too.
- Sip Ayurveda hot spice water cool to room temperature first. Or drink cool (not iced) mint tea.
- Eat fully ripe sweet, juicy fruits like melons, grapes, pears, and cherries.
- Favor cooling vegetables such as cucumber, asparagus, broccoli, peas, greens, and zucchini.
- Cook with cooling spices like fennel, mint, and coriander. Avoid hot spices like cayenne and chili peppers.
- Favor foods that are liquidy and cool or lukewarm, rather than dry (beans or breads for example) or hot foods (with hot peppers for example).
- Toxins create heat and inflammation, so choose organic when you can.

You get the idea—keep it cool. Enjoy summer but keep these tips in mind.

AYURVEDA ACTION
Cool Emotions with Breath

Summer can increase irritability in the summer, and fiery emotions disrupt digestion, so breathe mindfully once a day if you can. Cooling and calming the breath can help you see things from another point of view. Try Sheetali Pranayama:

1. Sit comfortably, hands resting in your lap.
2. Begin with a body scan. What Pitta qualities are emerging? Do you detect heat, aggravation, intensity?
3. Practice sheetali pranayama by inhaling through a curled tongue and exhaling through the nose. During exhalation, lightly touch the tip of the tongue to the roof of the mouth. This extends coolness to the upper palate. If you cannot curl your tongue, place your tongue tip between slightly open teeth and inhale through the sides of your tongue.
4. Continue for 1–5 minutes. Rest a minute when complete.

JUNE 30
RECAP AND WHAT'S AHEAD

In June, we got it going. You learned about pre- and probiotics to support deep, complete digestion. And you got Ayurveda insider knowledge about cholesterol and its role in repairing inflamed tissue and maintaining a healthy brain and heart. Ayurveda is less about diminishing symptoms and more about correcting causes. Inflammation comes from many things, but sugar, especially HFCS, is a major culprit.

We explored the miracle substance of raw honey, too. You learned different ways to use it and to never heat honey. In tea or other hot liquids, honey is added only when tea is cool enough to drink.

You also found out the important role of vitamin D for good health, and ways to cultivate happiness and joy. You learned about how to get better sleep, which can be challenging during the long summer days.

WHAT'S NEXT?

In July we will examine Pitta—its role and functions and how to pacify it. We want to find out how to reap the benefits of Pitta without falling into imbalance with heated bodies and emotions. Stay tuned!

MONTHLY REFLECTION TIME

What actions did you try and what was your experience? Did the new action feel worthwhile? Did you like it? Did you have any adverse reactions? Put a check in the third column for actions you plan to incorporate, whether daily, weekly, monthly, seasonally, or on occasion.

What New Actions This Month?	*Your Experience?*	*Habit Worthy?*
		☐
		☐
		☐

PITTA SEASON

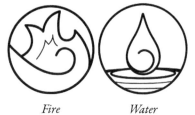

Fire   *Water*

JULY 1
PITTA FIRES US UP

Pitta is formed from the element fire with a small amount of water element, too. Pitta constitution-types are generally medium body size and have good muscle tone (think Denzel Washington, Madonna, Brad Pitt). They have a good digestion, good physical energy, and stamina. They tend to be smart in an analytical way, are determined, and are goal-oriented in work.

Pittas have good digestive fire and fiery personalities. Warm body temperatures are common, and they react to heat and light, such as too much sun, light in the eyes, or too much fire in the diet. They are goal-oriented and often successful but can be controlling. Physical toxins such as alcohol, cigarettes, or drugs, and toxic emotions such as anger, jealousy, and intolerance, create substantial imbalances for Pittas.

If you are Pitta constitution, or have significant Pitta in your constitution, imbalance will naturally arise and needs to be counteracted during the summer Pitta months. Environmental heat aggravates Pitta dosha, so it's important to cool your system. Agni (digestive fire) is easily agitated by external heat and pulls internal fire to the surface, resulting in skin conditions like rashes and prickly heat. Excess agni also can bring on bloodshot eyes, diarrhea, heartburn, and other digestive complaints. Aggravated Pitta can also show up as emotional heat, like excess anger, so it is worth pacifying Pitta to keep your cool!

Pitta qualities are:

- Hot
- Sharp
- Light
- Oily
- Liquid
- Subtle
- Mobile
- Clear
- Smooth
- Soft

Pitta season in North America is about July through October, though it varies depending on region. The Pitta months are hot and dry, wherever you live.

AYURVEDA ACTION
Check Your Pitta—See Much Influence?

Visit your Assessment 1 results again to see how strong your Pitta is. Most everyone needs to balance during Pitta season. Consider the strength and influence of your Pitta. How much Pitta balancing should you focus on over the next four months? (And remember, during Pitta season everyone's body heat can rise so that metabolism slows to help the body lower its overall temperature.)

JULY 2
FABULOUS PITTA FUNCTIONS

Pitta's primary functions are digestion, metabolism, and transformation. The seat, or home, is the liver, small intestines, and skin. Pitta governs your digestive agnis and is responsible for how sensory perceptions are metabolized. Pitta also determines how you discriminate between right and wrong. Pitta incisiveness leads to clarity and the capacity to process your experiences and emotions.

Transforming food into substances the body can absorb is Pitta's most important responsibility. Digestion takes place predominantly in the small intestine or duodenum, where the primary digestive enzymes reside. Pitta fires (agnis) digest or "cook" the food a second time, which is where nutrients are made available to be absorbed. Ayurveda believes that just as the planets revolve around the sun, your body revolves around the quality of your digestive fire.

All organs that work in conjunction with digestion are governed by the Pitta dosha. That means the spleen and pancreas are Pitta organs, along with the endocrine system. Pitta issues often show up as a malfunctioning liver.

Vision is also a Pitta function. If you cannot see in a dark room and light a fire, you have vision. Skin is interesting: its sensory aspect is Vata, but as an organ, skin is governed by Pitta. That's because skin reacts to sunlight to engage many bodily functions.

Out-of balance Pitta overheats the mind and body's internal fire, affecting body temperature, digestion, sleep, and emotions. A balanced Pitta has a joyful disposition, a sharp intellect, courage and healthy digestion. Hemoglobin formation requires Pitta heat, so the health of red blood cells is also governed by this dosha.

AYURVEDA ACTION
Create "Just Right" Digestive Fire

Balanced digestion is essential for lifelong radiant health. "Just right" agni is needed. Too much fire and food burns too quickly, along with nutrients. Too little fire results in incomplete digestion or indigestion. If you feel fatigued after eating, agni is weak. Eat a teaspoon of grated ginger with a few drops of lemon juice and a pinch of salt about 15-30 minutes before a meal. This blend activates salivary glands to activate digestion and support food absorption and energy assimilation.

When it's hot outside, metabolism slows to keep you cool. Increase fire with ginger only at mealtime to assure adequate fire to digest without overheating your system. Overheating lowers metabolism and cools body temperature.

JULY 3
PITTA PHYSICAL TRAITS

PITTAS ARE OFTEN medium build, lean, muscular and athletic. Adult Pittas could have weight issues from poor eating habits and imbalance, so your youthful body frame size is what to go by.

Pittas are intense, and often so are their body features. Facial features, such as the nose and jaws, might be more angular. Eyes are often medium-sized and light in color. Skin has a reddish tone, especially when exercising or when angry. If you are Pitta, your hands and feet are usually comfortably warm. Too much sun really bothers you.

Do you have lots of body moles, early graying of hair, red (or reddish) hair, or hair loss? Do you get angry when hungry? Generally, these signs point to Pitta.

AYURVEDA ACTION
Be Cool

- Get up early to meditate and walk in the cool mornings. Walk barefoot on dewy grass. Walks in the moonlight are cooling for Pitta. Avoid midday sun.
- Do abhyanga daily with cooling coconut oil to nourish your skin.
- Wear cool colors that reflect the heat, such as white, green, and blue. Avoid red, orange, and yellow.
- Practice cooling meditation and sheetali pranayama {June 29}. Meditation cools the mind. Use OM or your own mantra. Visualize cooling scenes on a lake or in the mountains.

JULY 4
PITTA SUBDOSHAS

Subdoshas are dosha intelligences that function in specific locations in our bodies. When I check clients' pulses, the most common imbalance I see is ranjaka Pitta. Ranjaka Pitta represents heat in the liver. This subdosha gets aggravated from the toxins and stressors in our culture. Let's look at all the Pitta subdoshas.

Ranjaka Pitta

Located in liver, gallbladder, spleen, and red blood cells. Ranjaka governs red blood cell formation and gives color to blood and stools. Toxins in the body from food, water, alcohol, drugs, and cigarettes overwhelm ranjaka. Ranjaka Pitta imbalance leads to anemia blood disorders, inflammation, anger, and jealousy.

Pachaka Pitta

Located in the lower stomach and small intestine. Pachaka governs digestion of food that is broken down into nutrients and waste products. It also regulates agni heat, rendering metabolism fast or slow, efficient or weak. Imbalance leads to heartburn, stomach acid, ulcers, etc.

Sadhaka Pitta

Located in the heart. Sadhaka governs emotion such as contentment, memory, intelligence, and processing of thoughts. Sadhaka Pitta imbalance leads to heart disease, memory loss, indecisiveness, and emotional disturbance such as sadness, heartache, and anger.

Alochaka Pitta

Located in the eye region, it governs visual perception and the reception and digestion of light from the external world. Alochaka Pitta imbalance leads to disorders related to eyes.

Bhrajaka Pitta

Located in skin. Bhrajaka governs your complexion's luster, color, and skin temperature. Bhrajaka Pitta imbalance leads to inflamed skin, discoloration, skin rashes, acne, skin cancer, and other skin disorders.

AYURVEDA ACTION
Cool the Ranjaka Heat of the Liver

Practice cooling yoga. Moon salutation is good, as are Camel, Cobra, Cow, Boat, Goat, and Bridge poses. Pitta can accumulate in the eyes, so exercise them as well. Rub the soles of your feet with cooling coconut oil at bedtime to bring heat down and out. Put coconut oil on your hair to nourish it. Spritz rosewater on your pillow.

Drink cool, refreshing drinks. Increase water intake, but make sure it's cool or warm, never iced. Add fresh lime juice to water. Coconut water is cooling, as are teas from peppermint, licorice, fennel, and rose. Drink aloe juice to cool the intestines. Minimize alcohol and caffeine, which especially aggravate Pitta when weather is hot.

JULY 5
PITTA MIND

Pitta dosha governs insight and intellect. The Pitta mind can be sharp, and out of balance, it can be cutting and judgmental. Pitta mind is associated with the brain's grey matter, involving muscle control, memory, emotions, speech, decision-making, and self-control. This is primarily where the brain's neuron cells reside, which are connected through a network of white matter. Structures in the grey matter process signals to sensory organs. That's a bit of the science, but bottom line, we want a healthy Pitta mind for our entire life!

A healthy Pitta mind leads to confidence, insightful vision, and nondestructive drive. A healthy Pitta's mind traits lead to natural leadership. They manifest a vision through work. They are often charismatic and enjoy engaging with others.

On the other hand, when Pitta minds becomes excessive, they can tend toward attachment to their vision over others', and too much control rather than healthy drive.

Excessive heat in the body moves upward and leads to a heated mind and out-of-balance expression of emotion. Draining periods of excessive work and ambition can put Pitta levels beyond balance. Eating too many hot foods can also elevate Pitta.

Hot weather aggravates Pitta, so cool it in the summer. Remember, everyone has some Pitta, which likely needs attending during Pitta season.

AYURVEDA ACTION
Sharpen Your Brain

Herbs are power-packed messengers of higher consciousness from the underlying field. Use these herbs for learning (dhi), retention (dhriti), and recall (smriti):

Brahmi

Choose the bacopa monniera variety as it is stronger, boosts mental clarity, and reduces mental stress. Or mix both forms 1:1—bacopa and gotu kola for a healthy brain tea.

Shankapushpi

Promotes brain circulation, improves memory and intelligence.

Ashwagandha

Reduces stress, enhances ojas, lowers cholesterol and blood sugar.

General dosage: 1/4 to 1/2 teaspoon one or two times daily on food or in drink

JULY 6
PITTA EMOTIONAL QUALITIES

Pittas are emotional. They are passionate, intense, focused, and expressive. You know where a Pitta stands. By keeping your Pitta healthy, your emotional expressions will be healthy.

Accumulated, unbalanced Pitta can lead to upward-moving heat that settles in the mind. This excess heat can lead to anger, judgment, resentment, envy, criticism, impatience, out-of-control drive, manipulations, and a rigid attachment to one's own vision. Pitta emotions can be fiery, and Pittas can become irritable, especially when hungry—or "hangry" as the term goes. Pittas can test their bodies with a ruthless drive for power and accomplishment when too much fire is stoked.

Healthy Pitta brings focused, respectful emotions and states such as compassionate insight into the human condition, enjoyment of others, enthusiasm, collaboration, and contentment. They can work hard, and they can surrender when it is time.

AYURVEDA ACTION
Chill Your Emotions

Heated emotions heat the body, the skin in particular. Emotions can fire up when you watch violent movies or if you hang around angry people. Breathe. Take time away. Rest. Pittas can cool and calm emotions by walking in the moonlight in the cool evening air. They can avoid hot, spicy food, which they generally love, and instead eat cooling foods like asparagus, cucumbers, and Ayurveda-recommended dairy products like kefir and homemade yogurt.

JULY 7
PITTA RITUCHARYA— PITTA SEASONAL REGIME

You change your wardrobe in summer—well it's also very important to change your diet and lifestyle. An Ayurveda adage is "as the macrocosm, so is the microcosm." This means that what happens around you in the environment affects your internal state. When the seasons change, we need to be properly adaptive to make the most of it and to avoid getting ill with the changes and new forces upon us. The variations are substantial, such as changes in daylight, temperature, humidity, and available foods. Making seasonal changes is ritucharya.

For climates cold in winter and warm in summer, Pitta season is generally July through October. When summer heat and dryness kick in, we are entering Pitta season.

Taking two weeks to shift your diet at each new dosha season is smart. At this time of year, we can take one week to transition out of Kapha actions and one week to hype up our Pitta actions. We want to expel the accumulations from the season we are leaving and one week to ease into the season we are entering. To transition out of Kapha, begin reducing consumption of beans, which are drying, and change from honey to raw sugars which are less heating.

The main idea of Pitta season is to cool it. Some important Pitta cooling actions are:

- Drink more water and especially coconut water.
- Reduce alcohol and caffeine drinks.
- Eat lightly sautéed greens and asparagus.
- Reduce hot peppers and heating herbs like ginger.
- Increase cooling herbs like coriander seeds, cilantro, and fennel.
- Go swimming and for walks in the cool evening, especially in the moonlight.
- Massage entire body with coconut oil.

AYURVEDA ACTION
Eat Microgreens

Microgreens have 4 to 6 times the vitamins and nutrients of mature greens of the same plant. Microgreens are supercharged and are one step up from sprouts. They are rich in vitamins, minerals, and beneficial plant compounds like antioxidants.

Vatas and Kaphas are generally aggravated by eating raw foods and even Pittas are some times. This is why Ayurveda often recommends eating cooked foods. Since microgreens and baby greens are so tender, they are more easily digestible than mature greens and are a good way to get the benefit of raw greens into your diet. Mature greens require you to chew through the dense cellulose cell wall structure to make the nutrients available, so those are better eaten cooked.

JULY 8
PITTA TIME OF DAY

THE NATURAL WORLD has a recurring ebb and flow. Dosha forces govern the tides of your life. They play out in the cycle of a life, a year, a day. Three, 4-hour time increments repeat every 12 hours in the morning and afternoon. Pitta influences are strongest at these times: 10 a.m. to 2 p.m. and 10 p.m. to 2 a.m.

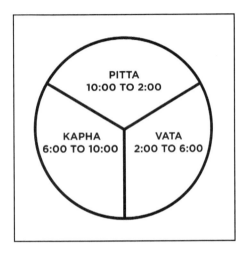

From 10 a.m. to 2 p.m. is when the sun is the highest and the most heat is generated. Pitta is the dosha of heat and transformation. Digestive fire is strongest midday, unless body heat is so high that metabolism has slowed to lower temperature. Generally, midday is the perfect time for the largest meal of the day.

Keep body heat under control by staying out of noontime sun. Pitta rules activity, so it is wise to go to bed and be ready to sleep before 10 p.m., in the Kapha zone of the daily cycle. If you're up past that hour, Pitta kicks in and you might get a second wind, making it difficult to fall asleep. The activity of Pitta hours should be internal, as that's when the body cleanses and repairs itself. If you are not sleeping, this healing work can't be done properly.

AYURVEDA ACTION
Eat Your Biggest Meal Midday

YOU HAVE SEEN this radiant-health tip before, but it is a big advantage for the Pitta time of the day. Eat your largest meal around noon, when digestive agni is strongest. Don't use this as an excuse to overeat, but do take advantage of heightened agni to take in most of your food energy midday.

If you eat meat, lunch is the time. If you must have dessert, again, midday is best.

JULY 9
PITTA TIME OF LIFE

WHEN YOU ARE looking to restore imbalances, consider your stage of life. Many factors determine what goes out of balance, and the underlying context of your time of life is a big one. Kapha is the time of youth (0-16 years) {Jan 25}. Pitta follows and can be life's longest stage, from age 16 to about 50 or 60. This is when your life is "digested" and "assimilated" through education, career, child-rearing, and other life work.

You develop your talents during this time and direct them into the world—very Pitta. This often is a fiery and goal-oriented time. You might find yourself feeling controlling and irritated in these years. Often, you are more identified with intellect. Overworking, a characteristic of our culture, can lead to stress and attempts to reduce it through alcohol and prescription or nonprescription drugs.

AYURVEDA ACTION
Take Time Off—Before You Explode

AWARENESS OF THE Pitta time of life can help you ease the pressure by doing things to keep stress managed. Take time to relax, indulge in leisurely walks, ground yourself, and eat cooling foods. Schedule vacations to get away from it all. You might need a few days on vacation before your shoulders relax and your mind calms.

Pittas have a hard time taking time off, but they need it. Pittas like to be successful, so tell yourself that rest will actually help you be more effective when you do go back to achieving your goals. It's true and it might inspire you to schedule that vacation.

JULY 10
PITTA DISTURBED AND BALANCED

Let's review what happens when Pitta is in and out of balance. Because Pitta is all about fire, out of balance signifies too much heat in the body—both physical and emotional heat.

This could show up as:

- Inflammation
- Loose stools
- Skin eruptions—rashes, prickly heat
- Bloodshot eyes
- Heartburn
- Indigestion
- Burning sensations
- Acid reflux
- Headaches
- Gastric or peptic ulcers
- Blood disorders
- Liver issues

Emotionally disturbed Pitta manifests as excessive anger and irritability. You might try to control people and circumstances to manage emotional angst. You may be more self-critical when Pitta is out of balance.

Specific diseases do not automatically emerge from a particular out-of-balance dosha. For instance, the source imbalance for skin eruptions or indigestion could be any dosha imbalance, but both tend to come up more frequently with Pitta imbalances.

Strong, balanced Pitta means strong intellect and powers of concentration. They are precise, sharp, direct, orderly, passionate, and romantic in healthy ways. Confidence and assertiveness come easily.

Pittas have sharp appetites and a naturally strong digestion. Healthy Pittas generally enjoy exercise and physical activities. When Pittas are balanced and strong, they make discerning, charismatic, and inclusive leaders with good stamina and a strong will. Pitta personality is light and bright.

AYURVEDA ACTION
Get Cooler with Coconut

Coconut water, revered in the Vedic tradition, is a very cooling drink for Pitta. Drink it daily in the hot months. FYI: The fatty acid composition of coconut changes as it matures. A young coconut, called a baal coconut, is 90–95 percent water, and this liquid is the purest, most hydrating, and most healing for ama. Over time, the liquid lessens and becomes milkier, and the coconut meat increases. Meat from mature coconuts is hard to digest.

JULY 11
BALANCING PITTA

In Ayurveda, vitiated (imbalanced) doshas (usually excessive) are balanced by introducing opposite qualities. Let's look at Pitta qualities and their opposites:

Pitta—Opposite

Hot—Cool
Sharp—Dull/Slow
Light—Heavy
Subtle—Gross
Mobile—Static
Clear—Sticky/Cloudy
Oily—Dry
Liquid—Dense
Smooth—Rough
Soft—Hard

The major quality of Pitta is heat, since it arises from fire and a bit of water vapor that is in things that burn. So mostly, when you need to pacify Pitta, you want to cool it. Pitta also has a tremendous drive and mobile quality. Too much drive and Pitta needs to settle and become a bit more static and comfortable in the present moment. Pittas need some heaviness to ground them.

Pitta also has an unusual tendency to be attracted to alcohol and other substances. They really need to watch out for this. Perhaps Pitta does this to calm down from all of the drive. Pittas and the Pitta in you can find other ways to calm and be at peace.

AYURVEDA ACTION
Balance Pitta with Diet & Lifestyle

Introduce opposite qualities in diet and lifestyle. To cool excessive Pitta, eat cool or moderate-temperature foods such as leafy green vegetables, asparagus, basmati white rice, and raw cow's milk. Pittas, with their strong digestion, are the only dosha that can benefit from cold foods like salads and sprouts. Alcohol and fermented foods should be avoided. Try cooling lifestyle activities like walks in the moonlight and noncompetitive swimming. Herbs like mint are cooling.

JULY 12
PITTA AND THE TASTES

PITTA IS AGGRAVATED by salty, sour, and pungent tastes, which should be avoided. Pitta is pacified by sweet, astringent, and bitter tastes (SwAB). Favor these.

The SWEET TASTE is composed of earth and water elements, which are cooling, grounding and soothing. Cooling has an anti-inflammatory effect, which is a tender issue for Pitta imbalance. Sweet is good for skin and hair. It cools burning sensations and pacifies mental "burning" of controlling and judging behaviors in the mind. Back off from sweet taste if you have excessive mucus.

The ASTRINGENT TASTE is composed of air and earth elements. This taste also cools, and so is good for a hot, imbalanced Pitta. Astringent dries and can help when too much oil or mucus is in the body. Pitta can be prone to diarrhea from fast-moving digestion, and astringent helps the colon retain the stool a bit. Slowing digestion helps secure more nutrients before elimination. Astringent tastes promote grounding, which balances Pitta's sharp mind.

The BITTER TASTE is composed of air and ether elements, and it cold and dry. Coldness alleviates excess heat in the body. Pitta has moisture in it, so some drying is okay, especially if oiliness is present in the skin or stool. Bitter purifies the blood and liver, which are the primary seats of Pitta. Pitta is more susceptible to toxins, so keeping blood and liver clean is good.

AYURVEDA ACTION
Eat for the Balancing Tastes

TO PACIFY PITTA, try these foods:

SWEET

Rice, dairy, dates, squash/pumpkin and pumpkin seeds, maple syrup, basil, cashews, cooked carrots, red lentils, mung beans

ASTRINGENT

Green bananas, pomegranates, cranberries, green beans, green grapes, parsley, cauliflower, chickpeas and most lentils/beans, coriander

BITTER

Leafy greens, turmeric, green/black tea, coffee, sesame seeds, dark chocolate, cumin

JULY 13
PITTA BALANCING DIET

If your constitution is Pitta, and for everyone during Pitta season, favor cool foods that are also grounding, like those listed below. Choose especially those with sweet {Feb 14}, astringent {Feb 18}, and bitter {Feb 19} tastes.

- Dairy: Raw cow's milk, butter, soft unsalted cheeses, ghee, sour yogurt, sour cream, and ice cream
- Sweeteners: Most natural, raw sweeteners such as date sugar, turbinado, maple syrup (honey and molasses are too heating)
- Grains: White basmati rice, quinoa, spelt, barley, oats, and wheat
- Fruits: Lighter, fully ripe sweet fruits in moderation, such as apples, avocados, cherries, coconuts, mangoes, melons, peaches, pears, pineapples, and pomegranates
- Legumes: Chickpeas, tofu, black-eyed peas, mung beans, and lentils
- Vegetables: Sweet and bitter vegetables are best, especially bitter leafy greens—also good are asparagus, broccoli, carrots, cucumbers, green beans, mushrooms, peas, parsley, salad greens, sweet green peppers, sweet potatoes, and zucchini
- Spices: Generally, reduce spices, especially hot peppers; basil, cinnamon, coriander, cardamom, dill, fresh ginger, and fennel okay in moderation
- Nuts: Soaked/peeled almonds; pumpkin, sunflower, and flax seeds; and coconut
- Meat: Chicken (white meat), turkey (white meat); clean river fish; some grass-fed non-GMO red meat
- Oils: Coconut, sunflower, olive, walnut, and grapeseed

AYURVEDA ACTION
Feed the Pitta Tiger

More than other doshas, Pittas need to eat regularly or they can "lose it." Pittas have a sharp appetite, and if that tiger is not fed it can start roaring. Eat the biggest meal in Pitta time, between 10 a.m. and 2 p.m., when appetite and metabolism are strongest. Don't skip meals. Try to eat in a peaceful environment, and slow down. Mindful eating helps you avoid overeating.

Select cooling foods, especially leafy greens, asparagus, summer squashes, and juicy fruits. Avoid hot, spicy foods and most oily nuts, which are heating. Pittas benefit from cooling garnishes like cilantro and parsley as well as cooling chutneys such as mint and coconut.

JULY 14
PITTA BALANCING LIFESTYLE

Remember the balancing qualities for Pitta? {Jul 11} Pitta qualities with the strongest influence are hot, fast, light, sharp, mobile, and subtle.

The principle of opposites means opposite qualities balance an imbalanced, excessive dosha. Some of the Pitta balancing qualities are cool, slow, heavy, and gross. Once you have balanced Pitta, you can engage in more Pitta preferences without thinking about it. Until then, it is wise to consciously participate in lifestyle activities to balance Pitta.

Lifestyle choices to balance Pitta should be slow, grounding, and cooling, such as:

- Spend time in Nature
- Meditate daily
- Walk in the moonlight
- Have a leisurely swim in cool water
- Eat slowly—or do anything more slowly than usual
- Do yoga, especially yin yoga
- Try grounding activities like gardening and building
- Enjoy daily rituals such as abhyanga self-massage and meditation
- Try nadi shodhana (alternate nostril breathing) or sheetali pranayama (cooling breath) {Jun 29}
- Rest...rest...rest
- Use cooling, calming aromatherapy oils like rose and sandalwood
- Surround yourself with cool colors like blue, green, and white
- Laugh and smile more often

AYURVEDA ACTION
Engage in a Sweet Lifestyle

Pitta imbalances are pacified by the sweet taste in foods. This applies to sweetness in lifestyle as well. Slooow down. Make time for meaningful conversations and experiences. Value time with others rather than thinking of it as time you could be working. Broaden your idea of success to include relationships and health.

Routines are helpful for Vata and also help regulate the Pitta drive. No daily routine is more helpful than getting to bed before Pitta time starts at 10 p.m. Otherwise, you might get a second wind and have difficulty falling asleep. Enjoy sweet sleep. Look forward to crawling into those sheets each night.

JULY 15
PITTA AND WEIGHT MANAGEMENT

You might think metabolism increases in the summer heat, but the opposite is true. The human physiology is built on the principle of homeostasis. One of the highest orders of homeostasis is body temperature. As internal temperature rises, the body needs to cool. Slowing metabolism is one of the first strategies the body uses to adapt to heat.

As metabolism slows, the digestive process is less effective because stomach acid reduces to avoid risk of overheating. This can add up to unwanted—and sometimes surprising—weight gain.

If you can keep your body internally cooler, your metabolism won't slow so much, and stomach acid will be sufficient. You have been reading about cooling tips for Pitta; here are some more cool tips to keep summer heat at bay so that Pitta stays balanced and metabolism stays strong: avoid midday sun, use sunscreen, invite gratitude into your emotions.

AYURVEDA ACTION
Check Pitta Weight Later

Pittas generally spend most of their life at a fairly good weight because of their robust metabolism. But if you are Pitta dominant and you find as the years role on you are putting on excess weight, it is more than likely from stress and demands that have you reaching for the ama producing foods like sugar and for alcohol to relax.

Pittas are used to eating a lot, which is okay in their youth when agni is naturally strong. But if agni has a wet blanket over it from ama accumulating over the years, a change in diet is needed. For one, the diet needs to be cleaner, including drinks. Secondly, in middle age when Pitta should be reducing how much they eat, they may not realize the need to do so. On go the pounds.

Big tip for unhealthy Pitta weight: eat cleaner, cleanse what is already going on in your body, and eat less.

JULY 16
PITTA SPICES

PITTA GOVERNS ALL transformations in the body, especially metabolism of food and experiences, and spices support digestion. Imbalanced Pitta leads to too much body heat. A digestive fire that is too strong and quick inhibits nutrient absorption. Pitta spices are cooling yet support digestion.

Pittas/Pitta season—Cook with cooling spices, like:

- Cardamom
- Cilantro
- Coriander
- Cumin
- Fennel
- Mint
- Saffron

Simultaneously, avoid certain heating spices:

- Black pepper
- Cayenne
- Chili peppers
- Dried ginger (fresh is okay)
- Salt
- Cloves

MAKE A PITTA CHURNA

- 2 Tbsp whole fennel seeds
- 2 Tbsp whole coriander seeds
- 2 Tbsp whole cumin seeds
- 1 Tbsp ground turmeric
- 2 Tbsp chopped fresh mint leaves (or 1 tsp. dried mint leaves)
- 1 Tbsp whole cardamom seed kernels

Grind together and store in an air-tight container. Add to dishes to balance Pitta.

AYURVEDA ACTION
Adjust Hot Spice Water to Cool

HOT SPICE WATER is fine even if you need to cool Pitta. However, adjust it to lower your heat by adding licorice root. Sweet and cooling, licorice root is good for balancing Pitta and adds great flavor. Licorice is not advised if you have high blood pressure.

As usual, put the seeds in boiling water to activate digestive and transport qualities—but then cool to room temperature before drinking to make it even more Pitta pacifying. You could also add mint to this recipe or drink mint tea that has cooled.

JULY 17
PITTA CHUTNEY

CHUTNEYS ADD DELIGHTFUL flavor to all kinds of foods, but have more to contribute when used correctly. Chutneys support agni and stimulate digestion. Most are heating and thus not good for Pitta, but here is one simple recipe that is cooling to get you started.

CILANTRO-MINT-COCONUT CHUTNEY

MIX INGREDIENTS IN a blender to your preferred consistency. I prefer mine a little chunky; some prefer a very smooth "sauce."

- 1 cup fresh cilantro
- 1 cup fresh mint
- 1/3 cup fresh coconut or 2 Tbsp dried (shredded or ground)
- 2 apples
- 1/2 tsp salt
- 1 Tbsp lime juice

AYURVEDA ACTION
Enjoy and Share Chutneys

YOU CAN SERVE chutney in a small bowl for dipping flatbreads or spooning over food. Only a teaspoon or two is needed to enhance flavor and meal digestion. Like all Ayurveda foods, chutneys—cooked and raw—are best served fresh. If you cook chutney, store it in the refrigerator short term, but it loses ojas each day. Try serving three chutneys at a meal—one for balancing each dosha, especially if you are dining with people who are tending various imbalances. See Kapha chutney {Mar 17} and Vata chutney {Nov 17}.

JULY 18
PITTA BREAKFAST

A Pitta-pacifying diet favors cool, dense, grounding, nourishing, and milder foods. It's not atypical for Pittas to skip a meal, but doing so does not play well for Pitta or those around them. Healthy Pittas often have excessive digestive enzymes and metabolize food quickly. They can get irritated when hungry.

And remember, even if you are not Pitta constitution or Pitta imbalanced, it is advisable for most people to favor Pitta-pacifying meals during this hot-weather season. Breakfast is a good start.

Consider these delicious breakfast options:

- Hot date nut milk—This scrumptious morning drink is velvety and nourishing. The sweetness that balances Pitta is filled with needed nutrients. Don't use cow's milk unless you can purchase it raw and unpasteurized. Otherwise consider nut milks. Cooling coconut milk is a good choice {recipe- Jan 21}. (This is my typical breakfast.)
- Fresh fruit bowl—If you are not too hungry, fresh juicy fruits are good. Eat enough fruit to satisfy Pitta metabolism. Chop and sprinkle with cardamom, fresh coconut, and chopped dates or raisins.
- Try soft boiled eggs, steamed greens with a bit of coconut oil, and sprouted grain bread
- Eat quinoa porridge with cardamom and soaked, peeled almonds (peels are hard to digest)

AYURVEDA ACTION
Nourish Your Liver with Fruit

Pitta imbalances often show up in ranjaka Pitta, involving a liver overtaxed with ama. Blueberries and strawberries nourish the liver, so include those with a fresh-fruit breakfast or as a snack. Remember, Ayurveda advises eating fruits alone, as they metabolize at a different rate than many other foods.

JULY 19
PITTA LUNCH/DINNER

Pitta fire is strongest at midday and thus, the best time for the largest, most nourishing meal of the day. Healthy Pittas, unlike Vatas and Kaphas, can do well with raw food. Even so, don't overdo it or you could overwhelm your metabolism. If Pitta is imbalanced, raw might be too demanding on digestion—limit raw to a side salad with a cooked meal if that's the case.

These cooling dishes can keep Pitta nourished but in check. Mix together a few of these to make a meal:

- Kitchari/mung dahl with coconut and cilantro {Mar 19/Mar 20}
- Sweet potato with kale and fresh ginger
- Asparagus and basmati white rice
- Carrots with thyme
- Carrots, zucchini, and rice
- Acorn squash with ghee and maple syrup
- Peas with mint
- Seasoned tofu with collard greens
- Veggie or turkey burgers with cheese

AYURVEDA ACTION
Explore Ayurveda Recipes Online

This book doesn't have a ton of recipes, but good Ayurveda recipe sites exist. Look for those with information on which dosha the recipe pacifies. Here are a few of my favorites:

- joyfulbelly.com
- food-alovestory.com
- franlife.blogspot.com
- healthy-indian.com/recipes

JULY 20
PITTA SUPPER

Supper is a "supplemental" meal. If the big meal was midday, make the evening meal light so you can be well on the way to digesting completely by bedtime. Of course, sometimes evening is the time to gather around a table for a larger meal, or you might be dining out. Joyful social-eating times are important, but try to make the last meal light when you can. Soups, which can be nourishing and varied, are a good way to do this. Cooked foods with small portions are easier to digest late in the day. A fruit plate is also a nice, light supper idea. You could try these Pitta pacifying supper ideas:

- Butternut squash soup
- Kale and carrot soup
- Coconut and beet soup
- Spinach soup with millet
- Fresh fruits (by themselves)

AYURVEDA ACTION
Select an Ayurveda Cookbook

An Ayurveda cookbook is helpful when you want to try new recipes and get additional cooking tips. A physical book you hold in your hands can be fun to sit with, page through, and get great ideas (like this book!). Here are some of my favorites.

- *Eat-Taste-Heal: An Ayurvedic Cookbook for Modern Living,* by Thomas Yarema, Daniel Rhoda, and Johnny Brannigan
- *Ayurvedic Cooking for Westerners: Familiar Western Food Prepared with Ayurvedic Principles,* by Amadea Morningstar
- *The Ayurvedic Cookbook,* by Amadea Morningstar and Urmila Desai
- *Heaven's Banquet: Vegetarian Cooking for Lifelong Health the Ayurveda Way,* by Miriam Kasin Hospodar

Reminder: When a recipe says it is good for Vata, that typically means it will lower or pacify Vata. If the recipe increases the dosha, the recipe should say so specifically, but normally food is used to lower excess dosha.

Bonus: To understand your deep relationship with food and eating habits, check out the wonderful *Healing Your Relationship with Food: The Ayurveda Answer,* by Meena Puri, a friend of mine. It contains delicious, foundational recipes as well.

JULY 21
PITTA BALANCING DRINKS

As with all Pitta-balancing strategies, cool is the idea. Making your own teas and other drinks can be fun, easy, economical—and ensures ingredient quality.

PITTA TEA

- 1 tsp hibiscus
- 1 tsp rose hips
- 1 tsp rose petals
- 1/2 tsp red clover
- 1/2 tsp skullcap
- 1 tsp fennel
- 1/2 tsp licorice
- 1/4 tsp cardamom
- Sprig of mint or a slice of lemon (optional)

Use whole seeds, leaves/roots, or powder as you prefer. Steep in boiling water and strain; if using powders leave them in if you enjoy the texture.

WATERMELON-MINT SMOOTHIE

- 2-3 cups watermelon, diced & seeded
- 1/4 cup fresh-squeezed lime juice
- 4-5 fresh mint leaves, plus 1 mint sprig for garnish (washed)

Blend ingredients to a smooth purée. Serve cool.

AYURVEDA ACTION
Avoid These to Pacify Pitta

We have talked a lot about what to do this month, but here are reminders on what to avoid with a Pitta constitution or Pitta imbalance, or during Pitta season:

- Alcohol, excess spices, and digestive irritants like coffee
- Sour and salty foods, which encourage the release of hot, irritating digestive fluids, including hydrochloric acid and bile
- Pungent foods that increase heart rate and blood flow—they can make you feel hot under the collar
- Strong, pungent spices and peppers; they make your body and digestion too hot and will also exhaust your liver

JULY 22
PITTA DAILY ROUTINE

A DAILY ROUTINE, called dinacharya, is an important way to support all doshas. When regular, your physiology anticipates the action and moves things in place to make the most of it. Because excess Pitta involves intensity, regularity calms.

IN THE MORNING

1. Choose a consistent time to awaken, even weekends and scrape tongue.
2. Eliminate.
3. Brush teeth. Do oil pulling {May 20}.
4. Wash and moisturize face.
5. Drink a large glass of warm water, which hydrates you more quickly.
6. Meditate or practice yoga.
7. Shower or bathe. Include abhyanga self-massage a few times a week.
8. Eat a Pitta-pacifying breakfast—fresh fruit or soft-boiled eggs with greens.

THROUGHOUT THE DAY

1. Balance work with time out to refresh. Do not overdo.
2. Eat lunch on time—don't skip.
3. Practice yogic breathing pranayamas {Mar 26} to keep cool.
4. Skip after-work cocktails. Try a relaxing tea or a bath. Water soothes Pitta.
5. Take a relaxing walk.
6. Eat a light supper early in the evening.

AT BEDTIME

1. Turn off electronics at least 30 minutes before bedtime.
2. Take a cool shower or wash your face and feet.
3. Apply light coconut oil to your skin and especially feet.
4. Brush and floss teeth.
5. Go to bed by 10 p.m., before Pitta time invites a second wind.
6. Take 1–2 triphala or triphala guggulu tablets or drink triphala tea.
7. Release tension with soft yogic breathing.

AYURVEDA ACTION
Adjust Triphala

WE'VE HAD A few discussions of triphala, but advice and recommendations for this triple-good herb bear repeating. If you do not eliminate in the morning, consider taking triphala {May 8} earlier in the evening. If constipated, increase the dosage. If you have a loose stool, decrease or eliminate triphala.

JULY 23
PITTA SUPER HERBS

Ayurveda recommends identifying an underlying cause before taking herbs to relieve symptoms. For instance, you might take cooling herbs if you know inflammation is present. However, if you consume a lot of sugar, herbs will only ease the symptoms and inflammation will remain. Even so, when you know you need to pacify Pitta, herbs can support healing while you address the causes of imbalance.

Pitta, composed mostly of fire and some water, can create heat and agitation when excessive. Cooling, soothing herbs help, along with a Pitta-balancing lifestyle. Do more research on these herbs or meet with an Ayurvedic practitioner to see if they are right for you.

SHATAVARI is one of the most powerful rejuvenation herbs, especially for women with reproductive and menopausal issues. Shatavari, nicknamed "she who possesses 100 husbands," also tones libido. The tastes are sweet and bitter, with cooling energetics great for pacifying Pitta.

BACOPA rejuvenates the nervous system and the mind. It also is called brahmi because of its esteemed role in supporting development of universal consciousness. Other herbs are also called brahmi, so be sure you are selecting bacopa. It also has sweet and bitter tastes and cooling energetics. Bacopa helps relieve anxiety, chronic fatigue, memory issues, and insomnia.

TRIPHALA is an herbal blend of amalaka, bibitaki, and haritaki. It contains all tastes except salty. The energetics are neutral balancing all three doshas. This formula pacifies all three doshas, and I recommend taking it as a nightly practice for most people. Triphala rejuvenates and gently detoxifies the body. It has a slight laxative effect.

AYURVEDA ACTION
Drink Cooling Tea

MINT AND ROSE petals are cooling for Pitta and make a nice tea. For added flavor, use licorice root, which is sweet, bitter, and cooling. Lemongrass is also cooling. Experiment and see what suits you while doing something good for your health.

JULY 24
PITTA WORK AND PLAY

Pittas love to work. They often are successful because they have sharp mental capacities, strong drive, and natural management skills. Pittas love challenges and making decisions. They are often insightful, quickly get to the heart of a problem, and figure out how to get around obstacles. Pittas are often in logical, goal-oriented professions and/or management positions.

At work, Pitta imbalances show up as stressful intensity, self-promotion, competitiveness, and controlling others. Pittas can become irritated and irritating when frazzled and fueled with too much drive, which can lead to burnout. To bring out the best in yourself and others, practice compassion. Try to laugh more at work and appreciate the playfulness that can be part of work.

By nature, Pitta play is competitive. If Pitta is balanced, then enjoy your competitive play. However, if Pitta is excessive, play in more relaxing ways. For instance, if you are in a yoga class, don't try to do a warrior pose better than the person next to you. Instead, move gently to the pose and relax into it. If you need to make it competitive, let the competition be with yourself. Extend your pose a little longer or breathe more deeply—or challenge yourself to ease up, enjoy, and do less! In this way you satisfy your Pitta's need for competition while cooling and relaxing the dosha.

Noncompetitive swimming is wonderful for Pitta because it is cooling. Relaxing walks in the moonlight are another good way for Pittas to play.

AYURVEDA ACTION
Dial Down Your Work Environment

Keep the temperature cool at work if you can, while still being sensitive to others' needs. How about a small fan? If you work from home, you have control. Don't skip lunch. Do a little pranayama before lunch and try mindful eating. This might be hard for "get 'er done" Pittas, but your digestion will thank you.

JULY 25
PITTA SKIN

PITTAS USUALLY HAVE soft, warm, radiant skin that flushes easily from exercise, stress, or alcohol. Pitta skin might have freckles and an abundance of moles. Imbalanced Pitta leads the physiology to push out toxins through the skin as the body releases excess heat. Pittas often see skin eruptions such as rashes, hives, and oily pimples.

Skin care, especially for Pittas, should be wholesome and toxin-free. Pittas are particularly reactive to toxins, so choose organic oils and skincare products. Look for high-quality Ayurveda natural skincare products or make your own.

Customize your skincare regime to keep it healthy. Kaphas, for example, might exfoliate every day, where Pittas only need to once a week. Pittas often have combination skin—oily and dry and usually sensitive. If your skin is oily, exfoliate more often. If dry, proceed with caution. Be observant of what is right for you.

Be cautious of commercial lotions, no matter how expensive. Avoid mineral-oil ingredients for sure. The best moisturizing oils for Pittas are coconut, sunflower, and grapeseed. Be your own laboratory. Assess what you need or get support.

No matter your constitution, your skin could need cooling in hot weather. Heating foods like chili peppers, spicy foods, vinegar, or sour foods can further heat and dry your skin. Alcohol is also drying, and especially for Pittas. Favor watery fruits, and melons in particular. Eat watery summer squashes, asparagus, and avocado.

AYURVEDA ACTION
Make Your Own Exfoliator

FAT-SOLUBLE TOXINS LIKE chemical residues, pesticides, and environmental pollutants settle in the fatty subcutaneous layer of skin. This ama (toxins) congests the lymphatic drainage system and inhibits surfacing of new skin cells. As we live longer, the process can become less vitalized. We can help by sloughing off dry, dead skin to reveal healthy, living skin. Start slowly to determine what treatment is best for your skin.

- 1 cup chickpea flour
- 1 Tbsp of any of these powders: triphala, sandalwood, arjuna, brahmi, shatavari
- Pitta Skin Types: Add 1/4 tsp powdered neem (not if pregnant) or mint

Mix into a paste with rosewater or slightly warm milk. Rinse off with warm water. Pat skin dry and moisturize; consider cooling coconut oil.

JULY 26
PITTA SPIRITUALITY

Pittas are strong even in spiritual pursuits. If you see yourself as a spiritual warrior rather than a peaceful monk, it might be your Pitta nature. Pitta fire is about transformation, including spiritual transformation.

The fire of kundalini Spirit is perfect for Pitta. As always, out-of-balance Pitta would be excessive drive and fire that could deter you from spiritual goals. Too much fire rages with ego desire. Too little fire and no transformation happens. Just-right fire is needed for optimum spiritual appreciation and experience.

Spiritual Pittas are like tigers. They are strong and committed to their sadhana, daily spiritual practice. They are the most disciplined yogis of the three doshas. They are also natural leaders and often use their spiritual power to help and guide others.

When balanced, Pittas fire their own spiritual development and lead others because their mission is service and not ego gratification.

My ultimate commitment to Ayurveda is to help sentient beings—that's you, gentle readers—hold the higher energies of spiritual transformation for enlightened living. It takes good health and balance for higher energies to move through you without knocking you off your feet.

AYURVEDA ACTION
Go from Active to Sitting Practices Over Time

If you have a strong Pitta nature, sitting meditation may be very difficult for you. To get there, start with more active practices such as kundalini yoga, then consider moving to walking mindful meditation before you sit for mantra meditation. None of these practices are a higher order on the path. See what works for you. As your Pitta comes into balance, choose other practices that harmonize with your current state yet lead to the edge of growth.

JULY 27
PITTA LOVE AND RELATIONSHIPS

In relationships, Pittas show up with fire. That means lots of passion and focus unless, of course, all that drive is focused on work. Promises are important to Pittas—ones they make and those that others make. If you tell a Pitta you are going to do something, they feel most in sync if there is follow-through, because basically, that is what a healthy Pitta does.

Pittas try to accomplish a lot, so avoid pressuring them for a lot of time. For those in relationship with a Pitta, communicate if you need more time to accomplish a task or you expect to be delayed in your arrival. A Pitta wants to know what is going on so they can utilize time. If you continually waste a Pitta's time, that could create a wedge in the relationship. Everyone needs to be who they are, however, so attempt to accommodate others' styles while honoring your own. Give and take.

Are you in relationship with a Pitta? Want them to feel good and connected to you? Here are ideas of what to do. (If you are a Pitta, ask for these treats for yourself.)

- Recognize and thank them for their contributions, even the small ones. Thanking others, even for mundane tasks, sweetens a relationship. "Thanks for emptying the dishwasher, Sweetie."
- Offer them a cooling drink like coconut water, or juice a watermelon and add mint.
- Massage their feet with cooling coconut oil.
- Spritz them with rosewater, especially at bedtime.
- Add cooling herbs like cilantro and mint to foods.
- Swim together in cool, natural waters.

AYURVEDA ACTION
Balance Pitta Energies = Happy Pitta Relationships

Pittas have strong emotions. When out of balance they can be tough on partners. A balanced Pitta is an awesome partner and can lead to very happy relationships for the Pitta and the partner. Balanced Pittas tend toward healthy, active sex and intimacy, engagement in shared passions, inspiring their partners, changing and growing with insight, and honoring alone time. Balance your Pitta and bring your best to significant others as partners, friends, and family.

JULY 28
PITTA CHILDREN

Pitta children operate with the same energies that have been described this month, but from a child's consciousness. They are in the Kapha time of life, so that is a major influence. Pitta children often have a moderate, athletic build and lots of energy. They are uncomfortable in hot weather. Like Pitta adults, they can get quite fussy if they miss a meal. Hunger hits them fast and they need to eat now, perhaps more than other children.

Pitta children like to learn with logic and visuals. They are often good in math. They tend toward perfectionism and need to be reminded that they do not need to excel at everything. Comparing themselves with others should be discouraged. Competition can energize them, and they can also feel down if they do not come in first. Although natural leaders, sometimes they put other children down as a way to elevate self. This is a good time for children to develop a sense of regard for others; wise adults can help guide Pitta children in this direction.

Pitta children flush easily when overheated or excited, and heat can lead to heated emotions. Pitta children may develop skin issues like pimples and rashes. They might experience diarrhea to release heat from the body

Pitta children should eat cooling foods {Jul 13} and participate in cooling activities like noncompetitive swimming. Mostly they need support in self-acceptance so their strong drive doesn't become perfectionism.

"Keeping it clean" is important for Pitta children, who are more affected by toxins in foods and the air. When possible, they should eat organically and avoid processed foods and sugars.

AYURVEDA ACTION
Have Healthy Pitta Kid Snacks Ready

Pitta children are likely hungry and worked up after school, or exhausted from their day. Eating the biggest meal at noon is unlikely for schoolchildren. Hungry Pitta children, especially, will want to snack after school, so have something good for them like fresh, juicy organic fruits, or a fruit salad with shaved coconut, a handful of soaked peeled almonds, cucumber slices, or sunflower seed butter on wheat crackers. Remember that hunger could also be thirst, so organic coconut water is a good choice.

JULY 29
PITTA AROMAS

More than anything, out-of-balance Pitta needs to be soothed, and aromas can help. The sense of smell triggers memories, emotions, and instincts, and it can influence the quality of your thoughts and experiences.

Sweet and cooling aromas to balance Pitta include:

- Rose
- Sandalwood
- Mint
- Jasmine
- Geranium
- Fennel
- Lavender

AYURVEDA ACTION
Ease with Aromatherapy

Neuro-associative conditioning links aroma to experience and memory. If you diffuse a certain oil when meditating, when you smell that aroma at other times, the meditative state is activated. Just drop about 6–10 drops of essential oil into a glass of warm water and allow the aroma to waft through the room. You can also use electric diffusers. Or place drops on a piece of cloth and take a few sniffs when you're feeling stressed.

JULY 30
COMMON CONDITIONS FROM IMBALANCED PITTA

It bears repeating: Ayurveda treats the individual, not the condition. Look for the source of imbalance that created the condition. The same imbalance could lead to different conditions in different people, and the same condition in any given group of sufferers may have different sources. That said, overheated Pitta can lead to common conditions.

Common Pitta conditions include ulcers, digestive weakness, heartburn, hyperacidity, skin eruptions, allergies, hot flashes, eyestrain, eye diseases, heartburn, and discontent. The heat can expel bad breath and body odors through sweating. Emotionally, Pitta imbalance can manifest as anger, irritation, and frustration, with tendencies toward judging and controlling behaviors. As you can see, you want to keep Pitta healthy.

AYURVEDA ACTION
Get Turmeric Every Day

Turmeric is one of the most highly regarded and researched (greenmedinfo.com) medicinal spices. It is beneficial to all doshas, but particularly Pitta. The most active component, curcumin, has been shown to have beneficial effects on purifying the blood. Turmeric also is an anti-inflammatory. {May 16}

Add more turmeric to your diet. Use fresh when possible. Here are suggestions:

- Add to eggs.
- Toss with roasted vegetables.
- Mix with greens.
- Use in soups.
- Add to a smoothie.
- Make a tea.

JULY 31
RECAP AND WHAT'S AHEAD

July, the heat and Pitta season begin. You learned about the heated nature of Pitta in digestion and emotions, as well as the conditions emerging from imbalance—like inflammation, heartburn, and skin eruptions.

Pitta is the dosha of digestion and transformation of food and emotions. Predominant Pitta qualities are hot, sharp, and mobile. Pitta fire burns hottest at midday, which is when the largest meal of the day should be consumed. "Cool it" is Pitta's best balancer, both in temperature and temperament. Sweet, astringent, and bitter tastes are cooling and are found in foods like dairy products, bitter greens, and beans. Keeping hydrated is important—drinking coconut water in the summer is especially cooling for Pittas.

Pittas do best to cook with cooling spices like cilantro, cardamom, fennel, mint, saffron, cumin, and coriander. They should avoid hot peppers, especially in the hot months. This is a great time of year to calm your Pitta with time in Nature, especially walks in the moonlight and leisurely swims.

WHAT'S NEXT?

August is often the hottest month for many of us and is in the thick of Pitta season. You will learn more ways to cool down, to hydrate, to select cooling foods from harvest season, and to take care of heat-stressed skin.

MONTHLY REFLECTION TIME

What actions did you try and what was your experience? Did the new action feel worthwhile? Did you like it? Did you have adverse reactions? Put a check in the third column for actions you plan to incorporate daily, weekly, monthly, seasonally, or on occasion.

What New Actions This Month?	*Your Experience?*	*Habit Worthy?*
		☐
		☐
		☐

AUGUST 1
MAKE YOUR OWN COOL

August begins, and the heat is on! That is tough on Pittas. But no matter your dosha constitution or your predominant doshic imbalance, most everyone needs balancing strategies for the Pitta season. In balance, Pitta is about drive, goals, generosity, courage, and passion. When out of balance, Pitta aggravates perfectionism, impatience, irritability, and the need to control.

August is a good month to do cooling physical and mental activities. Here are several to get you started:

- Walk in the moonlight.
- When you shower, turn down the temperature to tepid or even cool.
- Rub coconut oil on your scalp and the soles of your feet at bedtime (this helps with sleeping through the night).
- Eat cooling, sweet, bitter, and astringent foods such as asparagus, leafy greens, broccoli, carrots, cucumber, okra, spinach, melons, and milk. Generally, cooked foods are good for digestion but in summer, raw foods are fine on occasion. (Back off from raw if you get gassy.)
- Avoid heating foods like hot chilies and onions.
- Eat in a peaceful environment; honor your food and those around you.
- Spend time in Nature.

Stay cool, friends! It's about more than comfort. Keeping Pitta pacified supports your physical, emotional, mental, and spiritual well-being. It contributes to strong immunity, overall radiance, and longevity.

AYURVEDA ACTION
Do Your Daily Cool!

Here are reminder tips for pacifying Pitta:

- Meditate daily.
- Surround yourself with cooling colors like blue, green, and white.
- Appreciate others and express that appreciation.
- Use cooling, calming aromatherapy oils like rose and sandalwood.
- Take time to rest.
- Laugh and smile often.

AUGUST 2
SIZZLIN' HOT? TRY SOME REALLY COOL AYURVEDA

In the sizzlin' summer, Pitta fire runs the hottest. No matter which dosha dominates your constitution, or which typically is out of balance, Pitta dosha is assaulted by hot weather. Most people need to balance Pitta in these summer months.

HOW TO KNOW PITTA IS OUT OF BALANCE? LOOK FOR THESE SIGNS:

- Body heat is up.
- You have conditions such as heartburn, heat rash/prickly heat, bloodshot eyes, digestive complaints, or diarrhea.
- You feel increased aggression, irritability, anger, judgment, and jealousy, and you find yourself criticizing and/or losing your "cool."
- You're waking up between 2 a.m. and 4 a.m.

If you're experiencing one or more of these, your Pitta needs cooling.

AYURVEDA ACTION
Enjoy Watermelon, But Also Hydrate

Despite its name, watermelon is not hydrating. Although it can quench thirst temporarily, it is high in potassium, a diuretic, and is actually drying because it speeds up urine elimination. Watermelon rushes through your system, picking up toxins on the way, and you pee them out. If you have high Kapha and water retention, or want to flush your kidneys, watermelon can be good for you.

Drink more water if you eat a lot of watermelon, to compensate for the diuretic effect. Also, try to eat watermelon on its own rather than as part of a meal.

AUGUST 3

YOUR PITTA BALANCING SHOPPING LIST!

Back to one of the most basic Ayurveda principles: Like increases like and opposites decrease like. For example, if you are hot and you eat chili peppers, you will get hotter. If you are hot, and you eat watermelon, you will become cooler.

Pitta is fire. A major Pitta location is the stomach and a primary function is digestion. You balance Pitta when you cool the fires by eating sweet, astringent, and bitter foods. Here is your "cool" Pitta-balancing shopping list:

- Asparagus
- Broccoli
- Cucumbers
- Steamed greens
- Zucchini
- Cherries
- Grapes
- Mangoes

- Pears
- Pineapple
- Watermelon (always eat alone)
- Coconut
- Mung beans
- White basmati rice
- Milk (raw or VAT is best)
- Fennel, mint, coriander, cilantro, parsley

Avoid

- Hot spices, hot peppers
- Yogurt
- Sour cream

- Tomatoes
- Garlic and onions
- Alcohol and caffeine

AYURVEDA ACTION
Go Easy on the Raw

Even though you can eat more raw foods in the summer, it is important to eat a fair share of warm cooked foods for optimal digestion and good nutrition. That's true not only for Vata and Kapha types, but also Pittas. Instead of a big salad for dinner, consider cooked food and a side salad.

AUGUST 4
AYURVEDA SUMMER SKIN CARE

WHEN THE SKIN warms from hot weather or exercise, a natural balancing process activates to moisturize and cool it. However, when skin overheats too much or too often, its moisturizing functions are burned and become dysfunctional. This can cause early aging because there isn't enough moisture to prevent wrinkles and age spots from forming.

PROTECT YOURSELF FROM THE RAYS. Get a little direct sunlight every day for 15–30 minutes, but if you can, stay out of the sun during the hottest part of the day. During outings, wear a wide-brimmed hat, a shirt that protects skin, and good sunglasses. Hydrate, and eat a sweet, juicy fruit before going out in the sun.

TREAT SKIN TO ORGANIC ROSEWATER. Many health-food stores carry organic rosewater spritzer or rose hydrosol. Rose calms Pitta, and a little spritz is cooling.

DO ABHYANGA MASSAGE. The Ayurveda self-oil massage, abhyanga, nourishes and moisturizes skin deeply, and eliminates toxins from the skin and body. Sesame massage oil is typically recommended for dry Vata skin, but in the summer, coconut oil's cooling qualities are usually good for all doshas.

MILDLY SUNBURNED? Smooth on coconut oil or apply cucumber or aloe juice.

COOL YOUR EYES. A Pitta connection exists among skin, eyes, and emotions. In the evening, splash your eyes with cool water. Lie down for five minutes with cotton pads dampened with organic rosewater over your eyes. Do this daily to refresh your eyes and cool your emotions and skin.

AYURVEDA ACTION
Treat a Mosquito Bite Naturally

EVEN WITH USING natural protections, mosquitos sometimes sting. Here are a few of my favorite ways to treat mosquito bites naturally:

- Mix baking soda with water to make a paste and cover the bite. It sucks out the poison before it goes too deeply into tissues.
- Put ice on the bite to reduce inflammation.
- Dab equal parts tea tree oil and neem (not if pregnant) oil to swollen bug/mosquito bites. Neem oil also is a natural bug repellent. Note: These are herbalized oils, not pure essential oils that can irritate skin if used directly.
- Honey is naturally antibacterial and anti-inflammatory, so a little dab on the bite can soothe and heal.

AUGUST 5
CUCUMBERS FOR YOUR FACE

"Cool as a cucumber" is a saying for a reason. Applying cucumbers to skin is an ancient remedy to restore smooth texture and suppleness. Cucumber's natural ingredients tighten skin collagen, which can reduce fine lines and visible signs of cellulite. Juice on the skin promotes vibrancy and gives it a healthy, radiant glow. Use anywhere on your skin.

Cucumbers' cooling properties are especially beneficial in the summer, as skin around the eyes gets tired from wind, sun, or even eyestrain. A raw cucumber slice over each eye can reduce redness and puffiness. Applying cucumber externally to the skin has also shown healing effects on acne, eczema, and rosacea. Cucumbers have a high silica content, which may help fortify and nourish connective tissues in joints when eaten.

Facial Mask #1

A mask consisting of shredded cucumber, aloe vera and/or rosewater softens and also lightens skin color. Chill the mixture in the refrigerator before use for even greater effect.

Facial Mask #2

Another smoothing, hydrating mixture—1 Tbsp grated cucumber plus 1 Tbsp yogurt. Add green or white clay to stiffen and bind. Leave on for 15 minutes while you relax; then rinse with cool water.

FYI: You probably think of cucumbers as vegetables, but they are members of the melon family. Get organic cucumbers. Non-organic may contain pesticides, and the skins may be waxed. If you get non-organic, peel the skin.

AYURVEDA ACTION
Make a Cucumber & Honey Mix for Dark Circles

Shred cucumber and add raw honey in a 3:1 ratio for a soothing remedy for dark under-eye circles. Your dark circles will lighten over time with repeated applications.

AUGUST 6
ALOE VERA TO THE RESCUE

ALOE VERA IS summer's miracle plant. It is easy to grow your own to have on hand for sunburns and minor cuts. The plant is also good for nourishing skin, although it is a little tricky. Aloe vera is not a complete moisturizer. Because aloe vera gel is astringent, it can be drying if applied directly to skin. When properly combined with other ingredients, it becomes of great benefit to dry skin.

Here is how it works: For skin to feel moist, two conditions should be satisfied:

1. The moisture content of the skin needs to be sufficient, usually between 10 and 20%.
2. The skin needs the ability to retain moisture, which is easily lost through the course of a day due to dry weather, sun, chemicals, and poor (often sugary) diet. A well-nourished lipid layer helps skin retain moisture.

Aloe vera is 98.5 percent water, and the rest is loaded with more than 200 nutrients that nourish, soothe, and moisturize skin. But by itself, aloe vera is not capable of retaining the moisture, and its astringent qualities have a tightening, drying effect. Aloe vera is not drying when combined with emollients and humectants.

EMOLLIENTS fill the gaps between the scales of the skin, softening and smoothing them and reducing roughness and flakiness. The protective layer then helps prevent skin-moisture loss. Examples include oils such as grapeseed, sesame seed, jojoba, and shea and cocoa butters.

HUMECTANTS bond with water molecules to increase water content of the skin. Glycerin is a common humectant. Natural humectants include raw honey and skin's own elastin and collagen. In a humid environment, they draw water to the skin.

Never use petroleum products like mineral oil or petroleum jelly. These draw water from lower layers of the skin to the surface, which seems moisturizing, but is drying.

AYURVEDA ACTION
Go Natural with Aloe for Sunburn

BREAK OFF A piece of an aloe vera plant and squeeze the juice onto a sunburn for almost instant pain relief and healing. You can usually find aloe vera plants in garden centers and they're easy to grow. I have one that I have been keeping in a pot for more than 30 years. I take it outside each summer. It is amazingly hardy, and I have given many baby-aloe shoots to friends over the years.

Although aloe is healing to the skin, a little-known trait is that it can also be slightly drying: if you use it a lot, check out a moisturizer that balances aloe's dry quality {Sept 4.}. Or, simply mix it with a little coconut oil for skin hydration.

AUGUST 7
ROSES FOR PITTA (& YOU)

ROSES ARE ASSOCIATED with love and romance. Roses also balance Pitta, particularly sadhaka Pitta, a subdosha located in the heart that governs emotions. Sadhaka Pitta can go out of balance easily in summer.

Roses are cooling and yet they enhance agni (digestive fire). This double duty is unique, as usually heat is needed to enhance agni. Roses are known for soothing the heart and emotions, but they also soothe the mind. This combination is wonderful for intimacy. The scent of roses can balance the coordination between sadhaka Pitta and prana Vata, which governs the mind, sensory perception, respiration, and the brain. Roses can also regulate bhrajaka Pitta, the subdosha that controls skin biochemistry.

Rose aroma brings out your inner beauty and keeps your skin in balance. It's useful for treating Pitta-style headaches, nervousness, grief, and skin dullness. The sweet, astringent qualities of rose:

- Soothe digestion
- Balance emotions
- Nourish all seven dhatus (layers of tissues)
- Balance hormones
- Promote deep, restful sleep

AYURVEDA ACTION
Soothe with Rosewater

MAKE YOUR OWN rosewater. Boil six cups of organic rose petals in a quart of filtered water for 15 minutes. Cool, strain, and store in a glass jar in the refrigerator. Soak two organic cotton pads in rosewater and place over eyes to soothe burning. Or spritz your face with rosewater whenever you need refreshment and at bedtime.

Don't want to make it? Find a good quality rosewater or rose hydrosol such as those produced by essential oil companies that you trust.

AUGUST 8
SUMMER DRINKS

Yes water ... always water for hydration, but you can liven it up a bit in the summer. Stay cool in the Pitta season with tasty, refreshing drinks. Special drinks can help you to avoid the alcoholic choices, which are heating and have a more intense effect in summer.

Dehydration often causes "summer fatigue." We perspire and lose water, making it important to keep well hydrated. Do you have any signs of dehydration?

- Dry or sticky mouth, lips
- Little or no sweat
- Dry eyes
- Constipation or dry pellet stools
- Low urine amount or concentrated yellow color (clear urine might mean too much water; healthy urine is typically pale yellow)
- Low energy
- Irritability
- Sore muscles that don't recover
- Brain fog
- Overeating
- Constipation
- Under-eye bags and darkness
- Cracking and/or sore joints

AYURVEDA ACTION
Make a Spiced Coconut Smoothie

Coconut is very hydrating as well as cooling.

- Water and meat from one young coconut
- 2-3 Medjool dates, pits removed & chopped roughly (better yet, soak dates and peel the skin)
- 1/8 tsp ground cardamom

Blend all ingredients to a smooth purée.

AUGUST 9
A QUESTION ABOUT YOUR DIGESTION

Is there anything you cannot eat because it causes indigestion or even a violent reaction? **If so, you are not alone. In general, Americans and other Western cultures have woefully poor digestion. And the situation is getting worse, as evidenced by more and more specialty diets and the rise of allergies and chronic inflammation.

HOW DID WE GET HERE?

Seven decades ago we started a massive experiment: introducing processed foods, chemical toxins, artificial ingredients, and huge amounts of sugar into our food. This damaged our digestive systems to such an extent that many people cannot eat a full range of foods anymore. We have eliminated "hard to digest" foods because of our diminished digestive capacity, and in doing so have become deficient in a host of vitamins, minerals, and other food qualities that our bodies need. Many people have eliminated gluten, meat, nuts, seeds, or dairy to avoid digestive reaction.

Even if you have mitigated a digestive issue through an elimination diet, the remedy is probably temporary. In time, some other digestive issue will arise. We should be able to digest all real foods. With an Ayurveda diet, and with time and improved digestion, you should be able to reintroduce any foods you have temporarily eliminated.

BUT WHAT IF MY DIGESTION IS FAIRLY GOOD?

Even if the range of food you eat is broad and you have no digestive concerns, improved digestion can help you process and eliminate the environmental chemicals, toxins, and pollutants that are difficult to avoid, even when you try to consume only organic foods.

If your digestion is strong enough to digest a full range of real foods, it will be sufficiently primed to deal with and eliminate the omnipresent toxins you ingest. If you cannot ably digest all real foods, then environmental toxins will toss you around and have their way.

AYURVEDA ACTION
Make a Simple Sore-Throat Gargle

When missing essential nutrients, you are more susceptible to getting sick. Colds and sore throats seem even more unfair in summer. If you get a sore, irritated throat—here's a real quick remedy. Dissolve 1 tsp turmeric powder in hot water. Gargle with it, then spit out. Careful: turmeric can stain surfaces; a trash can might be the best place to spit.

AUGUST 10
COOL IT TO HYDRATE YOUR SKIN

Have you noticed that you have a shorter fuse, drier or inflamed skin, or digestive issues? These are all signs of too much heat in this Pitta season.

To combat these signs, it's important to stay cool and hydrated to nourish the radiant glow of healthy skin and to prevent Pitta aggravations from arising. These include heartburn, excessive body heat, sweating, anger, skin rashes, early graying of the hair, and excess stomach acid. Pitta pacifying beverages, food, activity, and state of mind/emotions can help you stay cool.

Drink cooling beverages. Drinking 6-8 glasses of water a day {Sep 2}, at a minimum (8 oz per glass), flushes toxins and replaces fluids lost to perspiration. Avoid iced or carbonated beverages because these disrupt your digestion. Room temp or slightly cool beverages are best in the summer heat (warm beverages other times of the year).

Sweet fruit juices such as grape, pear, or pineapple are Pitta pacifying. Boiled and cooled raw/VAT milk or natural milk alternatives with a pinch of cardamom soothes Pitta and nourishes skin. Avoid caffeine, sugar-laden drinks, and alcohol. These are toxic to the liver, and an overloaded liver can't effectively screen out toxins. While ads for colas make them appear thirst-quenching, they are dehydrating. Alcoholic drinks are even more dehydrating.

Eat foods that cool the body and hydrate skin. Purify and hydrate your skin by eating at least one sweet, juicy fruit a day, such as melon, pear, grapes, peach, nectarine, cherries, or plums.

Choose moist, cooling vegetables like zucchini and other summer squashes, broccoli, asparagus, cucumbers, and green leafy vegetables. Lightly sautéing is good. Make mung bean or red lentil soup to nourish and hydrate.

Try cooking with coconut oil—it's very cooling. Be generous with cilantro, sweet basil, and parsley in recipes. Cinnamon, cumin, cardamom, coriander, and fennel are good spices for the summer. Ghee and white basmati rice are great choices as well.

AYURVEDA ACTION
Choose "Cool" Exercise

Time on or around water is very cooling for Pitta constitutions and for Pitta season. Consider swimming or a gentle kayak/canoe outing. A leisurely stroll in the early morning or evening gets blood circulating while soothing Pitta. Ayurveda says a walk in the moonlight is just right for Pitta. Avoid activities like hot yoga.

AUGUST 11
PUZZLED BY SUMMER WEIGHT GAIN?

Summertime . . . and the living is easy . . . (to be sung, not read :-). Middle months are alive with sunshine to brighten your attitude. The rain waters gardens and cools. The lakes and rivers move us. And a huge range of vibrant fruits and vegetables is growing locally to nourish bodies and souls. The occasional thunderstorm startles us into appreciation of Nature's magnificence. Summer heat might be oppressive where you live and rain scarce. Then you must be even more vigilant about cooling.

Activity ramps up in the summer. Longer days invite more socializing. It's tempting to get into the spirit of things with rich and snacky foods and alcoholic beverages. These fun summer indulgences will aggravate Pitta. Alcohol is especially heating. If you have a Pitta constitution, keeping Pitta cooled in the hottest months is essential.

Pittas might have long-term ama build-up. The body's energy channels, especially around the stomach, may become clogged and create too much heat in the body. You would think fiery Pittas would have great digestion. However, if they do not regularly feed that fire, ama coats their digestive system and lowers metabolism. This can result in weight gain. Appetite and thirst could be excessive, and issues such as heartburn or irritability could erupt.

These factors, along with the body's automatic lowering of metabolism to keep cool {June 29} may lead to a surprise weight gain.

AYURVEDA ACTION
Balance Your Pitta with Cooling Foods

Eat three meals a day at regular times. Pittas get upset when meals are not regular—they become "hangry." A stewed apple {Nov 18} or oatmeal is good for breakfast. Try an herbal tea of 1/4 tsp each of coriander (detox), licorice (cooling), and fennel (digestion) through the day. You can let it cool to room temperature. Eat lots of sweet, juicy fruits. Squashes that are white inside (like zucchini), asparagus, and yellow split mung dahl are cooling and detoxing for Pitta. Quinoa and basmati rice are good. Cooling spices like fennel and small amounts of cumin and turmeric also balance Pitta.

AUGUST 12
SUNSCREENS—CAN NATURAL BE EFFECTIVE?

OVEREXPOSURE TO SUN carries risks, yet many are at risk from too little sun. Daily sun exposure delivers vitamin D from UVB rays—the good ones. The tally of ill health effects from insufficient vitamin D is growing. Vitamin D is crucial to radiant physical and mental health, and nearly all of your vitamin D comes from the sun.

Avoid UV exposure that is strong or of sufficient duration to result in skin burn. A pink glow, depending on your skin color, is just about right. With that caution, note that if you'll be in direct sun for a long period, sunscreen could be useful. UVB rays hit their peak about noon. A hat and shirt are the best sunscreen, but when you need UV protection what are the options? Check out the annual sunscreen guide posted online by Environmental Working Group (EWG), a nonprofit organization.[39] EWG tested 800 sunscreens and rated 25 percent acceptable in terms of effectiveness and safety from chemicals. Go to {Jun 6} to see some of the top ranked sunscreens.

Some naturalists suggest plain coconut oil is a good sunscreen. Oils have natural SPF, or Sun Protection Factor, values. Anthony J. O'Lenick, author of *Oils of Nature*, states that carrot seed oil has a natural SPF of 38–40. Other oils, like coconut oil, jojoba oil, and sesame, have lower SPF levels, ranging from 4–10.[40] Coconut oil is likely the most cost-effective. The key is to be sensible—stay out of noonday sun and wear protective clothing.

And don't forget about your hair. Run a little coconut oil through your hair before going outdoors.

AYURVEDA ACTION
Make Coconut Oil Sunscreen

- 1/4 cup coconut oil
- 1/4 cup shea butter
- 1/8 cup sesame oil or jojoba oil
- 2 Tbsp beeswax granules for water resistance
- 1–2 Tbsp non-nano zinc oxide powder (optional—dramatically increases SPF)
- Essential oils of your choice (lavender, rosemary, and/or peppermint—no citrus)

In a double boiler, melt the first four ingredients together. When melted, remove from heat and let cool. Whisk in zinc oxide if you are using it. Move mixture to the refrigerator for 15–30 minutes to set up. Remove from refrigerator and whip with a mixer until light and fluffy. Drizzle in a few drops of essential oils. Store in the fridge between uses.

AUGUST 13
YOGA FOR SOOTHING AND COOLING PITTA

Pittas may be drawn to hot yoga instinctively, but soothing yoga is more balancing, especially in summer. Remember, even if your constitution is not Pitta, summer is a good time to balance and soothe the Pitta you do have.

These yoga poses help Pitta sites such as the small intestines and liver: Fish, Camel, Boat, Cobra, Cow and Palm Tree.

In the summer, Pittas should avoid inverted poses such as shoulder stand and headstand. These poses pool excess blood to the thyroid and thymus glands and can provoke the eyes and brain in the summer.

Chandra namaskar, also known as Moon Salutation, honors moon energy. This restorative sequence can be done at any time of day, especially when you want to quiet the mind. Chandra namaskar in the evening is cooling and softening and quiets you for nighttime sleep. Moon salutation is a classic Pitta balancing sequence that keeps muscles, blood vessels, bones, and nerves toned and healthy while soothing Pitta. Find Moon Salutation sequences online or at your local yoga studio.

For Pitta, the spirit in which you do the pose matters. On the mat is a good time to lay down your Pitta drive and sense of competition. Let it go and enjoy your yoga practice. Move slowly and consciously, lengthen and extend. Be with what arises for you, even emotion.

AYURVEDA ACTION
Maintain Sweet Breath

- Fennel is a general toner for the digestive system. Chewing a teaspoon or so of fennel seeds after a meal stimulates digestive fire without aggravating Pitta—and freshens the breath.
- Chew cardamom or a clove (the spice, not garlic :-) after a meal.
- Chew mint, parsley or rosemary leaves.
- Enjoy a tea from fenugreek seeds.
- Scrape your tongue daily with an Ayurveda tongue scraper or the edge of a spoon.
- Drink plenty of water between meals, not during a meal.

AUGUST 14
PITTA COOLING FOODS – CLEAN & DIRTY

Organic is the best choice for any foods; however, organic options might not be feasible because of availability or cost. Check out this list of Pitta-balancing foods. Foods on the "clean" list are tolerable if you cannot find organic. Prioritize purchasing organic for foods on the dirty list.

Foods listed below will cool and nourish your hot Pitta. If you can't always buy organic, know when it is most important to do so. And of course, buy local if possible!

Clean Pitta Balancing Foods lowest in pesticides. Eat more of these:

- Asparagus
- Avocado
- Cabbage
- Mango
- Pineapple
- Sweet peas
- Cantaloupes
- Sweet potatoes
- Honeydew melon

Dirty Pitta Balancing Foods highest in pesticides.

- Apples
- Celery
- Spinach
- Sweet cherries
- Cucumbers
- Dark grapes
- Peaches

Pesticide ratings from the *Environmental Working Group's Guide to Pesticides in Produce*.[41]

AYURVEDA ACTION
"Butter" Toast with Coconut Oil

Spread coconut oil like butter on sprouted-grain or sourdough bread, which is more digestible because of the fermented sour ingredient. The coconut taste is lovely and coconut oil is healthy for you.

AUGUST 15
COCONUT BENEFITS

A FOOD THAT is so good for you, and so yummy, has to be one of life's little miracles. Coconut has been used reverently in Ayurveda for thousands of years. It's noted for immense health benefits and has recently emerged as the darling of the broader natural-health world.

Enjoy coconut's benefits from the top of your head to the bottom of your feet and almost anything in between. We can ingest it or use it topically. Coconut is used in many forms—the meat can be eaten or pressed to make oil or milk. The water from the core is sterile and nutritious.

All forms of coconut are cooling, so the hot days of August are an excellent time to go a little coconut-ty. Coconut is considered a divine plant in the Vedic tradition. Ayurveda's revered ancient healer, Sushruta, noted that "tender coconuts are 'bal means prana' in Nature, meaning they strengthen muscle, the cardiovascular system, and the seven body tissues.[42] Among coconut's many benefits:

- When pH levels deep in the digestive system fall—become too acidic—because of Pitta-induced toxins, coconut moves the toxins down and out to purify the system.
- Coconut can nourish the nervous system and reduce stress.
- Coconut fortifies hair with protein. Rub a little into your scalp and hair before washing your hair or before time in the sun. Enjoy the luster.
- Menopausal women benefit from the soma qualities of coconut, which is useful for healing hot flashes and stabilizing emotions.
- Coconut moisturizes the skin surface and deeper levels, healing wounds and preventing scars forming after injury.
- Coconut is one of the good fats that promote fat burning for energy. Cook with coconut oil or add it to your food for enhanced flavor.

AYURVEDA ACTION
Try Coconut Oil for Pets

COCONUT OIL MAY also be useful to add to your pet's diet for digestion and skin conditions. Start with very small amounts once each day, maybe 1/4 tsp, mixed with food. As with Ayurveda for humans, test a small amount in your pet's diet or on the skin in case your particular pet has a negative reaction.

AUGUST 16
COCONUT OIL CAN DO IT!

The benefits of coconut oil, ingested and on your skin, are astounding. Coconut oil:

1. Has a lower oxidation point, and so does not easily become rancid when stored.
2. Can be safely heated to higher temperatures—best oil for sautéing and frying.
3. Mixes with lime juice for a quick and nourishing salad dressing.
4. Gives stove-made popcorn a light, slightly nutty flavor.
5. Lowers cholesterol and stimulates fat metabolism if overweight and restores body fat if underweight.
6. Moistens an agitated liver. Replenishes a liver depleted in fats and cools an overheated liver, which also cools emotions like anger, jealousy, and the agitation of judging. Restores grace and kindness.
7. Has antiviral, antimicrobial, and anti-inflammatory properties.

AYURVEDA ACTION
Use Only Unrefined Virgin Coconut Oil

Choose only unrefined virgin coconut oil to receive its many health benefits. Most early benefit studies were conducted on partially hydrogenated coconut oil and had mixed results. Processing destroys the "home" of food. As more studies are done with unrefined virgin coconut oil, results are compelling for a wide range of benefits from skin health to digestion to cognitive function. Check out this astounding natural-healing research site for more: greenmedinfo.com.

AUGUST 17
COCONUT OIL FOR WEIGHT LOSS—REALLY?

Here's the benefit. Coconut oil breaks down quickly rather than being stored and is available for the energy we need. Eating this good fat can lessen your addiction to sugar for fuel.

And here's the science. Coconut oil contains saturated fats, and those have been on the "bad" list since the mid-20th century. Other foods containing saturated fats include animal products like lard and butter and tropical oils like palm. Saturated fats have been purported to increase cholesterol, reputedly a cause of heart disease. Yet saturated fat is an essential nutrient for proper cellular function.

Coconut has the highest amount of saturated fats compared with any other food—92 percent. However, more than half are medium-chain fatty acids (MCFA), which are metabolized differently than the long-chain fatty acids (LCFA) prevalent in most vegetable and seed oils. LCFAs are more difficult to break down and more easily stored as fat. Research shows that MCFAs in coconut oil:

- Convert directly into energy, lower cholesterol, and boost metabolism.
- Balance body fat, helping underweight people restore fat and overweight people metabolize the fat they have.
- Digest easily and quickly turn into energy without spiking blood-sugar levels, so insulin is not needed to digest them.
- Contain the most lauric acid of any plant, a potent antimicrobial that supports the immune system.

Try cooking with coconut oil or ingesting about a teaspoon daily. Some Ayurveds suggest that for weight loss, you may need to do this for three or four months.

AYURVEDA ACTION
Strengthen Your Liver with Coconut Oil

According to Ayurveda, an agitated liver becomes dry from holding ama. Coconut oil moistens a fat-deficient liver, which shows up as an excessive ranjaka Pitta subdosha. Coconut oil cools the liver just like it cools the rest of the body, and it can protect the liver from inflammation related to excessive alcohol use. Coconut oil can ease tensions, so it is a good massage-oil choice for Pittas, who sometimes fall to overheated emotions.

AUGUST 18
COCONUT WATER — LIQUID RADIANCE

Coconut water is the liquid you hear and feel when you shake a young, fresh coconut. Young coconuts are filled with water. Mature coconuts, which have the solid, white flesh known as coconut meat, have much less water. Coconut milk comes from grinding coconut meat and mixing it with water to create a product for cooking. (Note: coconut cream and cream of coconut are blended with sugar.)

The coconut meat and water are nutritional powerhouses, primarily because they are grown in mineral-rich volcanic and soils hydrated by sea water. Coconut water is:

- Pleasantly sweet and fat-free, low in sugar, and low in calories.
- Abundant in natural vitamins, particularly B vitamins that can be hard to get for vegetarians.
- Rich in minerals and trace elements such as zinc, selenium, iodine, sulfur, and manganese.
- Full of amino acids, enzymes, antioxidants, and phytonutrients that render free radicals harmless.
- A good source of electrolytes and natural salts, especially magnesium and phosphorus.
- A source of a plant hormone called cytokinin, which is anti-aging and anti-cancer.

Even though coconut water is sweet, recent research shows that it exhibits blood-sugar lowering properties.[43] It is one of the beverages most biocompatible to humans. This makes coconut water an excellent alternative to sports drinks, which increasingly are comprised of synthetic ingredients.

Coconut water has been used intravenously in remote regions of the world and by American healthcare workers in World War I when clean blood for transfusions was not available. That says something.

AYURVEDA ACTION
Replace Sports Drinks with Coconut Water

Coconut water has been billed as the world's safest sports drink. Many commercial sports drinks are loaded with sugar and other artificial ingredients. Take coconut water the next time you go bike-riding or running, or as you are out for a walk. Hydrate in the most natural way possible, calm your emotions, and take in nutrients in a pleasant-tasting way. Coconut water heals the digestive system and promotes better metabolism.

AUGUST 19
RESTORE TRANQUILITY WITH COCONUT

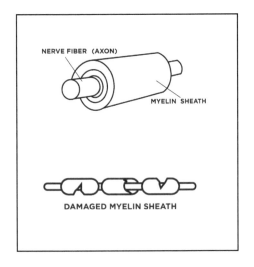

Frazzled nerves could be from the heat of summer or maybe just life. Either way, coconut can help soothe agitation and anxiety.

A fatty layer, called the myelin sheath, coats all nerves. The sheath directs nerve impulses and insulates the neuron from hyperactivity. When the fatty-sheath layer is dried out from stress, inflammation, or toxification, nerves become easily agitated and you may feel anxious—the connection between physiology and emotion!

In the eternal quest to regulate weight, many people have gone to no-fat or low-fat diets. This was, and is, misguided. The body needs healthy fats to nourish and maintain the myelin. When these sheaths are healthy you are less inclined toward physiological anxiety responses. When your chemistry is calm, you handle life better. Fat-burning creates a slow, calming energy. If you're burning sugar for energy, you are inviting a host of mental and physical problems.

A teaspoon of organic coconut oil daily is a neuron-comfort food that restores tranquility.

AYURVEDA ACTION
Take a Healing Bath with Coconut Oil

Add 1/4 cup coconut oil to your bathwater, along with 1/4 cup Epsom salts. If you wish, add a few drops of a relaxing essential oil, such as lavender. The Epsom salts will draw out toxins and the coconut oil will moisturize skin. Note: A hot bath can be drying. This is an upgrade.

AUGUST 20
COCONUT OIL TO BOOST BRAINPOWER

To boost brainpower, eat 1 tsp of coconut oil daily or use it in your food. Sauté veggies in coconut oil or make curries. The MCTs (Medium Chain Triglyceride) fats found in coconut oil are different in composition than most fats. MCTs have been found to boost cognitive performance in older adults, especially those with Alzheimer's and other memory conditions.

- The energy-hungry brain craves glucose. When glucose regulation is disrupted—common for most people to some degree—the brain's structure and function are compromised. Thanks to MCTs, coconut oil translates into a much-needed fuel source that "recharges metabolic processes within the brain, resulting in an almost immediate improvement in cognitive function."[44]
- Why is daily intake of coconut oil effective for cognitive impairments and diseases such as Alzheimer's? Glucose is the brain's primary fuel source. When insulin resistance develops in the brain, the brain's structure and function are impeded. The good-fat nature of coconut oil provides a healthy alternative fuel source to glucose. It recharges brain processes and improves cognitive function. Many fats are made up of long-chain triglycerides and are not easily absorbed. The MCTs have a shorter carbon-chain length, making them easier to absorb and more available as an energy source.

Coconut oil is one of the best sources of medium-chain triglycerides, and it is easy to add to your diet for a healthier, more nimble brain.

AYURVEDA ACTION
Squeeze Out Unhealthy Oils

Consider replacing your current cooking oils—which might be rancid and pro-inflammatory—with shelf-stable, healthy, unrefined coconut oil. The biggest culprits to replace ASAP are canola, soy, peanut, and grapeseed oils. Use coconut oil for cooking instead of olive oil, as it can better take the heat.

AUGUST 21
HOMEOSTASIS IS OUR INNER INTELLIGENCE

IF YOU EXERCISE vigorously for 30 minutes, your pulse rate will increase. When you cool down, your pulse returns to its "SET POINT," what is normal for you. Every process in your body has a set point that allows it to maintain a constant level of functioning, called HOMEOSTASIS.

Set points keep your internal temperature steady and regulate normal breathing. Your neurohormonal system has set points related to insulin, which govern how much energy from the food consumed should be available for your immediate needs and how much should be stored as fat. Your set points work remarkably well.

For example, your set point for weight works fairly well when you think about how many meals we eat in a lifetime and how weight could fluctuate if the system didn't self-regulate. HOWEVER, WHEN YOU REPEATEDLY OVERSTRESS YOUR RESOURCES AND UNDERNOURISH YOUR SYSTEM, YOU CAN CREATE A NEW SET POINT, THE NEW "NORMAL." This new set point can hold the pattern for high blood pressure, excessive weight, coldness in the body, over- or underproduction of hormones, diabetes, or other conditions, mild or serious.

Ayurveda, in essence, is about balance that keeps your nature in tune with all of Nature. Its principles and practices help you reboot to the right set point so that homeostasis is once again life-supporting.

AYURVEDA TIP
Restore Your Prakruti Set Point

AYURVEDIC PRACTICES WORK to return to your life set point, your prakruti, or original constitution by birth. Over the course of this year so far, you have worked with Vikruti to identify how your doshas are out of balance and establish practices to restore balance for radiant health according to your constitution.

When you are out of balance with Pitta for instance, you refrain from eating hot foods. But when your balance is restored, good agni is burning, and you are relatively clear of accumulated toxins, you can enjoy the hot peppers of the Pitta nature without negative effects. You live in harmony with how you were born. This is bliss. Now is a good time to look at Assessment 1 to reassess your Vikruti. See what changes you have made and what still needs work to balance your vikruti and get to your prakruti. Let the journey be a blast!

AUGUST 22
YOUR THIRST IS TALKING TO YOU

Proper hydration affects digestion, skin health, energy level, and mood. You lose about 10–15 cups of fluid each day through urine, sweat, bowel movements, a salty or dry diet, or kidney-flushing to get rid of toxins. Exercise, illness, and the weather can affect water loss. Water vapor in the breath is responsible for almost half the body's water loss.

WHAT IS THE TRUE THIRST SIGNAL? Losing fluid causes blood volume and blood pressure to drop, signaling thirst. Sometimes that signal is misread as hunger. In between meals, consider that feeling like you need to eat something might be thirst talking.

"I JUST DON'T FEEL LIKE DRINKING WATER." Dehydration is an early factor of many of the body's dis-ease conditions. Dehydration can start as fatigue, depression, poor digestion, or sluggish blood circulation. It can lead to more serious conditions.

HOW MUCH WATER? Like all of Ayurveda, it depends on you, your constitution, and your need to balance. However, I would say these are general guidelines for 8 oz glasses:

- KAPHAS typically need less water (6–8 GLASSES) because water is in the constitution and they easily retain water.
- VATAS are often chronically dehydrated, and they need to drink more water (11–12 GLASSES). However, just drinking water might not be efficient as it may encourage kidney flushing. Vatas should also eat watery foods and juicy fruits.
- PITTAS lose water and electrolytes easily through sweat, urine, and loose stools, so they need to drink a modest amount of water (9–10 GLASSES), perhaps more when they are exercising and sweating.

AYURVEDA ACTION
Calculate Water Needs

DR. CASE ADAMS SUGGESTS calculating water needs by dividing your weight by two.[45] This is the number of ounces of water you need each day. That's a lot, but hydration is important. About 20% of that comes from watery foods. Drinking water first thing in the morning has a bigger effect, as does water consumed about 30 minutes before a meal. Water taken hot and with herbs (teas) drives hydration deeper into the tissues.

AUGUST 23
SKIN HEALTH IN SUMMER

Summer can be very hard on your skin. Heat and dryness, exposure to wind, and often eating a bit more for fun and celebration than for health—all these take their toll.

First, do no harm whenever possible by not abusing your skin with lotions, creams, and makeup that have artificial ingredients. What you put on your skin metabolizes into your bloodstream, so only put something on your face or skin that is natural and healthy enough to eat. Look for simple ingredients for skin products. The best way to moisturize your skin is with a one-item ingredient list—think organic massage oils such as sesame massage oil or organic raw coconut oil.

Also, choose natural, organic fabrics to put next to your skin, such as those made with bamboo, hemp, silk, or responsibly sourced cotton.

Final tip—reach out. Giving and receiving touch each day is good for your health. A warm hug is grounding and stimulates receptors in the skin that invite deep relaxation. Whether or not you are in a relationship, look for ways to receive safe touch. Hug your friends or schedule a massage. Touch is important on physical, emotional, and spiritual levels.

AYURVEDA ACTION
Keep Your Nose Moist

Put a few drops of ghee or massage oil in your nose each morning. Simply dip your finger (wash hands or shower/bathe first) into the oil and massage the inside of each nostril. Oils keep the inner nose skin vibrant and functioning well to inhibit invaders from entering the nostrils and then the respiratory system. "Just a dab will do you."

AUGUST 24
YOUR SKIN INTRODUCES YOU

When you engage with others, they will notice your skin. Perhaps they are not looking at it directly, but their view will take it all in—and your skin tells a lot about you. Every inner disturbance is reflected in your skin. If your inner organs are dry, your skin will be dry. If your skin is red, your tissues or joints are likely inflamed. Take care of your inner world and your skin will reflect this.

Zinc is needed for radiant skin. Modern farming techniques rely on use and overuse of artificial fertilizers and pesticides, stripping our soil of natural nutrients. One nutrient that has become nearly unavailable in our food crops is zinc. Zinc has many functions in the body and is particularly essential in protein synthesis, enzyme function, and metabolism of carbohydrates. The added zinc we get in processed foods does not function like natural zinc. Minerals in real food have a relationship with all the elements of that food item and the functioning of that mineral occurs because of the interplay and balancing functions in those relationships. When you take a mineral or vitamin out of its home, it just is not the same.

Zinc is important for a strong immune system and immune health reflects in healthy, glowing skin. Pleased to meet you.

AYURVEDA ACTION
Eat More Zinc

Here are some zinc-rich foods to move into your diet:

- Oysters
- Ginger root
- Pecans
- Oats
- Split peas
- Egg yolk

AUGUST 25
THE EYES HAVE IT

KEEPING OUR SENSE organs healthy leads to many pleasures. But even the most health-conscious person can overlook eye health. As throughout Ayurveda, the whole and the part are inextricably connected and in fact are one. Overall good health leads to good eye health and good eye health contributes to good overall health. As with all sensory organs, overuse or underuse (or abuse) of the sense can contribute to disease.

We need to look both near and far at objects to strengthen our eye muscles. We are so used to looking closely at a computer, at a phone, at a book. Remind yourself of the importance of gazing at far objects. Nothing like a trip to the mountains to bring our distant gaze. Find a tree in the distance—be interested in really seeing it.

Misuse of the eyes can also mean looking at violent images on a screen or in our real life that incite our stress response. The eyes are governed by Pitta and the fire element.

When the body is heated or joints inflamed, our Pitta-governed eyes can be burdened with the extra heat. Inflammation, constipation, and blood impurities in particular lead to poor eye health.

Keeping your eyes cool helps tone the eye area and also helps reduce heat in your body in general. Summer is an especially good time to tend to your eyes.

AYURVEDA ACTION
Cool Your Eyes

ONE OF THE easiest ways to cool your eyes is to soak cotton swabs or pads in rosewater and place them on your eyes while you rest. For an even cooler effect, keep your rosewater in the refrigerator. Ahhh. Also, you can lightly caress your eyes by gently moving two fingertips over your eyelids.

AUGUST 26
SOUNDS GOOD!

EAR HEALTH IS also often neglected, even by the most health-conscious people. We sometimes imagine that we have no influence on the health of our hearing. The ears are influenced most by Vata and the air quality. Since Vata is cold and dry, we can keep ears healthy with warmth and moisture.

When you are doing your oil massage, do not forget to oil the insides of your ears. Or warm some sesame oil and put five warm drops of oil such as sesame massage oil into each ear canal. An especially good time to moisturize the ear with oil is when you are going to travel by air. Vata gets aggravated by the dry air in airports and planes which can dry out your ear membranes.

AYURVEDA ACTION
Listen to Pleasing Sounds

WHAT KINDS OF sounds do you hear in a day? Do you hear birds singing or do you hear the loud honks, wheels, and squeals of traffic? We cannot digest toxic sounds, just as we cannot digest toxic food. We all are necessarily exposed to many sounds that aren't pleasing during a day. Avoid what you can and accept what you can't avoid.

When you have a choice, choose pleasing sounds like chanting or classical music or wind chimes on your front porch. Consider a water feature for your home. Don't tune out pleasant sounds like children laughing or the wind blowing—listen for them. Take them in like the nutrients they are. Your hearing and your joy will improve.

AUGUST 27
HEALTHY SCALP

HAIR CARE IS important in Ayurveda. All the senses are located in the head and daily scalp massage keeps these senses in tune. Also, there are major marma points in the head that keep our energy body in tune as well. Marma in Sanskrit means hidden or secret, and marma points are the junctures where two types of tissues meet, such as muscles, blood vessels, tissues, ligaments, bones, or joints.

Head massage of marma points, then, supports sound sleep and can prevent tension headaches.

One of the important head marma points is the adipate marma. You can locate it by resting the wrist of your hand on the ridge of your brow bone. The adipate point is located inside the head below where your middle finger rests on your skull. There is a confluence of veins in this spot. Rub oil into that spot to stimulate the marma. Then rub or lightly scratch the entire scalp area. Leave the oil on for at least 30 minutes or longer and then wash your hair with very little shampoo.

AYURVEDA ACTION
Play with Your Hair

EACH HAIR HAS muscles attached to it that tighten when stressed. As you are watching a movie or reading a book, you could grasp small clumps of hair and twist in a clockwise fashion. The stimulation reduces stress and promotes the release of natural skin oils into the head.

AUGUST 28
HYDRATION PROBLEMS AND REMEDIES

HYDRATION IS ESSENTIAL for proper digestion because fluids are the medium for enzymatic activity. Without proper hydration, the stomach cannot secrete the two-thirds of a liter of hydrochloric acid typically needed to digest a meal.

Here are two common hydration problems and remedies.

DO YOU FEEL FULL AFTER DRINKING A LITTLE WATER? This could be weak digestion or insufficient acid production in the stomach. You need fire to get thirsty. Increase digestive capacity. Eat a slice of ginger with a squeeze of lime and a pinch of salt.

DO YOU HAVE DRY SKIN AND CANNOT QUENCH YOUR THIRST EVEN THOUGH YOU DRINK LOTS OF WATER? The deeper physiology is not getting enough moisture. This occurs when agni (digestive fire) is low and ama (toxin deposits) blocks the microchannels (srotas) that carry water to cells. Water passes through superficially.

To cleanse channels (srotas) and enhance moisture absorption, Ayurveda recommends boiling the water you drink. This activates the water with heat to bring out its sharp, penetrating qualities to cleanse even the smaller microchannels where stagnant ama can get stuck. Agni is further enhanced by adding digestive spices to the water. Once again, hot spice water is the superhero.

AYURVEDA ACTION
Hydrate in Many Ways

FEELING THIRSTY IS a sign that you are dehydrated—right now. Many challenging health conditions begin with chronic dehydration. Develop a few of these daily hydration habits:

- Drink Morning Lemon Detox {Jan 26} (after scraping tongue—always first)
- Drink 8 oz of room temperature water about 30 minutes before each meal (only drink 1/2 cup water with meal) to lubricate the stomach to receive food.
- Sip 16 oz or more hot spice water throughout the day.
- Eat brothy soups and dahls.
- Drink herbal teas hot or cooled to room temperature to take in healing Ayurveda herbs—brahmi tea, mint tea, or chai tea.
- Drink organic coconut water daily, especially in summer.
- If you need to snack, choose watery fruits like organic grapes, strawberries, and oranges.
- Add fresh lemon/lime slices or cucumbers to water for extra taste plus vitamins/minerals.
- Avoid alcohol, sugar, and processed foods, which are very dehydrating.

AUGUST 29
AYURVEDA LASSI FOR HYDRATION & DIGESTION

EATEN BY ITSELF, yogurt—especially highly processed, sugar-laden yogurt—can clog the channels of the digestive and elimination systems. When you add water and spices to make a lassi, it thins the yogurt and changes the molecular structure to aid hydration and digestion. Drink it before or with lunch (which should be your biggest meal of the day).

- Your lassi should contain plenty of probiotics. The probiotics are best when lassis are made with your own homemade yogurt so they are not sterilized out. Start with raw dairy milk. That can be hard to find, so vat/low temperature processed milk is an alternative. Your next best choice to homemade is plain, organic, full-fat yogurt with a "live and active cultures" seal.
- Probiotics are important because the body is loaded with good and bad bacteria. The good bacteria drive our immune processes. Ideally, the ratio is 85 percent good bacteria to 15 percent bad. But most people don't achieve that.
- Probiotics are found in varying amounts in foods but there are other ways to get probiotics if you cannot get a good quality raw milk or farm fresh yogurt. {Jun 9}.
- Mix all ingredients in a blender.

Sweet Lassi:

- 1 part yogurt
- 3 parts water
- Pinches of cardamom, raw cane sugar, rosewater

Digestive Lassi: This one has more digestive power

- 1 part yogurt
- 3 parts water
- Pinches of ginger, cumin, salt, black pepper

Drinking lassi is golden for your health.

AYURVEDA ACTION
Vatas, Go for Higher-Impact Hydration

VATA NEEDS TO keep hydrated all year long. Even in summer Pitta season, Vata needs attention. A wedge of lemon or lime in your water, along with a pinch of salt, helps Vatas retain more fluid for hydration. Try an herbal licorice-root tea; licorice is an antidiuretic and can help Vatas stay hydrated. Watermelon, on the other hand, is diuretic and helps with flushing toxins but could be too drying for Vatas.

AUGUST 30
SADHAKA PITTA

Processing emotions in a timely way gives you a strong emotional balance, the foundation for joy and happiness, and enlightened living. Some people process emotions quickly, which means they experience, let go, and move on. For others, the processing or "cooking" takes more time, allowing negative impressions more time to affect current thoughts and emotions.

Just as agni (digestive fire) helps us "cook" or digest food, there is an agni called sadhaka agni that helps "cook" and process emotions.

In modern terms, sadhaka agni is related to neurohormones in the brain and throughout the body, including the heart. When you have an experience, or recall an experience, the heart neurohormones send signals to the brain to register the feeling of the experience—sadness or happiness, for example.

You are born with low, high, or variable sadhaka agni. However, low sadhaka agni could also be caused by eating wrong foods, engaging in sadhaka-aggravating behaviors, or living in a non-supportive environment (environmental or emotional toxins).

And when sadhaka agni is low, it becomes a problem. You can lose discernment and find it hard to make choices about anything ranging from making a purchase to choosing relationships that serve. Chronic restlessness is also a sign of not cooking thoughts in a timely manner. Low sadhaka agni could prevent you from fully enjoying life's simple pleasures. When it is high, you experience, process, and let go.

How to increase sadhaka agni? Restore balance by adopting a healthy Ayurvedic diet, routine, and lifestyle and create a more profound connection between heart, mind, and consciousness.

AYURVEDA ACTION
Boost Your Physical & Emotional Heart

The herb arjuna supports and nourishes the physical and emotional heart. The herb promotes emotional balance, especially to those who are experiencing sadness or grief. In addition to "mending a broken heart," it is said to impart courage and purify will. Recommended doses are 1/4 to 1/2 tsp daily in warm water or nut/alternative milks.

AUGUST 31
RECAP AND WHAT'S AHEAD

August is a hot month, so Ayurveda emphasizes cooling Pitta and hydrating. Most people do not drink enough water.

This month you learned about coconut water as an effective, nourishing hydrator. Drink it daily in the hot months. Additionally, coconut oil is good for your skin, your digestion, and for lubrication of your tissues and organs. Find ways to add in a little coconut oil every day in the summer.

Hydrating is the big tip for August, but there are other ways to cool Pitta. Walking in the moonlight, leisurely swimming—especially in natural waters—and spending time in Nature are good. Also, eating cooling foods like asparagus, broccoli, cucumbers, greens, zucchini, white basmati rice, and grapes. An overheated metabolism slows to generate less heat, which can lead to summer weight gain. By keeping cool, you can keep metabolism strong and weight in check.

WHAT'S NEXT?

September is still the heart of Pitta season, so a focus on cooling and hydrating continues. Traditionally, September starts a new school year, but even if you are beyond those days, we can still get that rush to start good habits. We'll explore ways to do this effectively.

MONTHLY REFLECTION TIME

What actions did you try? What was your experience? Did the new action feel worthwhile? Did you like it? Did you have adverse reactions? Put a check in the third column for actions you plan to incorporate daily, weekly, monthly, seasonally, or on occasion.

What New Actions This Month?	*Your Experience?*	*Habit Worthy?*
....	....	☐
....	....	☐
....	....	☐

SEPTEMBER 1
STARTING FRESH IN THE FALL

Fall is a good time to take stock. Are your resolutions for the new year still swirling around you like hopeful suitors? Perhaps you have completely lost track of them. Or perhaps new notions for personal growth are coming back into focus. Four months are left in the year—maybe you're feeling time closing in on the growth and changes you had hoped for this year. The important action now is to find your way to radiant living. TODAY.

It could be helpful to get clear about the role of willpower. It might not be what you think. Do you believe willpower is abundant, limited, or a barrier to change? A Stanford University team of psychologists examined participants' beliefs about willpower, which they defined as "the ability to resist temptation and stay focused on a demanding task."[46]

According to Carole Dweck, one of the study's authors, "When you have a limited theory of willpower, you're constantly on alert, constantly monitoring yourself. 'Am I tired? Am I hungry? Do I need a break? How am I feeling?' And at the first sign that something is flagging, you think, 'I need a rest or a boost.'" That is when you might grab a sugar boost (my personal favorite is dark chocolate).

People who believe willpower is abundant and renewable are not constantly looking for those cues, and their actions are more sustained.

So how do we get to a belief of abundant willpower? Start with small, successful experiences and feel the resulting emotions to form new beliefs and habits.

AYURVEDA ACTION
Understand How to Change Habits

WHAT IS KNOWN about the habit mind:

- It is easier to start a new habit than to stop an old one.
- "Natural" willpower is strongest during the morning.
- Starting with a good first step in the morning can pivot your whole day in a good direction.
- Think of the domino theory in reverse: putting the first domino upright can start a virtuous cycle that continues to put dominoes upright throughout your day.
- In Ayurveda, the focus is not on stopping "bad" behaviors, but rather on adding "something good" that disrupts the old pattern.

SEPTEMBER 2
THIRSTY? IT IS ALREADY TOO LATE!

What would motivate you to drink more water? Drinking water keeps your organ systems moist, your skin plump, your body temperature regulated, and your blood flowing. All that and so much more. Water is the essential element supporting every one of the body's physiological, mechanical, and energetic functions.

Here's the science: Cells are composed of over 70% water by total cell mass. Cells also contain inorganic ions and carbon-containing (organic) molecules. Many cells hold a positively charged potassium ion within the water sac. Water outside the cell is teamed with positively charged sodium ions. These ions interact with electromagnetic polar affinity to create the sodium-potassium pump. In this little miraculous action, nutrients are transported into the cell and waste products are transported out.

We can eat the best food, but without proper hydration, nutrients will not get where they need to be. Water provides the transportation action. It is the medium for nearly every bodily function necessary to nourish and sustain our life systems.

HOW MUCH WATER DO YOU NEED?

THREE FACTORS DETERMINE how much water you need—body weight, water loss, and capacity for absorption. Many health professionals recommend about eight 8-oz glasses a day and Ayurveda has dosha specific recommendations {Aug 22}. Case Adams, a naturopath and author, believes that is not enough, because we have a base of losing 2–3 quarts of water daily. Case suggests 91 oz (11+ glasses) for women and 125 oz (15+ glasses) for men on average. If you are physically active or in weather that is dehydrating, you might need more. Case's recommendations are higher than most. A rough measure is to divide body weight by two—which equals the number of ounces needed each day.[47] That is Case's suggestion, but reflect on what is best for you.

Drinking that much water can be challenging. Be strategic. When and how you drink exaggerates water's effect. Enjoying lemon-detox tea {Jan 27} first thing in the morning, when the body is naturally dehydrated, has a greater benefit. Hot spice water has a bigger effect because boiling the water activates its spices. Drinking water with herbs (teas) also carries water deeper into tissues. Drinking 8 oz of water 30 minutes before eating has a larger impact, too. You don't have to get all your water from drinking. Eating watery foods is also good.

AYURVEDA ACTION
Confirm Your Water Intake

NOT SURE HOW much water you're drinking? Measure. Try filling a quart (32 oz) container with water. Can you drink that much at least two and perhaps three times a day? Here's to your radiant health—bottoms up.

SEPTEMBER 3
QUENCH! HYDRATE! HYDRATE!

Our bodies are composed of about two-thirds water. We move to the rhythms of water, and we're attracted to its simple and complete beauty. Water is our mate, the element we most closely match. Our thirst is quenched by drinking; we bathe in water to cleanse and soothe; and we dance in rain (even if only in our imaginations). As a primary source of health, water reminds us to be flexible, harmonious, and relaxed. Our attraction to water is mysterious, miraculous, and inexhaustible.

Proper hydration positively affects mood, skin, energy level, and of course digestion. Feeling overheated might seem like just an inconvenience, but that has health effects that add up over time. Recall {Aug 11} that when your body becomes overheated, your metabolism slows. And when metabolism slows, it creates incomplete digestion and weight gain. An overheated body also invites heated emotions—frustration, conflict, and angry outbursts.

Plain water is an excellent choice, of course, but you might want to alter it occasionally. Variety might even inspire you to increase your intake. A cooling Ayurveda drink can make regular occasions special and special occasions festive—without alcohol. Alcohol and sugar are very heating and drying.

AYURVEDA ACTION
Make a Healthy Pitta Mocktail

Celebrate: this delicious "mocktail" pacifies Pitta constitution and Pitta-season flareups. It will even help you sleep better at night. Aloe vera is cooling, and a major Pitta pacifier—supporting the gallbladder, fat digestion and breakdown of fat molecules. It also cleanses the liver and reduces inflammation. Pomegranate cools and builds the blood while stimulating digestion. Lime juice stimulates digestive secretions and reduces hyperacidity. Limes also aid in the breakdown and digestion of fats. Outside the body limes are acidic, but they have an alkalinizing effect when ingested.

- 1 tsp aloe vera gel
- 1 whole lime, juiced
- 2–3 fresh mint leaves
- 1 cup organic pomegranate juice
- 2 tsp raw honey or raw sugar

Combine ingredients in a tall glass—no ice, please! Crush the mint leaves with a spoon to release their flavor.

SEPTEMBER 4
KEEP YOUR COOL EVEN WHEN GRILLING

MEAT IS HEATING and involves fire, so it can agitate Pitta. Next time you grill outside, add balance by putting meat or veggies on top of basmati rice, which is cooling, and spoon on this cooling sauce.

MINT-COCONUT SAUCE

- 2 Tbsp ghee
- 1 Tbsp chickpea flour or 1/2 cup soaked (4-6 hours or overnight) raw cashews
- 2 Tbsp mild curry powder
- 1 1/2 cups organic coconut milk
- 3 Tbsp plain yogurt
- 1 cup chopped fresh mint leaves
- Salt and pepper to taste
- 1–2 tsp maple syrup (optional)

If using cashews, first blend the soaked cashews and coconut milk on high in a blender. In a saucepan, heat the ghee on medium-low. Add flour (omit if using cashews) and whisk to make a paste. Cook for 2 minutes, stirring constantly. Add the curry and stir for 2 minutes.

Whisking continuously and slowly, pour in the coconut milk (and raw cashews if using). Continue whisking until creamy. Remove from heat. Whisk in yogurt and mint, salt and pepper. Check taste and add maple syrup if desired.

AYURVEDA ACTION
Make Skin Moisturizer

COMBINE TO DEEPLY moisturize the skin. Here is a sample recipe using both an emollient and a humectant, but you can use these principles to customize with your preferred ingredients.

- 2 Tbsp aloe vera gel
- 1 Tbsp emollient: shea butter or coconut oil or both
- 2 Tbsp humectant: glycerin or honey

SEPTEMBER 5
FIRST THING IN THE MORNING

MORNING RITUALS ARE important in Ayurveda. Every good habit builds up ojas and resistance to disease. Use your natural morning willpower to start a new habit. Once a repeated action becomes a habit, it requires no mental energy—that is the beauty of habits. Before checking email, before giving over your day to others' demands, do one small, good thing for yourself and plan to do it every day.

1. Meditate—even if only for 5 minutes, even if you are still in bed.
2. Scrape your tongue with the round part of the side of a spoon or with an Ayurveda tongue scraper. Soooo refreshing!
3. After tongue scraping {Apr 20} and brushing teeth, do 10 minutes of oil pulling—perhaps while showering.
4. Exercise.
5. Start your day with a glass of warm water.
6. Breakfast gets you going—grapefruit with ginger and honey to cleanse and stimulate agni or hot grain cereal for nourishment. Set everything out the night before. I cook steel cut oats or cream of rice in a rice cooker. It cooks on its own while you get ready for your day.

Pick one thing to add to your morning routine.

AYURVEDA ACTION
Include Salt in Your Hydration Plan to Replace Electrolytes

EXERCISE IS RECOMMENDED as part of daily regime for all the doshas. Consider your needs to rehydrate. Electrolytes are needed for body systems to be fully functioning, so replenishing electrolytes is essential when you get dehydrated. Forget sports drinks. The best way to replace electrolytes is to take in trace minerals from good-quality natural mineral salts. Mineral salts, originally found in the oceans from which life originated (and now mined from the land where ancient oceans once were), are nearly identical to the elements in your body. The evidence is your salty tears and perspiration. Water and salt are the essence of life.

Sprinkle freshly prepared food with natural mineral salt. You could put a little salt in a glass of water if you are particularly dehydrated and need electrolyte replacement. Electrolytes are collections of minerals that we need for effective functioning. Choose mineral salts from good sources such as Ayurveda suppliers you trust.

SEPTEMBER 6
QUICK TIPS TO EAT HEALTHY ALL DAY

Once you get a good start to the day {Sep 5}, encourage yourself to keep it going.

Avoid sugar buzz.

Craving a sugar snack to keep your willpower going? Substitute a cup of tea with a teaspoon of honey. Honey is the only fat-burning sweetener.

What's for lunch?

Grabbing for convenience can lead you astray. Ayurveda recommends freshly prepared food, but leftover freshly prepared is better than processed. Try making soup or another dish that you can eat for three days. Invest in a quality thermos to carry healthier foods.

Suppertime.

Get rice going in the rice cooker and lightly sauté veggies for a quick meal. Or scramble some eggs and veggies for a light supper.

Late-night cravings?

Try a warm bath with Epsom salts. Sometimes you crave comfort, and food may be the first thing you turn to. Think of alternatives.

AYURVEDA ACTION
Treat a Cold with Tea

Colds happen, even in the summer. This Cold Soother Tea will help and tastes good.

- 1 Tbsp fresh ginger root, grated or sliced
- 1 Tbsp dried hibiscus flowers
- 1 to 2 sticks of cinnamon

Add 3 cups of boiling water. Simmer for several minutes; then strain. When cool enough to drink, sweeten with fresh orange juice or honey.

SEPTEMBER 7
INTERCEPT THAT HABIT

INTERCEPT: TO STOP, seize, or interrupt in progress or course.[48]

Take a habit you already have and intercept it by making a substitution to advance your new goal.

Example 1: Want to start walking in the morning? Place your walking clothes and shoes by your bed. When you get up, immediately dress for the walk. Or try the same with yoga clothes. Intercept your getting-out-of-bed habit with something that serves your new goal. It will be easier than trying to assert willpower an hour later.

Example 2: As part of your nighttime ritual, drape a string of dental floss over your toothbrush after you're done brushing. When morning comes, it's less effort to floss.

You get the idea. What strategies would advance your goals—large and small?

AYURVEDA ACTION
Cut Yourself Some Slack

HABITS CREATE STRONG neurological pathways. Cut yourself slack when you're working on changing a habit. It takes time. Try and try again. Would enlisting a buddy help establish your new habit? Supporting each other in something like exercise or reading more could be useful, whether you do an activity together or simply check in with each other: "I did it." You change habits by outgrowing those that no longer serve.

SEPTEMBER 8
CAN WE FEEL BLISS IN ANXIOUS TIMES?

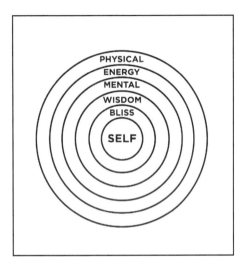

When you touch your innermost spiritual center, you contact bliss and joy. You can pass through that bliss field in any moment and know unbounded awareness. You experience Self, sometimes called Soul or Source, so that the light of bliss can shine. Your ego might feel reactive or compliant, but your Soul is trying to mentor you to more light, creative expression, and radiant health in your daily experience.

Political and social unrest and uncertainty can drive you into being reactive and anxious, and in opposition to others. Difficult situations can provoke anger, judgment, or the big freeze of being overwhelmed. Those are normal reactions. Suffering comes from getting stuck there. Relief comes from finding the higher mind of wisdom, calm, and centeredness.

Social and personal relational pressures serve a sacred purpose. Without pressure, you might feel less need to look at your stuck points and blaze a spiritual path. When pressure is great, return to your disciplines. They will serve you.

Can you live every moment in bliss? Well, not unless you're enlightened. The expectation of constant bliss will lead to suffering. Bliss is not a stagnant notion. The idea is to quickly stand upright each time you are knocked off center and to leave reactive space more quickly.

Ayurveda's broad science offers guidance to strengthen physical, energetic, mental-emotional, intuitive-wisdom, and bliss koshas (sheaths that surround you like Russian stacking dolls). Releasing old beliefs and our biased constructions of reality allow the light of pure consciousness to shine through more quickly and more often!

Welcome happiness and increase your capacities to generate, sustain, and share happiness by upgrading daily practices.

AYURVEDA ACTION
Cultivate & Embed New Healthy Experiences

Do not bemoan negative or difficult experiences. Accept the reality before you. Acknowledge, process, and act on those experiences rather than stuffing them, which never helps. Also cultivate and embed positive experiences. This does not happen automatically, so embed the positive consciously with a process like "gladdening the mind." {Jun 20}

SEPTEMBER 9
YOUR TOP EIGHT SUPER SPICES

In addition to delicious taste, spices increase Nature's intelligence in your meals. They help with digestion and assimilation in delivering more nourishment.

- CARDAMOM is sweet and pungent. It promotes digestion and is good for the heart. Cardamom improves the smell of breath and relieves gas and bloating. It also has been used as an aphrodisiac and to treat obesity.
- CINNAMON is a rich source of antioxidants, has anti-inflammatory properties, eases digestion, and may reduce blood-sugar and cholesterol levels. It stimulates blood flow and considered helpful for weight loss.
- CLOVES are antibacterial, anti-inflammatory, and antifungal. They have been studied for use in aiding detoxification from environmental pollutants.
- CORIANDER seeds have antioxidant and antibacterial qualities. Coriander soothes the stomach and relieves bloating. Coriander essential oil is used for arthritis relief.
- CUMIN is a diuretic (helps the body shed water), relieves diarrhea and bowel spasms, relieves morning sickness, and eases carpal tunnel syndrome.
- FENNEL SEED is loaded with powerful antioxidants and contains fiber, folate, potassium, and vitamin C. It boosts the immune system, reduces blood pressure, detoxifies, and is a mild appetite suppressant.
- GINGER naturally treats nausea from morning and motion sickness, and has anti-inflammatory properties for muscle and joint pain. It also has a diaphoretic property (causes sweating) and is good to detoxify, stimulate circulation, and ease bronchitis and congestion. Try a slice of fresh ginger in your hot spice water or cook with fresh grated ginger.
- TURMERIC, the best of medicinal herbs, promotes healthy cell replication and contains the flavonoid curcumin, known for anti-inflammatory properties. This spice may relieve the effects of chemotherapy, improve cognitive function, detox the liver, and boost immunity.

To activate the dormant intelligence of spices, lightly sauté them in ghee or coconut oil and add to recipes. Ayurvedic spices offer rich and varied aromas and flavor that stimulate digestive juices to enhance metabolism and balance the doshas. They can transform simple dishes into feasts for your senses, providing fulfillment and contentment from meals.

AYURVEDA ACTION
Even Pittas Can Eat Fresh Ginger

GINGER IS CONSIDERED the most sattvic (pure) of all spices. Dry/powdered ginger is drying, so is good for Kapha. Fresh ginger is better for Pitta and Vata. Fresh is neither as heating nor as drying. Fresh ginger is an anti-inflammatory thanks to its volatile oils. For Pitta season and for Pittas in general, stick with fresh.

SEPTEMBER 10
YOUR INNER PHYSICIAN

Our bodies are wise miracles if we give them a chance by practicing the wisdom of radiant living. Think about all the ways our physiology functions each and every minute. The intelligent version of your tissues and organs and processes can keep you abundantly healthy. Your inner physician knows how to engage the immune response—which chemicals to release and the proper timing. Your part in keeping healthy is to nourish that innate intelligence and to cultivate deep energy reserves.

Eating inappropriate foods (processed, leftovers, or wrong for your doshas) and carrying negative lifestyle habits both detract from health, blocking inner wisdom. Natural resources might be unavailable when we need them most. Your inner physician enables the body to repair, balance, and fine-tune itself to higher degrees of wellness and efficiency. With the knowledge of Ayurveda, you can make smart decisions to further your part in this miracle experience.

Ayurveda is helpful to treat manifest conditions, but it's most useful to prevent serious conditions from arising. As an Ayurvedic practitioner, my health has been better than ever, but it is not perfect. I recently had the ego-checking experience of needing to cancel an Ayurveda workshop due to a bout of the flu. Everyone is figuring this out as they go. Do a step here and there to upgrade your health. Small actions have big effects, especially when you rely on the long lever of Ayurveda knowledge.

"Give me a lever long enough and a fulcrum on which to place it, and I shall move the world."

—Archimedes

AYURVEDA ACTION
Eat Naturally Intelligent Foods

Food is medicine. Close to "three-quarters of the products sold in U.S. grocery stores contain genetically-modified ingredients {Jun 24}."[49] Artificial ingredients added to real food are bad, and processing means real food is no longer alive. It loses its intelligence.

Your body has the natural intelligence to process foods that come from Nature in their original form. This includes whole grains and organically grown fruits and vegetables. Eat more of these to improve your diet and reap the advantages of food's intelligence.

SEPTEMBER 11
SHOW A LITTLE LOVE TO YOUR LIVER

Your liver is the largest solid organ in your body, and it has a big job. About the size of a football in adults, it has more than 500 functions. Three of the most important include:

1. Cleaning the blood
2. Producing bile, essential for digesting fats
3. Storing glycogen, a form of sugar held in reserve and used for energy

You can see why a well-functioning liver is necessary for exceptional health.

Here is an overview of the science of the liver. During digestion, food, vitamins, minerals, and other nutrients pass from the intestines into the blood, which heads to the liver. Then the good stuff is transformed into forms your body can use. The liver also cleans blood by removing toxins. Once nutrients and toxins are separated, bile carries waste back into the intestines and urinary tract to be eliminated from the body. The filtered, nutrient-rich blood is then transported throughout the body.

The liver and gallbladder work together to help your body get the benefits from good fats. The liver produces bile, a thick, green, digestive juice, which is stored in the gallbladder until needed to digest fats and other lipids.

The body breaks down food carbohydrates into glucose. When stored in the liver, it is called glycogen. Glycogen provides backup fuel when blood glucose levels drop and the body needs a quick energy boost to stabilize.

AYURVEDA ACTION
Try Moonbathing to Calm Your Emotions

The liver (governed by Pitta) is essential to digest food. In Ayurveda, it plays an essential role in digesting emotions, especially those associated with the liver like hate, resentment, envy, irritability, frustration, impatience, and excessive ambition.[50]

Early on in my training, I was surprised at how often walking in the moonlight came up as a tip to cool Pitta. The moon is known in astrology for having a big effect on emotions. Make a practice of walking in the cool moonlight. This practice is especially powerful under a full moon, but do keep in mind an early evening walk so you can be in bed by 10 p.m.

SEPTEMBER 12
LIVER DISEASE FACTS

- The most prevalent liver condition is fatty liver disease, which affects about one-third of the U.S. population.
- Liver disease—including hepatitis, cirrhosis, and liver cancer—is the 12th leading cause of death in the United States.
- More than 20 liver diseases are currently diagnosed that have treatments, but many treatments only slow disease progression.
- One in 60 people have hepatitis C, and nearly two-thirds of those people don't know they have it. It is called the "silent epidemic" because infected people can live for decades without obvious symptoms.
- Hepatitis C is five times as widespread as HIV.
- Hepatitis C can be diagnosed through a blood test and is fully curable in more than 90% of patients.[51]

AYURVEDA ACTION
Drink Milk Thistle Tea for a Healthy Liver

How do you maintain or even restore effective liver functioning? Avoiding alcohol and eating real food (especially bitter greens) are high-impact strategies to support a healthy liver, but herbs can help, too. Milk thistle is perhaps best known as a liver tonic and contains antioxidants that fight liver disease and is antibacterial. You can make a tea with milk thistle powder or seeds. Add licorice root pieces, another antibacterial, to sweeten. Consider drinking this tea as a once-a-week ritual, say, on Sunday evenings or pick a day. Or drink the tea more often if you have concerns with liver issues.

SEPTEMBER 13
ALCOHOL, SUGAR, AND YOUR LIVER

A HEALTHY LIVER is the workhorse of our detoxification processes, maximizing digestion and eliminating dangerous toxins. Alcohol and sugar are the two biggest bullies when it comes to liver health.

ALCOHOL

ALCOHOL CONSUMPTION IS the primary cause of fatty liver disease. While it's normal for your liver to hold 5–10 percent of fat accumulation, more than that is a big problem.

Some research suggests that a modest amount of alcohol—about one drink daily—may help your heart. However, other research shows that one alcoholic drink per day can damage the brain, liver, and overall physiology. Ayurveda recommends little to no alcohol.

SUGAR

EXCESS FRUCTOSE IS the main cause of NAFLD (non-alcoholic fatty liver disease). Fructose is contained in ridiculously dangerous amounts in the high-fructose corn syrup found in nearly all processed foods. Fructose damages the liver in a similar way to alcohol. Unlike glucose, used by nearly all cells throughout your body, fructose is metabolized only in your liver. With fructose so prominent in the typical Western diet, this places a huge damaging burden on the liver.

My general notion is that joy also is one of our greatest health promoters. If occasional use of alcohol opens your social enjoyment and offers soothing relaxation, a drink or two a week might be right for you.

And if sweet treats bring you pleasure, enjoy natural sweets (but no high-fructose corn syrup) once in a while. The goal is health, not leading a sterile life absent of joy. Just keep leaning into better choices. Over time, your desires shift to that which best serves you.

AYURVEDA ACTION
Try an Alternative to Nightly Alcohol

IN AYURVEDA, ALCOHOL is understood to putrefy or rot the food we eat rather than allowing it to be digested. Beer, wine, or a cocktail once in a while is probably okay for most people, but consider using other special drinks to substitute. Try introducing an evening habit of drinks like chai latte, lavender lemonade, or fresh-squeezed fruit juice. Keep the ritual, change the content.

SEPTEMBER 14
HERBS FOR YOUR LIVER

THE LIVER AND brain are the only body organs able to regenerate or repair damage with new cells. Adding Ayurveda herbs to your dinacharya (daily routine) will help protect and regenerate your liver. Taking these herbs before drinking alcohol also has been shown to protect the liver from alcohol-related toxicity and help heal liver damage.[52]

BHUMYAMALAKI is a classic, most-revered Ayurvedic herb for the liver. It is very bitter and acts to cleanse, detoxify and strengthen liver functions. It also provides support for the gallbladder.

BARBERRY is extremely bitter and rich in vitamin C. It is used to protect the liver, increase bile flow, support healthy cell growth, and balance blood sugar.

TURMERIC is also bitter and the most studied spice for its many natural healing properties. Turmeric boosts the body's natural antioxidants. It has liver and brain-protectant properties to combat alcohol-induced oxidative stress. Turmeric helps clear the physical and subtle channels of the body.

GUDUCHI is referred to as "divine nectar" in the ancient Ayurveda texts. It burns off accumulated toxins in the liver. It also calms the mind. Guduchi supports production of powerful liver-protective enzymes, which are depleted when exposed to alcohol.

AMALAKI, or Indian gooseberry, is a small fruit rich in vitamin C and antioxidants. Amalaki is cleansing and supports healthy liver cells.

A typical dosage for any of the above is 1/4 to 1/2 tsp powder once or twice daily on your food or in water.

AYURVEDA ACTION
Make a Delicious Liver-Cleansing Soup

- 2 cups beets, thinly chopped
- 2 cups cabbage, thinly chopped
- 4 carrots, thinly chopped
- 1 potato, thinly chopped
- 2 Tbsp ghee
- 3 Tbsp raw apple cider vinegar
- 1/4 cup fresh dill, minced
- 1/4 tsp black pepper
- 1/4 tsp salt

Place all ingredients in a soup pot. Add water to twice the height of ingredients. Bring to a boil and simmer, covered, for 1 hour or more.

SEPTEMBER 15
IMMUNE SYSTEM—HOW IT WORKS

A STRONG IMMUNE system protects against threats from micro-organisms in the forms of bacteria, viruses, and parasites (protozoa). Each day, you inhale or ingest thousands of germs. Your immune system is at work 24/7. You don't notice all that effort until something goes wrong and an infection takes hold. Bacteria or viruses that make it past the immune system response can cause flu, cold, or food poisoning, among other things.

The immune system is a network of cells, tissues, and organs that work together to protect the body. White blood cells are produced from bone marrow and are carried in the blood to organs, where they develop and organize to launch responses against intrusion. White blood cells produce antibodies that can neutralize bacteria and viruses by attaching to infected cells and destroying them which enables the lymph nodes to filter out germs. When they do, the nodes can become swollen, a sign that the immune system is working.

In summary, your immune system:

- Creates a barrier to prevent bacteria and viruses from entering the body
- Detects and eliminates bacteria or viruses that get into the body
- Eliminates unwanted/infected cells such as cancer cells

All of us get sick. A goal of Ayurveda is to build a "strong-like-bull" immune system to prevent illnesses and to restore health quickly when illness does occur.

AYURVEDA ACTION
Build Your Immune System with Fresh Fruit

IN MANY PARTS of the world, it's apple harvest time. Fresh apples are rich in the antioxidants and soluble and insoluble fibers that build the immune system. Other juicy fruits—like pears, peaches, pineapples, and plums—are quick ojas builders that support a strong immunity. Pomegranate seeds and juices are also good because of their capacity to improve digestion, which in turn supports immune functions.

SEPTEMBER 16
TOP IMMUNE SYSTEM BOOSTERS

Ayurveda is designed to strengthen all the natural functions of your body. Cold, windy weather is on its way, and it's worth taking a few extra steps to boost your immune system so it can effectively do its job. Check out these tips.

HEALTHY DIET

Eat warm, freshly prepared food and drinks. Soups, stews, and cooked fruit can boost immunity strength. Select vegetables and grains to balance your dosha and also the season you are in. These are good for the immune system: white basmati rice and couscous; cooked apples or pears; vegetables like asparagus, zucchini, and other squashes.

Cook food with immune-enhancing spices such as ginger, cumin, fennel, coriander, turmeric, and black pepper to enhance agni (digestive fire) and reduce ama (toxins). Limit sugar and alcohol intake. Simple sugars impair white blood cell activity leading to a depressed immune system. Alcohol can impair white blood cells' mobility.

HEALTHY LIFESTYLE

The transition between seasons, along with the dryness and cold of fall, stresses the immune system and makes you more susceptible to illness. Take extra care to stay warm and moist during this time.

Take meals at regular times. Regular meals help prepare the body for nourishment by increasing appetite and enhancing digestion. Regularity decreases Vata, so it is good preparation for the start of Vata season.

Get enough sleep to allow organs to rejuvenate and for digestion to complete. In bed by 10 p.m. and up at or before sunrise is recommended. Vatas tend to get 4–7 hours of rest, Pitta 5–8 hours, and Kapha more than 8. Each dosha should aim for the average of 7–8 hours per night, though it is not "one size fits all." Feeling rested upon arising and having energy for your day is what's important.

Integrate exercise such as yoga and walking into your daily routine. Moving and stretching enhances circulation and moves toxins out of the body. Pranayama, a yogic breathing technique, is excellent for cleansing and strengthening the body and mind. Give yourself a warm abhyanga oil massage daily. Follow with a warm shower or bath.

AYURVEDA ACTION
Eat Greens for Strong Immunity

Try Swiss chard, mustard greens, and kale cooked in ghee with the immunity spice mix {Feb 27} to fortify your immune system. Serve on a bed of quinoa or barley for extra nutritional punch—a perfect immunity boosting meal.

SEPTEMBER 17
GET AWE-INSPIRED

AWE IS CLOSE to happiness, gratitude, surprise, love—and even fear—but it stands on its own. Awe has always played a part in spiritual, artistic, and transcendental experiences, but until recent years, it hasn't received much attention from researchers of emotion and psychology.

Awe is triggered by an experience so expansive (positive or negative) that it's a struggle to assimilate the vastness. In a state of awe, you have moved from contracted awareness to expanded awareness. Keltner and Haidt, two of the best-known researchers on the topic of awe, describe it as "in the upper reaches of pleasure and on the boundary of fear."[53]

I experienced awe as I climbed Machu Picchu in Peru with other yogis and my teacher Karina Mirsky. As is typical in an "awesome" experience, my attention turned away from self as I stood in the clouds at the peak and took in the pure, timeless beauty of Nature in her brilliance.

Also typical is to reevaluate what you believe to be true and real. I did this at the mountain peak and continue that integration to this day. In that place and time, I experienced a clear, innocent mind instead of my usual vigilant attention on protective constructs. I existed in the spaciousness between the conditions of my mind. What freedom! An awe experience is powerful, and recalling an awe experience is a strategy for receiving even more benefit.

Vastness expands your worldview and shrinks the ego. You get a feeling of a "small self" in a good way. Awe stirs a sense of oneness with others and opens a greater identification with the divine, eternal Self. Awe is a reminder that you are part of a much greater intelligence. Awe keeps egos in check. Awe helps you move through sadness to gratitude and acceptance.

AYURVEDA ACTION
Nurture Awe

- Spend time in Nature: Explore waterfalls and mountains and mushrooms. Nature is the big winner for awe.
- Meditate daily—another big one!
- Watch videos created to inspire awe—such as beautiful videos by National Geographic or inspiring messages by Jason Silva.
- Listen to music that moves you, especially music with dramatic highs and lows.

SEPTEMBER 18
EVEN MORE AWESOMENESS

WHAT DOES THE awe experience look like? It can involve deep stillness. You might get goosebumps, the jaw drops, eyebrows go up, and eyes widen. A deep breath helps in absorbing the experience. And even though awe has roots in joy, an element of reverence, fear, and trembling is present. Even if the awesome experience is beautiful and not scary, releasing our ego to the vastness of Nature can feel unnerving.

A common benefit of awe, according to researchers, is the mind-bending experience of time stretching out. What a benefit in a culture that often leaves you feeling time-starved. The shift in perception leads you to feel more time is available, a determining factor in your inclination to act more generously with time. You feel open to meeting new people, to being a compassionate listener, and to supporting the welfare of others. All emotions serve a purpose, and as Laskow believes, the purpose of awe might have something to do with drawing people together.[53]

Benefits of awe experiences include:

- Expanding a sense of time availability
- Inspiring creativity
- Giving you hope and helping you appreciate life
- Connecting to Nature
- Transforming your inner Self

Ayurveda is based on living closely to Nature, which is where you are most dependably able to experience awe. Consider cultivating awe with chosen experiences this winter.

AYURVEDA ACTION
Even More Ways to Nurture Awe

- Show up for inspirational speakers and teachers.
- Spend time creating or appreciating art.
- Walk mindfully around your neighborhood, as if it is the first time you have seen Nature around you.
- See another person, perhaps many others, with softness and compassion.
- Get out of your ordinary routine. Common experiences do not inspire awe. First-time experiences and a fresh disposition facilitate the ability to see things in a new, almost magical light. Prioritize adventure.

SEPTEMBER 19
YOUR HEART'S DESIRE FOR HEALTH—PHYSICAL

The beautiful, precious heart organ is the touchstone of your body temple. With each beat, it pumps oxygen and nutrient-rich blood to tissues and other organs, as it picks up waste and carries it away. The beat of the heart sets up an electrical wave that influences the rhythm of many of our physiological, emotional, mental, and spiritual rhythms. Your heart takes care of you—and you need to love and care for your heart.

According to the U.S. Centers for Disease Control:[54]

- Heart disease is the leading cause of death for men and women in the U.S.
- High blood pressure, excessive LDL cholesterol, and smoking are key heart-disease risk factors.
- Medical conditions and lifestyle also put people at risk, including diabetes, being overweight, poor diet, physical inactivity, and excessive alcohol use.

From an Ayurveda perspective, the most critical factor for heart disease is ama (toxins) collected in the blood vessels, tissues, and organs. Excessive ama makes your heart work harder. Diet is a primary culprit, along with the Western culture's emphasis on consumerism, disconnection, and a fast pace. Sedentary lifestyles, exposure to toxic chemicals, and a hunger for emotional/spiritual fulfillment are other challenges. You might not be plagued by all of these issues, but it can be difficult to avoid them all. An Ayurveda diet, moderate exercise, having a sense of meaning in life, establishing and valuing relationships, and meditation or prayer all lead to a healthy heart.

AYURVEDA ACTION
Use a Copper Cup

ARTERIAL PLAQUE IS ama (toxic matter) that collects in the blood vessels. Proper diet can decrease ama, and, as previously noted, Ayurveds recommend placing a copper cup of water next to your bed at night so it's available first thing in the morning. Copper cleanses and ionizes water. It is an antioxidant, and the water is more easily absorbed than "dead water" from treatment plants, which remove most of the trace minerals along with the vitality. Copper water balances all three doshas and supports digestion. Copper water can:[55]

- Stimulate brain function
- Boost bone strength
- Regulate functioning of the thyroid gland
- Combat arthritis and joint pain
- Boost skin health
- Regulate body fat
- Improve fertility
- Slow the aging process
- Improve cardiovascular health
- Act as an anticarcinogen

SEPTEMBER 20
YOUR HEART'S DESIRE FOR HEALTH—EMOTIONAL

THE HEART IS a physical organ and is also experienced as the seat of emotions. You want to experience emotions—rather than stuff, deny or identify with them—but also avoid dwelling on them. You might overwork the emotions thought of as negative, so balance is important. It's an art.

Mental and emotional balance, along with physical strength, is part of a "toned" heart. To have a healthy heart, we need a happy heart. Cultivating love, joy, and bliss is the best tonic for heart care.

Rather than use willpower to force disciplines that make you feel deprived or punished, engage lifestyle changes that promote well-being. An Ayurveda diet and lifestyle offer a foundational, nourished lightness for more delightful emotions. It takes energy to be happy. When your heart can circulate nutrient-rich blood, you reduce physical, emotional, and spiritual density and are lifted to radiate from the heart lotus in the daily pleasures of life.

AYURVEDA ACTION
Strengthen Your Physical & Emotional Heart

ARJUNA IS A revered herb for the physical and emotional heart, and strengthens the heart muscle, tones the circulation system, and supports healthy blood pressure and cholesterol levels. It also promotes emotional balance for the wounded heart, especially if you are experiencing grief or sadness. Arjuna is said to impart courage and strength. Typical dosage is 1/4 to 1/2 tsp powder daily stirred into warm water or warm alternative milks.

SEPTEMBER 21
YOUR HEART'S DESIRE FOR HEALTH—SPIRITUAL

The heart is the seat of consciousness, prana (life force) and Vata srotas (energy channels). Prana is synchronized by the rhythm of the heartbeat, along with the pace and nature of your breathing. The heart represents the lotus, where our soul resides. The heart is the jewel of the soul. When your heart is healthy and happy, the heart lotus receives Source light and will shine.

The heart draws and supplies blood to the body, which invites a sense of interdependency and integration. The heart is in service to the whole, literally and symbolically. When you are drawn to others, you think of a heart connection.

Ayurveda views the heart as your energetic center: Its physical energy is needed for all body functions. The heart chakra is also the seat of your subtle energies. Those who trace the evolution of consciousness say that we are entering a time of full development of our love capacities and heart chakra. Darkness is being revealed through purification. This can be tough to go through, but this process forms individual growth.

Like all of Ayurveda, balance is the key to heart health. When your consciousness is in balance, your mind, body, and senses become identified with the Unified Field of Energy, and you become radiant.

AYURVEDA ACTION
Take a Vacation with Novelty

Everyone needs to get away from it all sometimes. Plan time away from work and home tasks. Novelty is a key for joy. Travel invites fresh experiences and has a positive effect on your sense of self and your important relationships. Even a weekend away can be a big boost. Can't get away to someplace new? Try a "staycation": spend a weekend going places and doing things you always wanted to do, right where you live. Remember, the key is novelty.

SEPTEMBER 22
HIGH-IMPACT HEART HEALTH BY DOSHA

Excess mental and emotional stress challenges the heart, so it's important to manage these. The best choice for high-impact strategies relates to which dosha pushes your mental and emotional triggers, resulting in imbalance when stressed. You want to go beyond managing stress to nourish your emotional and physical heart. Nourishing heart connections keeps the heart from wasting away.

Pitta

According to long-held Ayurveda wisdom on heart health, Pitta's sharp, penetrating nature is often the instigator that first damages blood-vessel walls. Pittas put pressure on themselves and others to perform and to manage, well, everything. Eat a Pitta-pacifying diet and reduce toxins, which are particularly harmful for this dosha. Take a breath and let go of your need for perfection. Be involved in cooling, noncompetitive activities that can slow you down. Swimming or strolling in the moonlight is good.

Vata

Vata types can stress out all by themselves. They have worrisome minds that can lead to a sense of anxiety. Try relieving frantic, nervous energy through physical activity like yoga; then sit to meditate. Meditation is a go-to strategy for Vata. Creative expressions also help reduce Vata stress.

Kapha

Kaphas need to move to reduce stress, which often manifests as lethargy or depression. Because Kaphas are encouraged to action when there is a social connection, try a yoga class or make a date with friends for vigorous walking. It doesn't take much to deter Kapha activity, so have an alternate plan for walking if the weather is bad. Find a local mall, for instance, or climb stairs in your home or outdoors at public buildings.

AYURVEDA ACTION
Learn a Few Factoids from HeartMath

HeartMath[56] is a research center for the heart-brain connection (heartmath.com).

- A human heart's magnetic field can be felt several feet away.
- Negative emotions create nervous-system chaos; positive emotions do the opposite.
- The heart sends signals to the brain that can influence perceptions, emotional experience, and higher mental processes.

SEPTEMBER 23
KEEP YOUR HEART UPBEAT!

Stress is hard on the heart, so lean into one or two of these heart-healthy behaviors.

- Soothe—Try warm baths, abhyanga massage, time with friends, spiritual connections and experiences, and meditation. Some forms of meditation are proven to lower blood pressure, reverse arterial blockage, and invite bliss.
- Eat right—Attend to "what, when, and how" you eat. Reduce ama (toxins) with organic, freshly prepared foods and cook with a variety of spices. Eat more fruits and vegetables. Use spices to enliven "Nature's intelligence."
- Nourish the good times—Cultivate positive emotions. Learn what brings you happiness and do more of it—experience these times with mindfulness.
- Move it!—Exercise moderately and regularly. Find something that you enjoy doing physically. If you don't enjoy it, the commitment will fade.
- Keep it clean—Too much caffeine, alcohol, or sugar weakens the liver and digestive power, leading to accumulated ama that is not good for the heart. Reduce chemicals in your food and home. Arteriosclerosis is an example of accumulated and deposited ama.
- Invite restful sleep—It rests the heart and supports digestion of food and emotions. Go to bed at a regular time (ideally before 10 p.m.) to establish the anticipation and habit of sleep. Listen to soft music for 30 minutes before bedtime and keep the bedroom free and clear of clutter and electronics.

I suspect that none of this advice surprises you (especially if you've been diligently reading this book). Perhaps, however, repeating this information will remind and encourage you to establish yourself more strongly in heart-healthy habits.

AYURVEDA ACTION
Stew Fruit for a Heart-Healthy Breakfast

- 1 whole fresh, sweet apple or pear, cored & peeled
- 3 whole cloves or powdered blend of cloves, cinnamon & cardamom to taste.
- 1/4 cup purified water
- 1 tsp ghee

Core, peel, and slice or dice fruit. Add cloves or powdered spices, fruit, and water in a covered pot. Cook until apple/pear (or both!) is soft. Discard whole cloves if used. Sweeten with raw sugar to taste, if needed, or add 1/2 tsp raw honey when cool enough to eat.

SEPTEMBER 24
THE RHYTHM OF THE COSMOS

A CLEAR INTENT of Ayurveda is to relieve suffering and to promote radiant health. A more subtle and powerful intent is to lift the body, mind, and spirit to evolve in consciousness. Ayurveda is about receiving and holding these higher energies. Ayurveda is a path to lifelong radiant living and self-fulfillment.

The key is living in harmony with Nature's rhythms. The primary character of Nature is change. With Ayurveda, you learn to artfully adapt to change, restore balance, and minimize disturbance. We used to live closer to Nature than we do now. We ate what was in season, we adjusted to changes in temperatures, we used raw materials in the form they came from the earth, and we did not have an environment full of artificial chemicals. Humans possessed natural wisdom as a way of life. But now the wisdom of Nature has been collectively forgotten. Nature is the divine healer, and the closer you are to her, the healthier.

Nature is full of rhythms. Two of the most influential are day-to-night and the seasons. As the body adapts to changes, you align the microcosm (body) to the macrocosm (Nature/Universe). In the Veda texts, these laws of Nature are called Rta, which equates to rhythm in English. When your mind, body, and spirit rhythms are aligned with the Cosmos, you are living Ayurveda.

The earth knows to spin on its axis, a bird knows when to migrate, a carrot knows how to be a carrot, and a river knows how to flow. Even death is a rhythm of vibration, another form of experience. Each moment pulsates with a rhythm of consciousness that takes us into the next.

AYURVEDA ACTION
Practice Pranayama {Mar 14}

PRANA MEANS "LIFE force or breath sustaining the body" and ayama means "to extend or draw out." Together these words mean breath extension or control. The poetry of your breath is perhaps the simplest and yet most profound way to live in the truth of Nature's intelligence.

Here is a portion of a simple mindful breathing practice from Thich Nhat Hanh: As you breathe in, say to yourself, "I know I am breathing in." As you breathe out, say to yourself, "I know I am breathing out." Mindfulness is the opposite of forgetfulness. Mindfulness brings calm and joy and happiness.

SEPTEMBER 25
GO ORGANIC—AND WHEN IT MATTERS LESS

Use this list for what is best and to avoid in nonorganic choices. According to the U.S. Environmental Working Group (EWG), "dirty" foods contain harmful pesticides that persist even after washing and peeling. Clean ones are less likely to have persisting toxins on them. Strawberries had the most toxic residue, and avocados the least.[57]

Dirty—Clean

Strawberries—Avocados
Apples—Sweet Corn
Nectarines—Pineapples
Peaches—Cabbage
Celery Frozen—Sweet Peas
Grapes—Onions
Cherries—Asparagus
Spinach—Mangoes
Tomatoes—Papayas
Sweet bell peppers—Kiwis
Cherry tomatoes—Eggplant
Cucumbers—Honeydew melon and cantaloupe
Grapefruit—Cauliflower

AYURVEDA ACTION
Initiate Meal Time-Savers

The decision about what to prepare, shop for, and cook is often the biggest obstacle when trying to eat healthier. Ayurveda lifestyle is meant to make life easier, so don't strain. It is important to be flexible.

Here are time-saving hints I have found helpful:

- Use a rice cooker for rice and other grains. While rice is cooking, sauté a few veggies in ghee and spices.
- Come up with seven "go to" menus, including shopping lists. Keep the lists in your wallet or on your phone.
- Freshly prepared food is best, but a soup with a lot of veggies that you can eat over three days serves you better than eating processed fast food.
- When I like a recipe, I put it in a notebook so it's handy when I am thinking about what to fix for dinner.

SEPTEMBER 26
SCIENCE OF BREATH

YOGIS WHO ARE masters of "svarodaya" claim to be conscious of every breath they take. But most of us breathe without thinking. Breathing often reflects your state of mind. When you are stressed, breath becomes shallow and focused in the upper chest. You feel tension as your primitive brain is activated. This automatic functioning can result in thoughts and emotions of which you are unaware. In turn, this unexamined, subconscious thinking and feeling results in habits and programmed responses that might not even relate to any present circumstance. In contrast, breathing deeply into the lower lungs increases relaxation and leads to clarity of mind. Deep breathing is more likely when you commit to conscious, mindful breathing.

On inhale, air travels through the trachea (windpipe) to the lungs' bronchial tubes and smaller, limb-like bronchioles until it reaches tiny air sacks called alveoli. The lungs remove oxygen from the air and put it into the bloodstream. Oxygen and blood should be in balance. However, blood is unevenly distributed throughout the lung field, as the force of gravity results in more blood collecting around the lower lungs. When breathing is shallow, the deep pools of blood around the lower lungs don't get sufficient oxygen. If lungs are damaged, the blood-oxygen ratio is more inefficient.

What does this mean for physical, mental, emotional and spiritual health? When you breathe deeply, called diaphragmatic breathing, oxygen goes to the lowest part of the lungs, where the blood is most abundant and ready to release cellular waste and pick up fresh oxygen for transport. Shallow/chest breathing requires more effort to achieve the proper blood-oxygen ratio. It taxes the heart. Regular, slow, deep breathing is less stressful to the body and makes body processes more efficient.

AYURVEDA ACTION
Breathe for Higher Consciousness

DEEP BREATHING CALMS the nervous system and allows the brain's frontal lobe to engage more, which lessens the effect of the primitive brain. Try breath awareness strategies:

- As you sit to meditate, take a few moments for breath awareness. Notice your breath, the movement of your lungs, the feel of air on your nostrils.
- Practice yoga? Focus attention to the breath often. Breathe deeply as you move through asanas.
- While walking, become mindful of breath. What thoughts are you having? Move past the habitual, shallow breathing that engages the subconscious to deep breathing, which activates the higher, conscious mind. Become aware that with every breath, you are offering oxygen to enrich and nourish every cell of your body.

SEPTEMBER 27
BRAIN FOG—WHAT'S GOING ON?

Do you feel like your mind has become vague and wandering, perhaps soft around the edges? The brain is such a mystery, and it is often taken for granted. If you think nothing can be done for the brain, that over time it inevitably will decay—well, that could not be further from the truth. You can learn how to cleanse and nourish your brain. See also next. {Sept 28}

Keeping the lymph system clean and nourished helps keep your brain sharp. Ayurveda has long known the value of this, and now the arc of Ayurveda meets science.

TOXINS IN THE BRAIN—LYMPH IN THE BRAIN

About a decade ago, scientists used new microinstruments and technologies to discover lymph vessels hidden alongside blood vessels in the brains of mice. In 2015, scientists confirmed that lymph vessels are also found in the human brain. The lymph system clears toxins and delivers nutrients. Previous to this discovery, it was believed that the brain was exempt from the lymph system and relied only on the circulatory system to move nutrients and waste.[58]

This discovery changes everything. With an influx of indigestible (preserved) fats, toxins in food, heavy metals, and chemicals in the air, your brain is accumulating toxins like never before. Physiology can normally handle alien toxins, but when there are too many, or the digestive system has been overwhelmed and diminished, the toxins cannot be eliminated. They wind up in our brains and cause a host of problems such as brain fog, inflammation, and diseases like Parkinson's. Most people are in this state of overload.

Now that scientists have discovered the tiny lymph system in the central nervous system and brain, you can use strategies to keep the lymph clear and clean the brain.

AYURVEDA ACTION
Consider These Herbs to Freshen the Mind

Gotu kola

Enhances memory & concentration, supports the nervous system.

Bacopa

Calms and clears the mind.

Gotu kola and bacopa are also referred to as brahmi (very unusual for two herbs to be called by the same name) and often are taken together. A typical dosage is 1/4 to 1/2 tsp each in hot water. Strain and add raw honey when cool enough to drink if you wish.

SEPTEMBER 28
CLEANSING BRAIN LYMPH

THE BRAIN LYMPH system surrounds the brain sinuses in a large web of vessels in the skull from the forehead to the nape of the neck. According to Ayurveda, the innumerable and subtle lymph drains must be unclogged to properly eliminate toxins. About three pounds of toxins should drain from the brain lymphs each year.[59]

Lymph fluid gets pushed into the brain from a tight collection of blood vessels at the brain's base. The lymphatic fluid washes through the brain ventricles like a power washer, clearing toxic chemicals such as mercury, iron, and protein particles in the sinuses. From there they drain into cervical lymphs and into nasal lymphs. Brain lymphs that do not drain properly are connected to cognitive decline, anxiety, depression, and brain fog. Physical and emotional toxins can get lodged in the brain.

MOLECULES OF EMOTION

THE BRAIN CAN hide traumatic experiences, which allows us to function better. However, you might have recurrent, fragmented memories you can't shake. Childhood traumas are like deeply seated emotional toxins in the brain. We block awareness of that pain in the saggital sinus or brain lymph system.

Cleansing the brain lymphs removes physical toxins that contribute to deterioration, but you can also release molecules of emotions that influence your daily perceptions. You can cleanse the cerebrospinal fluid in the brain lymphs by doing Nasya, cleaning nasal sinuses with herbalized oil.

AYURVEDA ACTION
Do a Super Nasya Cleanse for Brain Fog

A SIMPLE NASYA is to tilt your head back and drop 1/4 dropper of special, herbailized oil into each nostril and inhale strongly to force the oil up into the nasal passages. Dr. John Douillard has a Super-Advanced Nasya cleanse. Details are on his website (lifespa.com), but here is a four-step summary:[60]

1. Massage the neck and head for 5 minutes, take a hot shower, and carefully inhale steam from a pan with boiling water plus a couple drops of eucalyptus oil. Apply hot towels or hot water bottles to the face and head sinuses for a few minutes.
2. Lie on a bed with your head hanging off the side, nostrils facing up and perpendicular to the floor. Take a few deep breaths through the nose and then drop 2–3 drops of Nasya oil into each nostril. With one big inhale, sniff the oil into the sinus cavities.
3. Afterwards, gargle with 2 tsp natural salt in 12 oz warm water.

SEPTEMBER 29
EMOTIONAL FLOW

AYURVEDA DOES NOT distinguish physical ama from emotional ama. Have you noticed that if you overload on sugar, your mood will spike and then deflate? You go from feeling energetic to lethargic, maybe even crabby. It all springs from the same connection.

As previously mentioned, physical and environmental toxins are stored primarily in fat cells. In Ayurveda, emotional toxins are stored in fat cells as well. Cleansing flushes out physical toxins as well as lingering, sluggish emotional toxins. According to Dr. Candice Pert, author of *Molecules of Emotions*, repetitive thinking loops get synced to patterns lodged in your fat cells in childhood. The patterns are like a tuning fork, which "hypnotizes" your raw emotional energy into the familiar. Thus, you find yourself repeating old patterns throughout adulthood.[61]

BALANCED MENTAL-EMOTIONAL STATE AND A CONTENTED SOUL

ONE WAY TO break up these patterns is through talk therapies and developing awareness of subconscious patterns and motivations. Another way is through toxin-cleansing diet strategies. Sound healing and or mantra chanting are other ways to disrupt old vibrational patterns.

According to Dr. John Douillard, who has written extensively on this topic, "The most effective way to convince the body that it is safe enough to release those toxins is to stimulate a fat-burning process. Once the body engages into a calm state of steady fat-burning, toxins stored within the fat cells and the pent-up molecules of emotions are released into the bloodstream."[62]

AYURVEDA ACTION
Emotional Cleanse

MEDITATION IS AN effective strategy for emotional cleansing. Each type of meditation has its purpose. For instance, concentrating on a flame fosters greater concentration. Mantra meditation supports emotional cleansing. It uses the mantra's sound and energy to break down constructions of the mind.

Stresses released in meditation are the old emotional patterns. To release emotional toxins, set aside time to meditate. One thing that has helped me be consistent is a change in language from "I've got to meditate for 20 minutes" to "I get to meditate for 20 minutes." I feel a sense of gratitude for meditation rather than seeing it as an obligation.

SEPTEMBER 30
RECAP AND WHAT'S AHEAD

SEPTEMBER IN MANY countries begins an academic year—or perhaps just provokes that memory. Either way, we seem to get a second wind for self-improvement, perhaps because the year is heading into the home stretch, or because cooler weather is coming.

We looked at supporting and improving the health of big organs like the liver, heart, and brain. In Ayurveda, physical and emotional health are integrated. Clearing ama is important. The liver, in particular, is affected by alcohol and sugar. With mainstream science's discovery of a micro-lymph system in the brain (Ayurveda always knew), cleansing the lymph system becomes even more important. Ama in the brain lymph can lead to a host of issues related to mental health and aging.

Building a strong immunity system was another September focus. The fall often brings more colds and flus, partly because we may begin to have more stress in our lives, and because we are around groups of people in more confined spaces. September is a great time to fortify your immune system. Using fresh ginger daily is a good way to do this.

WHAT'S NEXT?

OCTOBER BRINGS US to the final month of Pitta season. This is a good time to consider a fall cleanse. See cleanse entries. {index} After spring, the fall is the most important time to cleanse. We will dive into understanding the six stages of disease and how to halt its progress early on. The nights are getting longer, and sleep may be more inviting. You will learn how to get a better night's sleep. And we'll examine teeth, which we often think about only when there is a problem. Teeth are alive and need real attention!

MONTHLY REFLECTION TIME

WHAT ACTIONS DID you try? What was your experience? Did the new action feel worthwhile? Did you like it? Did you have an adverse reaction? Put a check in the third column for actions you plan to incorporate daily, weekly, monthly, seasonally, or on occasion.

What New Actions This Month?	*Your Experience?*	*Habit Worthy?*
		☐
		☐
		☐

OCTOBER 1
SIX STAGES OF DISEASE AND PREVENTION

Let's look at how disease manifests from an Ayurveda vantage, beginning with a review of the six stages in disease progression.

Ayurveda enables you to recognize and correct imbalances that lead to disease before symptoms occur. In conventional medicine, a disease isn't diagnosed unless the patient has specific symptoms, or lab tests indicate a health issue. Ayurveda can determine what is going on *before* illness manifests. Prevention through balance is the first priority. If that is not successful, Ayurveda attends to the cure.

Pathogenesis is the field of science that studies how a disease develops over time. Understanding this slow-moving process helps you intervene and correct before health issues become severe and possibly irreversible.

The six stages are listed below, and we will dive deeper into each one on subsequent daily readings.

1. ACCUMULATION—A dosha increases and accumulates in its seat at a rate that is more than the body can expel.
2. AGGRAVATION—If accumulation is not stopped, the dosha becomes aggravated and symptoms become noticeable.
3. MIGRATION—The aggravated dosha moves from its seat and spreads into tissues.
4. RELOCATION—When the traveling, imbalanced/aggravated dosha finds tissue weakness, it deposits there.
5. MANIFESTATION—The imbalanced dosha settles in the weak spot. A resulting problem or disease could start out minor, but unattended, will likely grow.
6. CHRONICITY—The excessive dosha disrupts system integrity and disease or conditions are evident.

AYURVEDA ACTION
Alleviate Accumulation & Aggravation of a Dosha

When you self-assess, or a practitioner gives you feedback that a dosha is out of balance, it's time to do something. Begin to calm Vata, cool Pitta, or energize your Kapha. This is a good time to take Assessment 1 again. Has anything changed? Which dosha is out of balance for you today? Engage at least one lifestyle strategy and change your diet to pacify the out-of-balance dosha. If you catch imbalances when they are small, they're easier to tame.

OCTOBER 2
STAGES OF DISEASE & PREVENTION—ACCUMULATION

A DOSHA CAN increase and accumulate in its seat at a rate that is more than the body can expel. There is a seat for each dosha in the gastrointestinal track—illustrating the importance of good digestion. For Vata, the seat is primarily the colon; for Pitta, the small intestine and stomach; and for Kapha, the stomach and lungs. You might notice accumulation as discomfort, or you might not notice it at all. If Vata is moving out of balance, you could experience more air in the form of gas. Pitta accumulation might show up as heat around the belly button or yellowish discoloration around the eyes or in the urine. Kapha accumulation is indicated by lack of hunger, slow digestion, or feeling full.

The doshas are principles of intelligence. Through imbalanced diet or lifestyle, as well as personal and environmental stressors, imbalance in doshas starts the disease process. Dosha imbalances can be identified through self-observation or working with an Ayurveda practitioner, who uses pulse, tongue, client concerns, and observation assessment.

This first stage is minor imbalance, and likely you are feeling fairly healthy. You might instinctively eat the opposite/balancing tastes of the accumulated dosha. Trust your instincts here. If you are drawn to what is good for you, it is easy to find balance.

AYURVEDA ACTION
Detox Daily

DAILY DETOXIFYING IS the most helpful strategy for preventing disease. Even if you eat organically and use nontoxic cleaners, you're still exposed to plenty of toxins. Everyone should cleanse and detox every day.

My favorite detox strategies are:

- Drink hot spice water {xvi}.
- Scrape your tongue first thing every morning {Apr 20}.
- Eat fresh ginger or have fresh ginger tea every day {Feb 4}.
- Take triphala or triphala guggulu tablets or drink triphala tea before bed every night. {May 8}.

OCTOBER 3
STAGES OF DISEASE & PREVENTION – AGGRAVATION

If the accumulation is not stopped, the dosha becomes aggravated and noticeable. Vata aggravated may result in increased gas and constipation. You might notice pain in the back or flanks (sides of the torso just below the ribs). Pitta aggravated may show as heartburn, acid indigestion, or aggression. Kapha aggravated may increase mucus in the lungs or be experienced as bloating or lethargy.

Ayurveda uses the term "vitiation" to indicate when there is a qualitative change in a dosha. The term means the dosha has "become abnormal" or "spoiled."

At this phase, you're typically disturbed enough that you begin to be attracted to foods and behaviors that will make the condition worse. Now you cannot trust your instincts, as you could during the accumulation stage. Once you start this path, you need conscious effort to get back on track.

Using the law of opposites, when a dosha becomes excessive, you add the opposite. Too much Pitta—cool and calm it. Too much Vata—ground it. Too much Kapha—move it.

AYURVEDA ACTION
Eat Lightly

This is a good time to eat lightly and commit to breaking bad eating and lifestyle habits. For instance, are you starting to eat on the run, grab for chocolate, stay up late? Make minor adjustments back toward balance.

OCTOBER 4
STAGES OF DISEASE & PREVENTION – MIGRATION

The aggravated dosha moves from its seat and spreads into the tissues. You might sense that something is wrong, but you cannot quite pinpoint what. The problem is on the move, looking for a place to settle. Symptoms are occurring, but they may not be distinct. The situation is still reversible if you attend to it with committed awareness and action.

Vata, the dosha of movement, is always involved. This is the state of the vitiation moving to find a vulnerable place to settle. It could move to the ears, skin, bones, or thighs. Watch for dehydration during this phase. You might develop a craving for more dryness, such as dry, crunchy foods.

Pitta might move to the stomach, eyes, skin, and heart. You may find yourself craving hot, spicy food.

Kapha will move to the lungs and host congestion in the lungs, sinuses, or the lymph system of the head, resulting in headaches. You have a craving toward sugary foods.

Again, those cravings are not serving you at this stage of progression.

AYURVEDA ACTION
Reverse Direction

If you're aware, halt and reverse the direction of the imbalance progression right here. If Vata is vitiated, eat warm, cooked foods, invite regularity in your schedule, and hydrate! If it is Pitta that is moving around, pacify it with sweet, cooling foods like dairy products. And if Kapha is disturbed, warm up Kapha with spicy foods and more activity.

OCTOBER 5
STAGES OF DISEASE & PREVENTION—RELOCATION

When the migrating, imbalanced dosha finds weakness in tissue, it will deposit there. This weakness may be:

- inherited
- a predisposition
- caused by injury
- a result of past-life actions
- left over from previous illnesses
- from physical/emotional trauma
- part of addiction
- unresolved emotions
- a result of over- or underuse of some part of your body, mind, or spirit

When the dosha excess enters this weak spot, it changes the tissues and its qualities. The tissues become dull.

A battle ensues between the agni (digestive capacity) of the tissue and the aggravated dosha. If the dhatu (tissue) agni is weak, vitiation will win. The dosha will change the qualities of the confronted tissue, which eventually disturbs proper formation of mature tissue.

For example, excess Vata might make the tissue it affects cold and dry. Excess Pitta might bring heat and oiliness. Excess Kapha could result in stagnation and pooling of toxins, as well as congestion.

AYURVEDA ACTION
Get Serious About Balancing Your Dosha

Look at what is holding this imbalance in place too long. Make decisions to reduce the stress, or avoid exposure to toxins, or whatever is the issue.

If you rebalance (or pacify) the excessive dosha before it goes beyond this stage, you can prevent lasting damage. Continue with daily detox routines. This is the time to get serious with menu planning and embedding good lifestyle habits. Rest is very important, too.

OCTOBER 6
STAGES OF DISEASE & PREVENTION–MANIFESTATION

The imbalanced dosha has settled in the weak spot. It could be minor at first, but left unattended, the problem will grow in intensity. The problem might start as minor aches from Vata that have settled in the joints, or excess mucus in the sinuses from settling Kapha, or a Pitta imbalance that has settled as a skin irritation.

The excessive dosha has won over the dhatu. Symptoms will be overtly, clearly observable, and you will know there is an issue. The seeds of the disease are taking root. Vata dryness in the joints becomes cracking, painful joints. Pitta heat in the tissues becomes inflammation. Kapha congestion will create swelling.

AYURVEDA ACTION
Try Panchakarma to Turn It Around

An Ayurveda approach to manifested disease could include herbal remedies and panchakarma (purification strategies) as well as diet and lifestyle changes. In addition to regular herbs taken for maintenance, an herbal remedy may need to be customized for the more serious condition that has arisen. This is a good time to work with an Ayurvedic practitioner or visit an Ayurveda healing center to participate in a panchakarma treatment. Keep good habits going. Ayurveda is generally a slow but sure process.

OCTOBER 7
STAGES OF DISEASE AND PREVENTION – CHRONICITY

The excessive dosha has disrupted the system's integrity, and disease or conditions are evident. Minor aches have formed arthritis in the joints; sinus tissues may become congested; that little skin irritation may manifest as eczema; and the symptoms have now emerged into a chronic condition. The dosha-targeted tissue and its surrounding area are stabilizing in a state of illness. At this stage, it is important to do more than just treat the disease.

Vata vitiated in this stage can be severe dehydration or even emaciation. Chronic Pitta imbalance could reveal as stomach ulcers, hemorrhaging, or bleeding disorders. Severe and chronic Kapha imbalance could show up as tumors and lipomas. We may need to use medications if the condition is in the advanced stage, however, you now know that it is important to rebalance the out of balance dosha that is the source of the problem so that healing is possible and the doshic triggers that keep the condition active can be withdrawn.

Allopathic treatment, also known as conventional medicine, primarily treats disease and its symptoms. This treatment might take care of the symptoms in this location, but the disturbance may spread or lie dormant to reappear. Ayurveda practices aim to work with the cause of the problem by determining the imbalances and then rebalancing them so that the natural state of health returns.

AYURVEDA ACTION
Work with Allopathic Treatment

Decide the best approach for you. Allopathic medicine is amazing in emergencies and offers testing capacities to identify what is happening with your physiology. As an Ayurvedic practitioner, I never suggest stopping medication or not seeking allopathic treatment. I was on the faculty of a medical school for three years. At that time, students received almost no instruction on nutrition. That was many years ago and now I see some medical schools are doing better in this regard.

As you work with your allopathic healthcare team, know that Ayurveda is great at building strength so your immune system will be robust enough to take over after major allopathic treatments do their work. It will be up to you and your natural-health team to help you restore your health as best as possible once a disease has become chronic.

Herbs might be useful here to kick-start balance restoration. You can do it one step at a time. Again, when situations are chronic, work with a competent Ayurveda or other natural health practitioners as part of your health care team.

OCTOBER 8
BENEFITS OF RAW APPLE CIDER VINEGAR—PART 1

Vinegar for therapeutic benefit goes back thousands of years, possibly to around 5000 BC. Raw apple cider vinegar (ACV) is the most available therapeutic vinegar. For full benefit, use organic, raw, unpasteurized, and unfiltered.

ACV contains trace minerals such as potassium, magnesium, calcium, sodium, phosphorus, and copper. It has multiple forms of the B vitamins, as well as vitamins A, C, and E. A daily dose of ACV provides antioxidants that inhibit molecule oxidation and block formation of cell-damaging free radicals.

Organic ACV is made by exposing apples to yeast, which begins fermentation and turns sugars to alcohol. Alcohol in this fermented form is healthy. Helpful bacteria are added as the brew continues to ferment. Thin strings of living, beneficial bacteria create sediment in raw vinegar known as the "mother," which is beneficial to health.

Myriad benefits of ACV are included here and in the following date. Precautions: ACV is not recommended for pregnant women or those breastfeeding, if you have GERD (gastroesophageal reflux disease) issues, or if you are on blood thinners. If you have these issues, consult with your primary care healthcare[allopathic] provider.

BALANCES PH

Humans are designed to burn fat for energy, but fat has been demonized, and we have been conditioned to grab sugar for energy. Many diets include processed, food-like substances, and meats and grains that are acidic when digested. Eating like this disturbs the body's pH balance, which can lead to bone-density loss, inflammation, and heart and mental conditions. While ACV (and lemon juice) is mildly acidic outside the body, its structures change to alkaline through the digestive processes.

BOOSTS STOMACH ACID PRODUCTION

Too much acidity has negative repercussions, but the stomach needs sufficient acid to break down food for proper digestion. ACV is rich in acetic acid, which boosts stomach-acid production in folks with low levels of HCL (hydrochloric acid), one of the three stomach/gastric acids. The ACV becomes more alkaline once it's been digested in the stomach and the ascetic acid decomposed.

AYURVEDA ACTION
Drink Apple Cider Vinegar Daily

Start with 1/4 tsp of ACV to see how that goes for you and then you can build up to 1 teaspoon of ACV two or three times daily for a maximum of one tablespoon. Taken in warm water daily, ACV can establish proper acetic acid levels.

OCTOBER 9
BENEFITS OF RAW APPLE CIDER VINEGAR—PART 2

Here we go—there are plenty more benefits of taking ACV daily.

Promotes Healthy Cholesterol

The ascetic acid in ACV lowers bad cholesterol levels (LDL) that can build up in the blood stream and lead to heart conditions.

Supports Healthy Blood Sugar

Research has shown that ACV reduces blood-sugar spikes after eating. The ACV could prevent the complete digestion of sugars and simple carbohydrates and in this case, passing these through without complete digestion can be good. Balancing blood sugar reduces cravings, and increases satiety, and supports weight loss.

Acts as a Powerful Antioxidant

ACV is rich in antioxidants and can reduce the effects of stress.

Improves Skin

ACV can be applied directly to skin. It has antimicrobial properties and is sometimes used to treat head lice, warts, and mild eczema. The Medicinal Botanical Program at Mountain State University recommends a 50/50 solution of water and ACV applied to skin[63] to provide relief for minor issues. For sensitive skin dilute more—one tablespoon to one-half cup water. You can also add a half-cup of ACV to bathwater.

Inhibits Candida

Candida bacteria reside in the gut. However, candida can overproduce and overwhelm gut balance, causing issues like yeast infections, toe fungus, and more. A daily drink of ACV diluted in water can restore natural balance.

Lowers Blood Pressure

ACV increases calcium absorption from the large intestine, which is linked to lowering blood pressure.

AYURVEDA ACTION
Test Doses of Apple Cider Vinegar

Take 1 teaspoon to 1 tablespoon with 8–12 ounces of water 15–30 minutes before meals or drink the Ayurveda simple detox drink {Jan 26} with some added beneficial ingredients {Jan 27} first thing in the morning. Test small amounts of ACV for internal consumption, and test small areas on skin for external applications. ACV is a strong substance so do indeed test what works for you and I invite you to do more research on this topic to find your comfort zone.

OCTOBER 10
SWEET DREAMS ARE MADE OF THIS!

Would you like to feel energized with abundant vitality? Would you like your skin to glow from inner radiance? Would you like to own your strength and endurance? Would you like to feel rested and grounded and fully alive in ways that open you to authenticity and love?

LAST QUESTION: HAVE YOU BEEN SLEEPING OKAY LATELY?

Some people are great sleepers—they could nod off on a train or in a thunderstorm. Others are challenged to get their nightly ZZZs. I am one of the latter, so I have a keen interest in this topic. Sleep issues can stem from long-standing doshic tendencies, a doshic imbalance, and time of life. It also could be seasonal with more daylight and activity in summer (Pitta) and more disturbance and dryness in the fall (Vata).

Sleep is one of the three pillars of good health in Ayurveda. (The others are proper digestion, and proper lifestyle.) If sleep is compromised, that creates conditions for poor health.

When you have a lot to do, it's tempting to burn the midnight oil and forgo sleep, but it is the *last* thing you should do. Sleep reconnects you with Source—the underlying field of intelligence. Source intelligence restores energy, builds cells, regulates weight, and strengthens immunity.

Sleep also is a time to digest emotions and daily experience. During sleep, your brain performs specialized sorting, stabilizing, and filing tasks. It culls, reinforces, and stores memories from the day. Lots of essential restorative activity happens during sleep.

Restful nightly sleep is the key to peak performance for individual tasks, an entire day, or long term. Ayurveda offers simple, effective tools to invite deep, restful sleep.

AYURVEDA ACTION
Do This When You Aren't Sleeping Well

1. Close down all media at least 30 minutes before bedtime.
2. Do not take your phone into your bedroom.
3. To relieve chronic insomnia, take 1/4 tsp or up to /2 tsp ashwagandha powder in warm raw milk or milk alternatives at bedtime. Grate in a little nutmeg (1/4 tsp) to invite deeper sleep.

OCTOBER 11
IS NAPPING OKAY?

IN GENERAL, NAPPING is not recommended by Ayurveda, because sleeping during the day can impede your ability to easily fall asleep at night. There are exceptions, however: sometimes a nap is warranted.

- The very young and the elderly need more rest and a nap may serve well.
- When it's hot in the summer and you feel exhausted or depleted, a short nap can be helpful.
- Rest or a nap after sex can help you restore lost energy.
- Certainly, if you are ill then more rest is needed.
- If you are grieving the loss of a person or a dream or a security, then extra sleep may help; however, be careful not to fall into depression with too much sleep. Kaphas are more prone to this, as they love to sleep and generally do sleep well. They typically do not need naps.

BUT NOTE: Napping more than 30 minutes during daylight hours, before nighttime melatonin is engaged, can increase your tamas guna, which leads to dullness.

Ayurveda uses the term "satmya" to mean the body's acclimation to something that would not normally be considered healthy. If you are in a place where napping is a part of the culture, such as Mexico or some countries in the Middle East, then you get a free pass—as you are actually in tune with the Nature of where you live.

AYURVEDA ACTION
Try Meditating Instead of Napping

NAPPING MAY BE right for you under some of the conditions noted above. But you might consider meditation for 20 minutes rather than napping for 20 minutes to see if that restores your energy. Meditation increases melatonin, which enables more restful sleep at night. Meditation also helps you release repetitive limit-setting thoughts—often what interferes with falling asleep at night. If you are feeling fatigued during the day, try meditation. There are so many more benefits than from just rest.

OCTOBER 12
FIVE RITUALS TO INVITE REPLENISHING SLEEP

The body physiology needs a pattern that invites sleep. What you do all day affects the quality of your sleep, and restful sleep is vital to every aspect of health, from the health of your organs and hormonal processes to healthy cell development. Travel, holidays, and environmental conditions—life—can cause disruptions in your usual sleep pattern. If you get off track, gently return to sleep rituals.

And if you don't sleep well a night or two, well, that happens. Worrying and dramatizing your thoughts about needing sleep will likely awaken you more. Tell yourself it's okay and that you will get through the next day. Then, try these tips to support restful, nourishing sleep. You might be surprised with the results.

Warm milk and nutmeg nightcap: Nutmeg is one of the best medicines for calming the mind. Use raw milk if you can get it, or low temp vat milk, almond milk, or rice milk. Raw milk contains peptides (proteins) that calm nerves and reduce anxiety.

Take a hot bath before bed: To relax muscles and soothe Vata. Add Epsom salts to clear toxins and a favorite essential oil, such as lavender, for aromatherapy. However, if it's a hot day or your emotions are hot, try a cooling shower or bath instead.

Do abhyanga massage: Use sesame massage oil to soothe Vata or coconut or sunflower oil to soothe Pitta. For Kapha dry brush or use a small amount of sesame oil. If you're short on time, do a mini-massage focusing on scalp and feet.

Do some yoga: Starting your day with yoga can lead to better sleep at night. Doing stretches in bed can relax muscle tension.

Balance your dosha with diet: Favor foods that balance your sleep dosha imbalance. Difficulty falling asleep and restless sleep—that is Vata. Early morning awakening (2 to 4 a.m.) is Pitta. Sleeping but not feeling refreshed upon awakening is Kapha.

AYURVEDA ACTION
Increase Melatonin Naturally

Here are ways to naturally invite evening melatonin, which is necessary for sleep:

- Close down artificial light in the evening.
- Turn off your computer and phone screens, which emit 35 percent blue light—too much. Natural light is only 25 percent.
- Be in some sunlight every day.
- Eat melatonin-rich foods like goji berries, pineapples, oranges, tart cherries, walnuts, and almonds.

OCTOBER 13
FIVE MORE RITUALS TO INVITE REPLENISHING SLEEP

MEDITATE OR DO A RELAXATION PRACTICE: Once in bed, an easy breathing practice is to inhale to a count of three or four and to exhale double that count. Doubling the exhale releases the body tension so you can let go into relaxation. Want to go a step further? Use 1:2:4 breathing and take 8 breaths lying on your back, 16 breaths on your left side and 32 breaths on your right side.

MAKE YOUR BEDROOM SIMPLE, COOL, AND DARK. Use your bedroom only for sleep, sex, and meditation. Keep it sparsely decorated. Light exposure reduces the release of melatonin needed for deep sleep. Unplug any light-emitting devices.

DRINK HERBAL TEA. One to three times during the day will help avoid accumulating stress. Passionflower is a good herb for chronic insomnia. Tulsi and brahmi make great-tasting nervine/calming teas that promote restful sleep. Avoid caffeine after midday; it can stay in your system for 12 hours. Alcohol is a depressant. It might initially induce drowsiness, but it suppresses REM sleep (when dreams occur) and causes restless sleep after it metabolizes.

GO TO BED BY 10 P.M.: This is Kapha time and energies are slower. Pitta time is 10 p.m. to 2 a.m., so if you stay up after 10 p.m. you might get a second wind.

NOURISH YOURSELF: Here's an interesting phenomenon—sometimes you cannot sleep because you do not have enough energy to do so. It takes energy for the body to engage the proper responses to allow sleep and nighttime restorative processes such as re-energizing cells and cleansing waste from the brain.

If you cannot sleep because you are rehashing conflicts of the day, try breathing in an attitude of respect for yourself and the other person. Consider what lesson the experience might have for you. What might you choose to correct? Look for an opportunity to communicate with the person(s), or with someone who could open your understanding of the situation.

AYURVEDA ACTION
Try One of the Best Sleep Snackzzz

EATING TWO KIWI fruits 1 hour before bed for a month helped adults fall asleep 35 percent faster and sleep 13 percent longer.[64] The reason? Could be the high concentration of antioxidant vitamins C and E, which regulate sleep-related neurotransmitters in the brain, or the rich amount of serotonin found in kiwis. Ayurveda does not generally recommend snacking at night, but if you like having a snack and sleep is an issue too, try this tip.

OCTOBER 14
PRESCRIPTION SLEEP AIDS?

How are you sleeping? According to the U.S. National Sleep Foundation, good sleep health is strongly related to sticking to a regular sleep schedule:[65]

- Only 47 percent of adults report waking and feeling well rested.
- Maintaining a consistent sleep schedule and feeling well-rested are related; those with most regular and consistent weekday sleep schedules are about 1.5 times more likely to report feeling well-rested compared to their counterparts.
- When sleep schedules vary by more than an hour, about 40% say it affects their productivity.
- Women are more likely than men to have emotional and physical tolls on their sleep.
- Younger adults are much more likely than older adults to say less sleep affects them physically,

PRESCRIPTION SLEEP AIDS

Dr. Rubin Naiman, a clinical psychologist specializing in integrative sleep medicine tells us, "Sleeping pills don't work nearly as well as people believe." A meta-analysis of Trazodone, an antidepressant used to promote sleep, found it works about equally as well as a placebo. The study also found that it decreased the time it took to fall asleep by only about 15–20 minutes and increased total time sleeping by only 20 minutes.[66]

A surprising result is that sleeping pills tend to "result in amnesia for nighttime awakening." As an alternative, Dr. Naiman suggests regular use of a melatonin supplement and occasional use of other herbs to invite sleep. Melatonin supplementation is important, he says, because melatonin production is shut down by light. In our modern society, artificial light extends light-exposure time far beyond what our bodies evolved to understand. Try natural ways to increase melatonin first. {Oct 12} With time and a few Ayurveda strategies, you may invite sleep naturally.

AYURVEDA ACTION
Learn the Weight & Sleep Connection

According to a recent University of Stanford study, the less sleep people got, the heavier they were.[67] Insufficient sleep boosts ghrelin, a hormone that makes you feel hungry. Ever notice how you reach for the sugary foods to power through a day, when you have not slept well? The double whammy is that insufficient restful sleep also suppresses a hormone called leptin which makes us feel full. Science says lack of sleep causes hunger cravings and weight gain.

OCTOBER 15
HERBS FOR SLEEP & DETOX FROM SLEEP AIDS

About 4–5 percent of the U.S. population regularly take sleep medications. More women than men medicate for sleep, and sleep-medication use increases as people age. Even if effective in the short term, prescription medications lose their effectiveness over time. Sleep is more than being unconscious or passing out—a lot goes on. It is an active journey of physical and emotional digestion, an ordering of daily experiences, building of the immune system, repairing cells, and deep rest.

The liver processes sleeping pills, and they can toxify it. If you have been using sleep medication and want to reduce or stop, first clear your system and then use herbs that invite sleep. These can be made into teas or used in warm cow's milk or alternatives like coconut or almond milk. Withdrawing from prescription medications should always be discussed with your health provider.

HERBS TO DETOXIFY THE LIVER FROM SLEEPING AIDS

- Milk thistle
- Siberian ginseng
- Dandelion
- Turmeric

NATURAL ALTERNATIVES TO INVITE SLEEP

Western Herbs

- Valerian
- Kava kava
- Lemon balm
- Passionflower
- Chamomile
- St. John's wort

Ayurveda Herbs

- Jatamansi (Indian valerian)
- Ashwagandha
- Brahmi
- Triphala
- Neem (not if pregnant)
- Shatavari

In general, herbs should be used consistently only short term—try six weeks on and two weeks off—to help your system make proper adjustments. Typical doses are 1/4 to 1/2 teaspoon daily.

AYURVEDA ACTION
Drink Warm Milk for Better Sleep

IF RAW OR low-temperature vat pasteurized milk is unavailable, drink warm almond or coconut milk at bedtime. Give your milk an upgrade by adding one of these: chopped dates, chopped/skinned raw almonds, shredded coconut, ghee, saffron, or cardamom. Ashwagandha added to warm milk calms the nervous system.

OCTOBER 16
FALL CLEANUP WITH AYURVEDA!

FALL INSPIRES A time of gathering and bundling fallen limbs, raking leaves, last chance to clean your windows, and maybe even cleaning out a closet or two. Ayurveda says this is a good time to do internal cleanup as well.

Ama, the Ayurveda the term for toxins, is the sticky waste product of incomplete digestion, whether physical or emotional. Ama builds in the digestive track or seat of your emotions when digestion is weak or overburdened by the wrong foods or experiences. Unless cleared, ama travels through the body and settles to cause problems. An Ayurveda change of season presents an opportunity to cleanse ama from your system to prevent illness and charge up radiance.

Fat-soluble ama accumulates in fat cells. Stress tells the body it is in an emergency situation, and the brain sends messages to store fat for future energy. Stress-fat laden with toxins gets stored mostly around the belly and lower body. You crave stimulants, sugar, and carbohydrates. How much you eat is a factor, but weight and shape issues also can be about the capacity to properly digest food and the state of the environment in which we eat.

Good eating and lifestyle habits prevent ama from collecting. Purification strategies can eliminate it. Even small changes for a personal Ayurveda fall cleanup will reward you with energy, clarity of expression, and strengthened immunity.

AYURVEDA ACTION
Raid Your Pantry for Radiant Health

- CINNAMON warms and circulates blood, relieves pain, and benefits those with diabetes.
- GINGER boosts immunity, soothes queasy stomach, helps to expel mucus/phlegm, and helps some colds and the flu.
- WALNUTS strengthen the kidneys, combat chronic coughs, and help relieve pain in the knees and back.

OCTOBER 17
EVERYDAY DETOX & HEALTHY TRANSITION OF SEASONS

Detoxification is a daily experience in Ayurveda. Two of the easiest ways to detox: 1) sip hot spice water every 15-30 minutes throughout the day, and 2) allow three to six hours between meals without snacking so complete digestion can occur.

Effect of snacking

Snacking means the body will constantly burn the new foods taken in, resulting in no opportunity to burn stored fat—a container for much of the ama we host. Unless you are hypoglycemic or have other conditions that could be exacerbated, avoid snacking for regular detox. It is good to be hungry at mealtime. If you are salivating with anticipation, the digestive juices are ready to do their job.

More ways to detox

Eat more liquidy meals, such as brothy soups. Blending soups makes them easy to digest. One recommended detox soup is made with mung beans {Mar 20}. In Ayurveda, mung beans are considered to act like a magnet, drawing out ama. Kitchari, made with mung beans or lentils, rice, and veggies, is also a good choice for a detox meal.

The change of seasons brings on different environmental and psychological forces. Pitta season soon will transition to Vata season. Doing a conscious cleanse between Ayurveda seasons helps you drop some of your current unhealthy habits and begin more healthful practices.

For a seasonal detox, try focusing on a week-long diet of foods recommended in the Detox Diet {April 3} or other cleansing days. {index}

AYURVEDA ACTION
Eat Cooked Prunes for Breakfast

Another way to detox is to eat cooked prunes for breakfast, especially if you are constipated. If the stool becomes too loose, cut back or stop. Most other cooked juicy fruits are excellent cleansers, too. Really constipated? Prune juice is more intense.

OCTOBER 18
VITAMIN SUPPLEMENTS VS. HERBS

Wondering about vitamin supplements? Vitamins are in herbs! Ingesting herbs is a way to get vitamins and minerals naturally, in real food. Many people take vitamin and mineral supplements daily to fortify their well-being, but a number of recent studies question the capacity of synthetic, isolated forms of vitamins to offer nutrition that can be absorbed by the body.

When active ingredients are taken out of their food and herb "homes" and put into supplements, they lose much of their bioavailability. Some research suggests that synthetic vitamins may be doing harm. High doses could even increase cancer risk.[68]

Most synthetic vitamins contain artificial ingredients such as silicon or titanium dioxide, talc, dyes, waxes, artificial sweeteners, animal parts, and carcinogenic chemicals. If you take vitamins, check the ingredient list.

If you need more vitamins and minerals, food is the best source. Eat more fresh vegetables and a small amount of fruits. If you still need to supplement, choose quality over quantity.

Chyawanprash is an ancient Ayurveda jam that includes organic fruits and herbs that are natural sources of some vitamins and minerals. Chyawanprash is known for high vitamin-C content. Although not a complete source of daily vitamins and minerals, it is great to have an organic, whole-food product that supplies some of these nutrients in their natural form. The body can more easily absorb them. Put a teaspoon or so on your morning hot-grain cereal.

Here are high-vitamin herbs to include in your diet (they are also rich in minerals).

- Cilantro: Vitamin A, B6, C, K
- Kelp: Vitamin A, B1, B2 & B12, C, D, E
- Lemongrass: Vitamin A, B-complex, C
- Oregano: Vitamin A, C, K
- Parsley: Vitamin A, C, K
- Rose hips: Very high in Vitamin C, some A and B
- Watercress: C, D, E

AYURVEDA ACTION
Get Your Vitamin P

Okay, there isn't really a vitamin P. But if we imagined it to be so, it would be the vitamin of pleasure. When you eat in a settled environment and find pleasure in your food and company, you are doing wonders for your health.

OCTOBER 19
KITCHARI—THE AYURVEDA CLEANSING RESET

Kitchari is a quick reset if you are feeling sluggish after too many treats or if you have been traveling or stressed and your digestion is off. A three-day mono diet of only kitchari is a good, quick cleanse between seasons. Kitchari {Mar 19} is easily digestible and often referred to as Ayurveda's perfect meal. It is great to get into your regular diet and a wonderful way to get back on track.

Kitchari offers a delight to your body and senses. It can be the centerpiece of a cleansing mono-diet. One to three days a month of eating kitchari for every meal would be an easy way to cleanse regularly. This time-tested meal is a complete protein and rich in fiber.

If the taste of your kitchari seems bland, and you do not have issues with inflammation or ulcers, add more spices. Include veggies that are good for pacifying your excessive dosha. Top with toasted nuts or coconut to add crunch. Ayurveda believes disease begins in the digestive tract. Kitchari is your medicine.

White basmati rice is preferred for kitchari. It is easily digestible because the husk has been milled off. Other long-grained white rices are more nutritious than short-grained and have a lower glycemic index. Brown rice will supply more nutrients than white rice but is harder to digest. During a cleanse, the metabolism slows and agni decreases, so eat what is easy to digest.

Kitchari is cooked with a legume, sometimes garbanzo beans (Kapha pacifying), but traditionally split yellow mung beans. The husk of mung beans is hard to digest, but when split, the husk naturally falls off.

AYURVEDA ACTION
Try Coconut Oil Plus Chia Seeds to Boost Energy

Coconut oil is composed of healthy medium-chain triglycerides. Combining it with chia seeds can give you an energy boost. Mix 1 tablespoon coconut oil with 1/2 tablespoon chia seeds. Eat as is or spread on sprouted-grain bread.

OCTOBER 20
A PERFECT PROTEIN – RICE AND BEANS

Rice and beans make a perfect protein. What does this mean? Let's start here:

- Twenty amino acids combine in various configurations to make proteins the body needs.
- The body can produce only 10 of them on its own.
- The other 10 are essential amino acids and the body does not make these—your food can supply them.

Animal proteins are termed "complete" because they contain all 10 essential amino acids in forms we can assimilate. Plant foods, however, need to be combined to form a complete protein. Most grains, including rice, are low on lysine, a major building block for protein. This is one we get from food, and it is fundamental for normal human growth, proper cell function, and a strong stress response.

Legumes and lentils have lots of lysine but are low in other essential amino acids, specifically methionine, tryptophan, and cystine. Grains are high in these. Beans and rice together: a perfect combination and a staple for vegetarians. This combo is great for a cleanse because it keeps blood sugar stable so the body can burn fat, which is where most toxins reside. If you do not eat them together at the same meal, but on the same day you still get most of the benefit.

Juice- or water-only cleanses result in unstable blood sugar. People run into trouble with completing their cleanse and often crave sugars during and after. An Ayurveda cleanse with a foundation of mung beans and rice is a stable, effective solution. Fat metabolism is the goal of a cleanse, which won't happen if the body is stressed from blood-sugar instability.

AYURVEDA ACTION
Add Hing to Take Out Beans' Air Quality

Hing, also known as asafoetida, must be the original Beano. Hing is effective at removing excessive air quality from beans. It is powerful—you only need a pinch. Although it smells potent in the jar, once incorporated into a recipe it is moderate, like adding a bit of onion. Hing is a digestive aid and can reduce the growth of unhealthy flora in the gut, especially candida. It is known for significantly reducing gas. It is a powerful antispasmodic and is used to treat coughs and asthma.

Hing is hot and stimulating. It clears stagnation in the circulation and treats low libido.

Sauté a bit, less than 1/8 teaspoon, in ghee and add to your dish. Experiment from there to get the right amount for you.

OCTOBER 21
HEALTHY TEETH

I NEVER THOUGHT much about the liveliness of my teeth, but in the back of my mind I must have assumed that once fully formed, they were solid masses like piano keys. Not true! They have life circulating through them. And like other parts of the body, teeth are constantly breaking down and replacing their cells in a slow regeneration.

With proper nutrition from vitamins, minerals, and enzymes, along with good hygiene, teeth stay healthy. And surprise—damaged, decayed teeth can regenerate.

The primary focus in dentistry has been that sugar and acids on the teeth cause decay. It is a factor, but according to Nadine Artemis, a leader in natural dental care, the primary cause of decay is ingested sugars and processed foods that suppress the endocrine system. Therefore, the key to tooth health is keeping the inner tooth core vitally supplied by the hormone-regulated dentinal lymph fluid system that transports nutrients and hauls away toxins.[69]

- The dentinal fluid moves from inside the tooth outward, in a centrifugal fashion. When a tooth is compromised, more fluid rushes to repair the tooth.
- However, when the flow is interrupted or not strong enough because of poor digestion and toxins in the bloodstream, the movement reverses and becomes centripetal. That is, fluids containing bacteria, acids, and fungi are drawn into the tooth from the mouth.
- The pulp chamber becomes inflamed and oxidized. Slowly the enamel surface begins to demineralize and salivary enzymes break down the tooth. Bacteria takes hold, causing further decay. So yes, sugar sitting in the mouth will be sucked in and will interact with the bacteria in plaque to start decaying the tooth, but the changing direction of the fluid movement is the source.

This concept changes the understanding of the Nature of tooth health and what you can do to promote healthy teeth. Poor digestion and malnourishment are the originating causes of tooth decay. Ayurveda always proposes solutions to correct problems at their source.

AYURVEDA ACTION
Use Strawberries to Whiten Teeth

STRAWBERRIES CONTAIN MALIC acid, which helps remove stains and whitens teeth. Eat a bunch of strawberries or mash up a strawberry with a little baking soda and apply the paste to your teeth. It will fizz a bit. Leave on for five minutes; then brush and rinse.

OCTOBER 22
FLASH THOSE PEARLY WHITES

The key to a healthy flow of dentinal fluid is a nutrient-dense diet rich in minerals and vitamins—basically a healthy Ayurveda diet. Strong teeth grind and break down food, which improves digestion. Good digestion builds stronger teeth. Another virtuous cycle. However, brushing teeth daily with low-abrasive and even nourishing toothpaste keeps tartar at bay and establishes a healthy pH for our mouths. Here is a DIY toothpaste.

DRY TOOTH POWDER—USE ON ITS OWN IF YOU LIKE

- 3 Tbsp organic baking soda (mild abrasive)
- 1 Tbsp finely ground sea salt (mild antibacterial, whitener & good for gums)

Optional: 1/2 tsp. finely ground organic dried sage (sage is antimicrobial but has a strong taste)—or I use powdered organic neem

TOOTH OIL—ADD INGREDIENTS TO TOOTH POWDER TO MAKE DYI TOOTHPASTE

- Organic virgin coconut oil, softened but not liquified
- Few drops peppermint, spearmint, anise, clove or cinnamon-bark essential oil, according to the taste you want (be sparing, they are very strong)

DIRECTIONS: Grind natural mineral salt in a small coffee grinder to make it fine, otherwise it is abrasive. Mix in all dry ingredients. You can use this as a tooth powder if you wish. To make a paste, mix in a teaspoon of coconut oil at a time until you find the right consistency. Put into a small, sealable jar or squeezable container and keep in a relatively cool place. Brush. Don't forget to floss!

AYURVEDIC ACTION
Find Out—Is Baking Soda Good for Teeth?

Mild abrasion is important to eliminate plaque and stains. Baking soda is an old folk remedy for cleaning teeth, but is it safe? A scientific report produced by the FDA compares the abrasion factor of a number of toothpastes plus baking soda.[70] A value of 200 is the recommended limit. Here is a sample of findings:

07	straight baking soda
49	Tom's of Maine Sensitive
70	Colgate Total
93	Tom's of Maine Regular
110	Colgate Herbal
200	Colgate 2-in-1 Tartar Control/Whitening

OCTOBER 23
OIL PULLING

OIL PULLING IS a process of swishing oil in your mouth for 10–20 minutes before spitting it out. Benefits include loosening particles stuck in the teeth, reducing plaque and bacteria, and supporting gum health and oral hygiene. Because oil can blend with oil, it can attract and pull other oils and fat-soluble toxins out of tissues.

Bacteria in the mouth are the same as found in the plaque that forms in arteries. It makes sense to eliminate these bacteria as soon as they enter the body, before they have a chance to migrate into the bloodstream where they can do more harm.

Most over-the-counter mouthwashes are alcohol based and wipe out both good and bad microbes. Research on oil pulling has shown its capacity to deter bad bacteria and plaque while toning gum tissue.[71] Mouth health also is related to healthy joints and jaw muscles.

In addition to improvements in the gums and sinuses, oil pulling freshens your breath. When you regularly oil pull, you are supporting healthy microbial populations and limiting volatile sulfur compounds (VSCs), which gets to the source of bad breath.

Each morning after scraping your tongue {Apr 20} and brushing teeth, take one tablespoon of oil into your mouth and swish for 10–15 minutes. Thoroughly move the oil around. It could be helpful to do this in the shower. Commonly recommended oils are organic sesame or coconut oil or a combination of the two.

The oil becomes thin and whitish when it has done its job. Spit it out in the trash or the toilet, not the drains, to avoid clogging. Do not swallow the oil. You don't want to ingest the bacteria and plaque the oil has pulled.

AYURVEDA ACTION
Use These Oils for Oil Pulling

SESAME OIL IS traditionally used for oil pulling. As it is warming, this would be a good oil for Vatas and Kaphas or during those times of the year. Coconut oil is also good and is more cooling for Pitta. Coconut oil is also antibacterial and antiviral. Remember, the oil is pulling out toxins, so spit it out afterward.

OCTOBER 24
NATURAL TEETH WHITENING WITH TURMERIC

THE TEETH-WHITENING INDUSTRY alleges that common ingredients used—carbamide and hydrogen peroxides—are safe. However, even the American Dental Association expresses caution. I am suspicious that anyone should consider them either safe or okay "with caution," and I was happy to learn that turmeric, a yellow spice that stains everything it touches, actually whitens teeth.

I have tried brushing with organic turmeric. Sometimes I follow the turmeric by brushing with a little baking soda, salt, and organic neem (not if pregnant) powder. The combination works well!

Turmeric whitens your teeth, but stains everything else, so you might want a dedicated toothbrush. Be very careful to wipe away any drops of turmeric on your countertop, because it can stain and the stains are difficult to remove.

IMPORTANT: TURMERIC HAS A SLIGHT ABRASIVE EFFECT, SO DON'T MAKE THIS A DAILY HABIT. Start with once or twice a week until teeth are whitened and then stop until you notice you need to whiten again.

AYURVEDA ACTION
Whiten with Turmeric

YOU CAN CHEW fresh turmeric root or use organic turmeric powder. Wet your toothbrush and dip it in the turmeric powder and brush as usual. Let the turmeric sit on your teeth for 5–10 minutes. Spit it out; then brush and rinse a few times.

OCTOBER 25
BE READY TO MAKE THE TWIST AND TURN!

You want good prana, or your internal life force, to flow freely and nourish so you can have healthy relationships, effective and satisfying work, and a delightful sense of playfulness. A change in the season signals a time for you to change, too. Unless you are paying attention, external forces can have their way with you. Illness could result.

Let's understand the dynamic of this seasonal turn and why action is essential.

- Over the summer, most people get heated internally, unless they were conscious about Ayurveda strategies such as eating cooling foods and using cooling herbs. Once Vata winds arrive, lingering internal summer heat turns to dryness, which intercepts complete digestion and snags toxins. The downward spiral begins.
- Autumn winds blow in dry, cold, rough, and light qualities. Without adjustments, your internal conditions might match these external changes, which could lead to coldness, dryness, roughness, stress, immune-system aggravations and weight gain.

If you get sick, and we all do at times, know that the illness builds and informs your immune system for the future. No guilt necessary!

Here are four high-impact strategies to meet the new season so that you can release accumulated summer heat and add moisture to your tissues. These will give you a good start for a healthy autumn Vata transition:

1. Reset digestion.
2. Purify tissues.
3. Boost the immune system.
4. Shift to a Vata diet.

These strategies will be detailed in the next four day entries. Don't feel pressured to do every strategy offered above. Do what feels right and know your intention is to take some discerning control and not just ride the bronco. Intention goes a long way.

AYURVEDA ACTION
Make Your Own Lip Balm

When the winds come, so can chapped lips. Combine 2 tablespoons coconut oil with 2 tablespoons beeswax and 1 tablespoon shea butter. Warm slowly in a saucepan. Use a small funnel to put in containers. Let set until solid.

OCTOBER 26
RESET YOUR DIGESTION

Have you seen the saying "When mama is happy, everybody is happy"? Healthy digestion is mama, generating good prana intelligence that informs the building, expressing, and eliminating life forces within you.

Here are a few quick ways to do a digestion reset:

- Start each day by drinking hot lemon water. This stimulates your liver and kick-starts your digestion.
- Remove hard-to-digest foods from your diet for seven days, including processed foods, breads, soy, gluten, meats, and sugars.
- Eat whole foods, including lots of vegetables and some whole grains.
- Eat a mono-diet of kitchari [Mar 19] for 1–3 days.
- Do not snack between meals or after supper for seven days. Allow your digestive system to rest between meals.
- Hydrate between meals but drink no more than 1/2 cup water, preferably hot, with your meal. Too much water with food weakens the digestive juices.

AYURVEDA ACTION
Try a 1-Day Mono-diet Reset

For one day, eat the same thing at every meal. It could be kitchari or vegetable juices. Fresh, juicy, whole fruits are good too—but a fruit-juice diet is not recommended because of the sugar content. You could do this reset one day a month or maybe one day a week, but not more often. Never take on a digestive cleanse when you are weak or your health is unstable, or if you are pregnant or nursing. If your health is not good, it is better to eat a mix of foods, but you could lean toward watery, brothy soups that are nourishing and easy to digest. When in doubt, get guidance from a health professional.

OCTOBER 27
PURIFY YOUR TISSUES

LINGERING INTERNAL HEAT from the hotter months can mean tissues are dry, and the winds of this season bring dryness as well. Your body, the great homeostasis instrument that it is, creates reactive mucus to moisturize the dry tissues. Excess mucus is a breeding ground for bacteria, which can generate seasonal illnesses.

To stay healthy at this seasonal turn, cleanse old toxins lodged in dry tissues. Under guidance, or if you are experienced, consider a dramatic cleanse. {Apr 4} However, a moderate daily cleansing to clear your shrotas/channels is another option.

A few quick ways to cleanse tissues:

1. Drink lemon detox tea each morning. {Jan 27}
2. Drink hot spice water throughout the day {xvi}.
3. Take 1-2 tablets triphala or triphala guggulu at bedtime or make powder into tea. Triphala cleanses the villi in the intestinal tract, allowing nutrients to reach tissues, and guggulu pulls deeper toxins from joints {May 8}.
4. Drink brahmi/gotu kola tea or tulsi tea each day to clear brain tissues and ease the agitated mind {July 5}.
5. Use turmeric in cooking, make turmeric tea, or take 3-4 tablets of turmeric 3 times a day between meals to reduce heat and purify blood {Mar 9}.
6. Hydrate. Drink lots of water, especially hot water, which is more cleansing. Take the shatavari herb to hydrate your tissues {Feb 4}.
7. Eat stewed apples {Nov 18} to dispel heat from your body. Stop if stools become too loose.

AYURVEDA ACTION
Meditate—It's the Great Purifier

THE BENEFITS OF meditation have been time tested through research and enlightened experience. Meditation reduces the patterns of beliefs, attachments, and negative protective self-talk. "Monkey mind" leaves you anxious. If you have wandered away from meditation, now may be a good time to re-establish a practice. If you haven't been given a mantra, try the universal mantra: OM.

Sit quietly for even five minutes to start. Take a deep breath. Then slowly say, or sing, or listen for the mantra. If you have a thought, the mind is detoxing. Once you only witness a thought, you are in Self, which is not monkey mind. When witnessing, you have dropped the enmeshment and can return to the mantra. Remember, having thoughts is not getting in the way of meditation. Awareness is part of the process. Just return to the mantra.

OCTOBER 28
BOOST YOUR IMMUNE SYSTEM

Ayurveda immunity means resistance against the loss of integrity, proportion, and interrelationship among an individual's bioenergies (doshas) and tissues (dhatus).

The Ayurvedic concept of immunity is intricately interwoven with the concepts of nutrition, agni (digestive fire), and tissue formation. Your immune system might be more unstable at the change of season, when the dosha balance is naturally transitioning to be more adaptive.

HERE ARE TIPS.

Cook with immune-boosting spices: Turmeric has an immune-modulating effect. It is detoxifying and enhances the intelligence of the immune cells. Cumin burns ama. Black pepper clears the energy channels so ojas can reach the deeper tissues.

Eat immune-boosting foods: Apples support the immune system because they contain antioxidants and both insoluble and soluble fiber, which cleanse the bowel. Leafy greens such as Swiss chard, kale, mustard greens, and spinach, when cooked with spices, are great immunity-boosters because they provide iron, calcium and other nutrients while cleansing the bowel. Other good foods include broccoli, cabbage, cauliflower and quinoa.

Drink immune system strengthening tea: Add a 1-inch piece of fresh ginger (sliced), a stick of cinnamon and 2 black peppercorns or trikatu powder (a combination of black pepper, long pepper, and ginger) to a quart of boiled water. Put in a thermos. Drink throughout the day. Add 1/2 teaspoon of raw honey, if desired, when ready to drink.

Hydrate: Sip hot water throughout the day, which is more hydrating and goes deeper into the tissues than an equivalent amount of room-temperature water. Avoid cold/iced water.

AYURVEDA ACTION
Remember Your Inner Intelligence

The human body has hundreds of different cell types and 50 to 75 trillion cells. Each cell knows who you are and where it has to be in order for it to be part of you—and to be able to communicate to all the other cells. This is called inner intelligence. In the world of cells information must flow, and ama blocks the flow of this information. Take a moment to be in awe of the intelligence operating within you at this very moment.

OCTOBER 29
SHIFT TO A VATA PACIFYING DIET

As Vata season approaches, most folks will benefit from a Vata-pacifying diet—or at least leaning in that direction. Generally, Vata season starts in November, but now is the time to get ready. Here is quick guidance for a Vata-balancing diet. Favor:

- Warm cooked foods, especially brothy soups
- Good fats like ghee and avocado, sesame and olive oils
- Grains, especially quinoa (highest in protein) and white basmati rice
- Root vegetables such as beets and carrots, and moist veggies like squashes and sweet potatoes.
- Nuts (not peanuts)
- Warming organic spices including cardamom, cumin, ginger, cinnamon, salt, cloves, fenugreek, mustard seed, and hingvastak (a blend containing hing)

AYURVEDA ACTION
Drink Vata Water

Perhaps you have been drinking your hot spice water but now as Vata season arises you may be aware of some Vata imbalances emerging like dryness or anxiety. Consider a change-up from hot spice water to Vata water: To a thermos of hot water, add three mint leaves, 1/2 teaspoon fennel seed, and 1/2 teaspoon marshmallow root.

Mint is sweet and pacifies all doshas. It is good for digestion and respiratory health. Fennel enkindles the digestive fire and supports digestion; it also calms the nervous system. Marshmallow root relieves irritation by coating inflamed surfaces. It is moisturizing to dry skin when taken internally.

OCTOBER 30
TRANSITIONING TO FALL

We are leaving Pitta season (July–October) and entering Vata. Depending on where you live, September and October could be a mix of summer and fall, with Pitta and Vata influences combining. But now we are solidly entering the fall Vata season, dry and cool. Everyone should adjust for a new dosha season, but especially those with Vata imbalances. Attend to this transition or the windy, cool Vata weather will throw you for a loop. Here are ideas.

DIET

Transition from cool, raw, light foods and drinks to those that are warm, cooked and grounding. Eat cooked, leafy bitter greens to help you to clear out accumulated Pitta from the hot weather. Root vegetables and brothy soups are great right now. Kitchari makes a balancing fall meal, and if you add fall squashes, your Vata will be happy. Add some sour taste. A great addition would be eating sauerkraut or kimchi to get Vata-pacifying sour taste as well as the probiotic {Jun 8} benefit of fermented foods.

Cook fall apples with a little water, ghee and spices like cinnamon to please your Vata. Raw apples aggravate Vata. Quinoa is a good grain for Vata season, and it is loaded with protein. Nuts and seeds are wonderful for the fall, especially almonds, cashews, brazil nuts, hazelnuts, walnuts, pumpkin seeds, sunflower seeds, and sesame seeds.

HERBS AND SPICES

Clear Pitta heat from the small intestines with triphala tea or tablets taken at night. Move from cooling summer drinks to hot teas. Always sip hot spice water daily, but consider tulsi tea or fresh-ginger tea. Use cinnamon and cardamom to flavor your food or in teas. Mild pepper spices like black and white pepper are good, but avoid hot chilies and horseradish—these are too drying for Vata.

LIFESTYLE

Fall winds can blow you off your mark. This is a time you might feel more anxiety and pressure to get it all done. Stick with or get back to routines such as daily meditation and yoga. Do abhyanga with sesame oil or almond oil. Be kind to yourself.

AYURVEDA ACTION
Make a Fall-Blend Tea

There are many tea recipes in this book. Here is another for transitioning to Vata season. Mix fresh ginger with crushed cardamom seeds and cinnamon pieces. You can use powdered ginger and cinnamon, but I prefer the pieces. Boil water, add spices, and steep for five minutes. Strain and enjoy. Add raw honey when cool enough to drink. Adjust spices to make tea the strength you like.

OCTOBER 31
RECAP AND WHAT'S AHEAD

In October you learned about the six stages of disease and the capacity of Ayurveda to prevent disease when the imbalance is at the early accumulation or aggravation stage. After that, you are treating the disease. The earlier you can make minor adjustments the better. The seasonal transition is a time to make minor changes, because the new dosha season brings environmental factors that affect you.

You also learned about the benefits of raw apple cider vinegar, one of Nature's little miracles. It is abundant in vitamins and minerals and is a strong antioxidant for dispelling harmful free radicals. ACV can balance pH and support the production of stomach acid needed for complete digestion. Check important precautions. {Oct 8}

Sleep is for resting, but is also a time to digest and build new cells and to clear the mind. Sleep hours are active and important for vital brain and body functions, so proper sleep is essential. One of the most important tips for improving sleep is to go to bed at a regular time—10 p.m. according to Ayurveda. Other ways to foster good sleep: increase melatonin naturally by getting more sunshine, drink warm milk with nutmeg or ashwagandha, and do a warm oil abhyanga massage. Here's to good ZZZs.

Ayurveda recommends cleansing between dosha seasons, advised in October and November as Pitta season transitions to Vata. A simple cleanse this time of year is to eat more liquidy meals like soups.

You also learned about healthy teeth. Keeping the teeth healthy is more about what gets into your tummy and how you digest it than what sits on your teeth.

WHAT'S NEXT?

In November we will learn how to navigate the dryer, colder Vata season. You will learn how to balance and ground Vata with warm cooked foods and by establishing routines.

MONTHLY REFLECTION TIME

What actions did you try? What was your experience? Did the new action feel worthwhile? Did you like it? Did you have any adverse reactions? Put a check in the third column for actions you plan to incorporate daily, weekly, monthly, seasonally, or on occasion.

What New Actions This Month?	*Your Experience?*	*Habit Worthy?*
....	....	☐
....	....	☐
....	....	☐

VATA SEASON

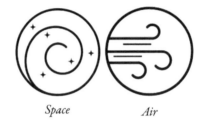

Space *Air*

NOVEMBER 1
VATA MOVES US

November: up, down, here, there, calm, stormy—a month of variable weather and sometimes variable moods. The natural heat and fire of Pitta season has moved on, and Vata season has arrived. Vata season generally runs November through February in the northern hemisphere, but it could be different where you live.

The Vata dosha is about movement and change, including breathing, digestion, and nerve signals. If Vata is dominant in your constitution, you are likely to have bursts of energy and high activity followed by fatigue. Vatas are quick about everything. They understand quickly, especially more ethereal topics, and they also forget quickly. "What did you say your name is?"

When your Vata is in balance you enjoy a creative mind, playful energy, enthusiasm, and lively conversation. When Vata is out of balance you experience anxiety, worry, insomnia, restlessness, constipation, dry skin, painful menstrual cramps, and other nervous disorders. More gaseous air in your system could be experienced in the form of burping or flatulence especially when you eat raw foods.

Vata dosha is responsible for more than half of illnesses because it typically goes out of balance first, especially from stress—and can lead the other doshas out of balance and cause early stages of disease. Balancing Vata is important for everyone. Everyone has some Vata. However strongly it is represented in you, it will be more susceptible to imbalance in Vata season. Vata is the dosha of life's later years—after 55 or 60. Even if Vata is not strongest in your constitution, it is wise to understand it.

Vata-types tend toward thinness and playfulness in action and spirit. They need to get sufficient rest and not overdo. Eating warm, cooked foods and staying warm are important. Vatas can be "flighty," so a regular lifestyle routine helps balance.

AYURVEDA ACTION
Adopt a Seasonal Routine to Pacify Vata

Routine is the operative word—Vata is soothed by regularity. Daily self-care is especially important to calm and nurture Vata. What are you doing now for self-care? Consider these tips for adding high-impact Vata balancing during Vata season:

- Daily, warm oil self-abhyanga massage. {Dec 6} Sesame oil is particularly balancing for Vata.
- Listen to calm, soothing music.
- Drink fresh ginger tea daily.

NOVEMBER 2
VATA FUNCTIONS

Vata is responsible for physical and mental movement, elimination of wastes, sensory input and nervous-system impulses, respiration, communication via speech, and other functions relating to movement. Its main site is the colon. If you experience bloating and gas, these may be early signs of *Vata* aggravation. Also watch for dry skin, constipation, irregular appetite, loss of sleep, stress, and tiredness. Internal drying can aggravate organs and disrupt the fluid functioning of your systems.

Fall, in the influence of Vata season, can be a time of anxiety. Vata is made up of the air and space elements, and emotionally stimulates racing thoughts and pounding-heart anxiety.

AYURVEDA ACTION
Balance Vata with the Principle of Opposites

As Vata season begins, focus on the qualities opposite of what cold weather brings. Think grounding, warming, and routine. Generate internal fire and warmth by eating more cooked foods and by grounding with yoga, massage, and meditation practices. Feed enthusiasm by connecting with others. Use more oils in cooking and on the body to moisten yourself during this dry season. Doing all of these as a daily routine soothes Vata back into place.

Be ready to invite in the good qualities of Vata—playfulness, good spirit, movement, and insightfulness! Making a few adjustments will invite your Vata autumn experience to be filled with healthy Vata and all the liveliness that brings.

NOVEMBER 3
VATA PHYSICAL TRAITS

Vatas' constitutions tend toward lightness in weight and delicate features. As noted, even if your birth constitution is Vata, imbalance issues of any dosha can lead to significant weight gain. Think of your body type when you were a child. Did you tend toward being thin? If so, your constitution could be Vata.

The face may be thin and oblong. A person with Vata constitution may have small eyes and a relatively small nose—the nose bridge, in particular, might be narrow. As with other features, the lips may be thin.

Complexion can be dull and tends toward dryness. Vatas do well to keep their skin oiled. When Vata is out of balance, hair loss could be an issue, and dandruff from dryness.

Bones with Vata constitution are usually long and narrow, but Vatas may also have irregular-shaped bones that are especially long or short. Bones can seem to stick out, too, as Vata bodies are not particularly muscular. Fingers can be long, and nails can be dry with ridges, or brittle.

AYURVEDA ACTION
Nourish Your Senses

Occupy your body. Bring it alive. Touch, taste, hear, smell, and see what is around you today. Nourishing your senses will bring you back into your own form as you experience your environment fully. Own it!

NOVEMBER 4
VATA SUBDOSHAS

Each dosha has five associate subdoshas, or intelligences. The names may not be important to you, but it can be helpful to know what is going on in your mind-body system with each dosha.

PRANA VATA

Located in brain, head, throat, heart, and respiratory organs. Prana Vata governs respiration, the mind, and perception through the senses. It is the force of magnetic attraction. In balance, *Prana Vata* draws in health, harmony, and well-being. Imbalanced leads to anxiety, insomnia, fears, neurological and respiratory disorders.

UDANA VATA

Located primarily in throat, navel, and lungs. *Udana Vata* is responsible for action and expression through speech, and enthusiasm. Imbalance leads to throat and speech issues, dry cough, and fatigue.

SAMANA VATA

Located in the stomach and small intestine. Samana governs peristaltic movement in digestion and represents the force of absorption. It carries nutrients from the intestines into the circulatory system and from your senses into the central nervous system. In balance, Samana supports sensory stimuli. Imbalance leads to improper digestion, gas, diarrhea, and malnourishment from food or experience.

APANA VATA

Located in the pelvic region. Apana governs impulses related to downward flow—urination, elimination, menstruation. It is dedicated to eliminating wastes. Imbalance leads to constipation, menstrual, and prostate issues.

VYANA VATA

Located in the heart and circulatory system. It governs blood circulation and heart rhythm. Vyana moves nutrients from the intestines into the circulatory system and sends signals from the nervous system to a muscle or organ. Imbalance leads to high blood pressure, irregular heart rhythm, loss of muscle tone, and stress-related autoimmune disorders in the muscles and nerves.

AYURVEDA ACTION
Use Yoga to Balance Vata Subdoshas

According to the Banyan Botanicals blog, these are yoga balancers (breathing and movement practices) for each subdosha:[72]

- Prana—Nadi Shodhana and Bhramari pranayama
- Udana—Nadi Shodhana and Ujjayi breath
- Samana—Kapalabhati and Bhastrika
- Apana—Yoga in general
- Vyana—Nadi Shodhana

You can learn more about these yoga techniques in local yoga classes or online.

NOVEMBER 5
VATA MIND

Recall that Vata is composed of air and space. These elements' qualities lead to understanding Vata mind. As it governs the nervous system, your mind experience can make it evident what is going on with your Vata. Out-of-balance Vata mind wanders; thoughts are unstable. You might feel easily irritated and have a general template of anxiety in your approach to life. The fight-or-flight response is quickly triggered. Vata's ungrounded nature can lead to feeling disassociated from the body, which leaves the sense of security disturbed.

Vata mind is quick to learn and also quick to forget. You might be intensely alert one minute and easily distracted the next. The Vata brain type is prone to impulsivity and sensation-seeking. Responses to external conditions might lead to bursts in attention, focus, and energy. The autonomic response may be strong and you may feel less controlled by your own motivation.

But Vata balanced? This gives you a beautiful sense of creativity and enhances your capacity to feel at home in the spaciousness of Spirit. Strong and healthy Vata is intuitive and often makes decisions that "work out well."

AYURVEDA ACTION
Establish Routines for Grounding

Learn to be still. Vata is aggravated by excessive movement and feelings of insecurity or fears. Take time to meditate or do gentle yoga, or establish other quieting, self-care routines. Eat at regular times.

NOVEMBER 6
VATA EMOTIONS

A FEAR RESPONSE is triggered easily when Vata is imbalanced. Phobias can arise. This can lead you to distance from others, with accompanying loneliness and anxiety. Vatas tend to be undernourished, and this lack of substance can bring feelings of sadness and even depression. Flightiness in the Vata-imbalanced mind could make it difficult to process emotions—which may be left unsettled and "up in the air." Mood swings might be dramatic. The air quality can affect communication like a windstorm, with rapid thoughts leading to rapid speech.

A healthy Vata is upbeat and full of optimism, enthusiastic, energetic, and playful.

Greet Vata with a smile for the energy and movement it can bring to your life.

AYURVEDA ACTION
Feed Creativity and Minimize Stress

STRESS AFFECTS THE Vata dosha much more than the other two. Yet Vata is often drawn to overstimulation, working too much, or stressful situations. An "up" Vata might make too many commitments, which isn't helpful for you. Keep an eye on this—don't overcommit.

Spend time nurturing the strength of your Vata, which is creativity. When setting priorities and making decisions about how to spend time, allow and value time for painting, writing, or another inspiring activity. Also create time for intimacy. Reduce Vata drag and increase Vata nurturance.

NOVEMBER 7
VATA RITUCHARYA— VATA SEASON REGIME

Vata season has taken hold, and autumn winds blow in dry, cold, rough, and light qualities. As noted earlier, Vata season is generally November through the end of February, but adjust for your location. In recent years, climate change has caused more variance in seasons, which affects doshic transitions as well.

Without adjustments, your internal conditions will match these external changes, leading you to coldness, dryness, roughness, stress, immune-system aggravations, and possible weight gain. This is the time to fortify balance so that you don't get blown over into Vata aggravations.

We see the leaves blowing wildly, we hear the wind howling, we feel a chill against our skin, and we notice the earth beginning to harden. You also spend more time indoors, which can mean warm, dry forced-air heat. This exacerbates Vata.

Vata season is characterized by light, dry, rough, hard, mobile, cool, and irregular. These qualities will be pushing against your doshas. Besides paying attention to your typical out-of-balance dosha, account for the pressures of the dosha season you are in. This is especially important for Vata season. Since Vata is mobile, Vata qualities are easily pushed around unless you fortify yourself.

AYURVEDA ACTION
Enhance Your Hot Spice Water for Vata

Still another great tea. Variety is the spice of life.

- 1 tsp fennel seeds
- 1 tsp cumin seeds
- 1/2 tsp coriander seeds
- 1/2 tsp fresh grated ginger
- 1 squeeze lemon juice
- Raw organic sugar, turbinado sugar, raw honey, or sucanat to taste

Place in 4 cups of boiled water and steep 2-5 minutes. Ginger is heating for cold Vata and lemon is sour to also pacify Vata.

NOVEMBER 8
VATA TIME OF DAY

The Vata time of day is 2 a.m. to 6 a.m. and 2 p.m. to 6 p.m. Vata principles of movement and lightness are most active during these 8 hours. Your nervous system is engaged and sensitive. That can work against you or work for you if you're conscious of these influences.

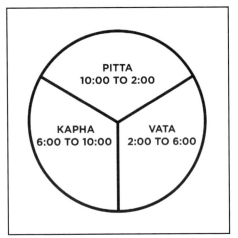

Vata-pacifying routines are helpful during the Vata times of the day. For instance, keeping routines and digestion regular helps Vata stay tamed and productive. If you skip a meal, which Vatas are prone to do, the brain scavenges for stored glucose and blood-sugar levels can plummet. If you gravitate to a sugary snack, especially between 2 p.m. and 6 p.m., your brain might be calling for fuel. You would be better served to eat a larger meal at noon (Pitta time), so that you have glucose available in the afternoon when Vata is peaking.

The latter half of the Vata hours, between 2 p.m. and 6 p.m., is when Nature stills and cortisol levels begin to decline. This is an ideal time to meditate, perhaps a second meditation of the day.

In the middle of the night, between 2 a.m. and 6 a.m., your sleep might begin to lighten, especially when the fire of Pitta (10 p.m.—2 a.m.) comes up against Vata lightness at 2 a.m. If you tend to awaken around 2 a.m., you likely have a Pitta imbalance with a Vata influence.

AYURVEDA ACTION
Get On Up by 6 a.m.

If you are able to arise by 6 a.m., you are getting out of bed at the optimum time, before Kapha influence starts. Once Kapha arrives, you may find it more difficult to make the move. Arise during Vata time, before 6 a.m., to start the day with energy.

I have a beautiful heart shaped salt lamp on a timer in my bedroom. It is set to 6 a.m. so I can awaken to light. Plus, there are detoxing benefits to the salt emission in the room. You could explore the benefits of salt lamps online if you wish.

NOVEMBER 9
VATA TIME OF LIFE

The senior, or wisdom, or elder years, after about age 50 or 60, is Vata time of life. With the benefits of Ayurveda, these can be the relaxed, wise, sage years! You will be guided by both your strengths and vulnerabilities. The air and space elements have more influence at this time. Enjoy those benefits and also be conscious about grounding and nourishing.

A sense of mastery often emerges at this time, especially when it comes to spiritual development. You could also find that you're not as resilient. Your energy bounce back might not be as quick. But you have more grace to accept life and the reality in which you live, so you might feel less stressed.

Now is an important time to listen to your body. Keep it nourished with intelligent, real food. Keep your body limber and tissues moist. Ayurveda provides the guidance you need to make this the best time of your life!

Even if self-care has always been important to you, now is the time to ramp it up. Go get that massage, take that yoga class, and spend more time with family, friends, and pets.

AYURVEDA ACTION
Do Daily Nasya

Vata qualities naturally increase after about 55 years of age—the Vata time of life. Keep body tissues moist to support tone and flexibility. You can do nasya daily. Nasya is a practice of applying medicated oil to the nostrils. Tilt your head back while standing or lie down on a bed with your head tilting over the edge. Drip four or five drops of nasya oil in each nostril, trying to cover the entire inner surface. Take a big sniff in to get oil into the nasal passages. You can also use your finger to spread the oil.

Medicated nasya oils are formulated for this purpose, but you can also use other oils like abhyanga massage oil, ghee, or even organic olive oil.

NOVEMBER 10
VATA DISTURBED AND BALANCED

Look for these signs that could indicate your Vata is out of balance:

- Nervousness
- Anxiety
- Difficulty falling or staying asleep
- Panic
- Fear
- A weakened immune system
- Constipation
- Skin dryness, chapped lips
- Emotional conflict
- Inability to make decisions
- Impulsiveness
- Fast and disconnected speech or difficulty speaking up
- Gas bloating

If one or more of these presents, your Vata needs balancing. Vata is the most common imbalance, presenting over half the time there are symptoms of any imbalance. Due to its subtle elements, it is always the first dosha to become imbalanced. As you live longer, Vata increases in your system. And fall is Vata season—a good reason to do something now.

In balance, Vata is creative, joyful, enthusiastic, lean, quick, lively in conversation and activity, flexible, agile, and spiritual. Balanced Vata means a toned nervous system, and your responses to life's stresses are coordinated and appropriate. You feel spacious and own your movements. With a few adjustments, your autumn experience may be filled with healthy Vata and the liveliness that brings.

AYURVEDA ACTION
Spark Joy

Marie Kondo's method of clearing clutter famously asks whether what you own sparks joy. For many people, it has been a successful strategy to separate from possessions that are overwhelming their space.

We have psychological clutter, too. Deep, focused engagement is an element of fulfillment and enjoyment. If you are busy, busy, busy, that settled space which Vata needs in order to be grounded and creative is absent. Better to have a limited number of things, activities, and thoughts you care about deeply. Your Vata will thank and serve you.

NOVEMBER 11
BALANCING VATA

Every day you react to change and find a new balance. The body uses doshas to buffer changes and prevent disease. When you maintain a dosha ratio similar to your original constitution, homeostasis results in good health. When weather conditions change, or stressors erupt, or your comfort is challenged, doshas are the first responders to become aggravated or elevated.

Making seasonal adjustments helps keep balance and health. During Vata season, be more focused on generating your internal fire and warmth, eating more cooked foods, grounding with yoga, massage, and meditation practices, and using more oils in cooking and on your body to moisten yourself in this dry season. Feed enthusiasm by connecting with others.

You have been learning about Vata pacifying actions. Here is a summary of the most strategic actions to pacify Vata:

- Follow a Vata-pacifying diet—Cook with ghee or avocado oil, use spices like cinnamon, cloves, cumin and ginger; eat a warm breakfast of cooked quinoa or cream of wheat or rice; eat more soups and kitchari; and enjoy nuts like walnuts, almonds, and cashews. Minimize raw foods and salads. Avoid iced and cold drinks.
- Sleep well—Drink warm raw cow's milk or nut milks with a pinch of ground nutmeg or turmeric to take you into slumber.
- Establish routines for grounding—Be still. Vata is aggravated by excessive movement and feelings of insecurity or fears. Take time to meditate, do gentle yoga or other quiet self-care routines. Eat at regular times.
- Enjoy a daily self-massage—called abhyanga {Dec 6}.
- Nourish your senses. Touch, taste, hear, smell, and see {Jan 12}.

AYURVEDA ACTION
Balance Vata with Food

Vatas do best with regular mealtimes and warm, cooked meals prepared with fresh, organic, and whole foods: Zucchini is good, as are brothy soups and light dairy products such as paneer cheese. Hot spice water supports Vata pacifying, as do fresh ginger and cardamom.

NOVEMBER 12
VATA AND THE TASTES

Vata is pacified by the "S" tastes—sweet, sour, and salty. Vata is aggravated by PAB—pungent, astringent, and bitter tastes.

What are these balancing tastes—sweet, sour, and salty? Well, salty we know for sure—that shows up in salt itself and also seafood that comes from salty water. We have a sense for the other two, but there is also some mystery with them.

The sweet taste is composed of earth and water, and you can see how this could balance Vata's air and space nature. Earth and water are moist, grounding, and heavy—just what Vata needs. Sweet tastes include some of the wet, heavy fruits like melons, ripe bananas, and dates. Grounding vegetables like beets, cooked carrots, and sweet potatoes nourish an imbalanced Vata. Dairy is especially pacifying for Vata—think raw milk and soft, moist cheeses. Eggs are also good, along with spices such as basil, cardamom, cinnamon, fennel, mint, and saffron.

Sour taste is composed of earth and fire—grounding and heating for Vata. Qualities are liquidy, unctuous, and heating. The sour taste causes the mouth to pucker, which moistens and builds bulk in the tongue tissues. Sour taste would include lemons, limes, and grapefruits, also sour cream and yogurt. Vinegar and most fermented foods like sauerkraut and kimchi are considered sour. But butter, cheese, and sourdough breads are also considered sour. The sour taste awakens the mind, gathers scattered energy, and stimulates the senses. Sour is good for liver detoxing.

Salty taste is composed of water and fire—good for balancing dry and cold Vata. This taste stimulates appetite, which helps Vata's light appetite and need for nourishment. The salty taste helps moisten and build tissue and supports a toned nervous system The salty taste is there in soy sauce, sea vegetables/seaweed, and cottage cheese. Surprisingly perhaps, celery and celery seed are considered salty.

AYURVEDA ACTION
Use Mineral Salt

I recommend land-mined mineral salt because I no longer trust the cleanliness of sea salts. According to Dr. Mercola, 90 percent of sea salt contains plastic microparticles.[73] Salt in the diet protects against heart disease. Without adequate salt, your body pulls sodium from bones. In the Western diet, super-salted processed foods have been a problem for some time. But if you are eating real food, you can comfortably salt your foods for taste.

NOVEMBER 13
VATA BALANCING DIET

A Vata menu is predominantly warm, cooked, moist foods. Most everyone can benefit from Vata pacifying during the Vata season. Focus on a diet that introduces the qualities opposite of what Vata season brings. Think grounding, warming, and routine. Here are foods to favor:

- VEGETABLES. Cooked asparagus, beets, carrots, winter squashes, sweet potatoes, and zucchini are good. Cucumbers are also good.
- DAIRY. Most dairy is good, although I recommend only raw cow's milk if you can get it. Otherwise, consume milk alternatives like almond or hemp milk. Soft cheeses like paneer and cottage cheese are better than hard cheeses.
- BEANS. Some beans are astringent and too drying for Vata season. If you have a "jones" for beans, select small lentils or add the spice hing (also called asafoetida) to reduce beans' air/drying quality.
- GRAINS. White basmati rice is good for Vata because it is easily digested.
- SWEETENERS. In moderation, all natural sweeteners work for Vata—remember—in moderation. Try whole cane sugar, turbinado sugar, and grade B maple syrup.
- FRUITS. Sweet heavy fruits like oranges, bananas, melons, berries, peaches, mangoes, grapes, and even raisins soaked in water overnight.
- NUTS. All nuts are fine, since they are oily and moistening – Except peanuts which are legumes and not really nuts.
- SPICES. Try adding cardamom, cumin, ginger, salt, cloves, cinnamon, fenugreek, hing, and mustard seeds to your food. You can make teas as well.
- OILS. All oils pacify Vata but especially ghee, sesame, and olive oil. Never heat olive oil, only use at room temperature.

AYURVEDA ACTION
Soup It Up to Pacify Vata

THE BIG VATA diet tip: Eat more brothy soups to pacify Vata. They make an ideal supper. Soup is certainly moist, as well as warm and grounding—exactly what Vata needs. If you are eating while traveling or you are at work, you may be able to find a restaurant that makes homemade soups daily. Go for it!

NOVEMBER 14
VATA BALANCING LIFESTYLE

As with food, Vata's air and space qualities need to be balanced with lifestyle practices that are the opposite. Here are the opposite qualities you need:

Heavy—ground and nourish

Warm—warm yourself physically and emotionally

Oily—loving and softening

Smooth—soothing, graceful

Stable—steady, secure

Gross—tangible results, obvious communications

Vata can be flighty and nervous when out of balance. Routine grounding and quieting activities will serve nervous/anxious Vata well. Rest when you need to and don't overcommit. A daily routine could include yoga, meditation, walks, reading, massage, and sipping tea. Your Vata might want to do it all, but pick just a few things you can stick to. This will calm your Vata more than anything—in addition to a warm, moist Vata diet.

Moderate exercise is good, and smooth, graceful exercises like yoga or tai chi are fabulous. Slow, deep breathing is good for Vata too. Consider pranayama practices. Overexertion exhausts Vata. Whatever you do, hydrate when you exercise and allow time for recovery.

AYURVEDA ACTION
Enjoy Guided Meditations

Need to slow down? The app Insight Timer offers thousands of free guided meditations, and other meditation apps are out there as well. The guided meditations on Insight Timer are on topics like sleep, love, and stress. Some of my favorites from the app are by Karina Mirsky, Jennifer Piercy, Bethany Auriel-Hagan, Kenneth Soares, and Cory Cochiolo. Explore. Many wonderful meditations are out there and one of them could be right for you.

NOVEMBER 15
VATA AND WEIGHT MANAGEMENT

VATAS ARE OFTEN appropriately thin, but not always. They can be too thin and require additional nourishment. Eating warm, cooked grounding foods such as winter squashes and practicing a daily rasayana like chyawanprash, an Ayurveda rasayana jam, nourishes and fortifies. Vatas aren't immune to excessive weight gain. Their susceptibility to stress can lead to emotional eating of sweet, sugary foods. When ama is thick, even Vatas can become overweight.

Each season has a distinct purpose in nurturing and sustaining physiology. In Vata season fortifying foods fuel, nourish, and build. In general, you need to eat more food—it is the Nature of the year-long cycle and of health. Spring is a season to cleanse and lighten. But for now, power up.

How do you eat more nourishing food without significant weight gain? I always acknowledged my own five-pound "winter weight gain" with a sigh of acceptance. In truth, a temporary, small weight gain in winter is common and normal. However, you do not need to overdo it.

In the winter your physiology is active with warming, building tasks that need extra energy. In the effort to sufficiently nourish, it's tempting to get the energy with sugars and carbs. The holidays, although enjoyable, can also be stressful with travel, increased social time, and rich foods.

Overeating and selecting the wrong foods can be an effort to satisfy energy needs for the building phase seasonal demands. But you can be smart and power up in a way that does not pack on pounds. Get a little more protein and eat more nutrient-dense foods during this transition to colder temperatures.

AYURVEDA ACTION
Avoid Raw, Cold and Dry

RAW FOODS EXACERBATE mobile and air qualities, which aggravate Vata and often result in flatulence and burping. Vata's fire isn't strong enough to break down and digest completely raw foods. Since using a number of Ayurvedic principles in preparing food, I rarely experience gas; it doesn't have to be a natural part of eating. What a nice benefit for you—and others.

It is best to avoid cold and iced beverages, along with coffee and alcohol. Dry foods are tough for Vatas to digest as well. Skip foods like popcorn, chips, rice cakes, and crackers.

NOVEMBER 16
VATA SPICES

Vata needs spices that ground, nourish, and warm the light winds of Vata. This list contains spices that are Vata-pacifying. Use them daily. Your food will be flavorful while doing the important work of balancing Vata.

- Garlic
- Ginger
- Hing (asafoetida)
- Mustard seed
- Nutmeg
- Oregano
- Parsley
- Peppermint
- Salt
- Thyme
- Turmeric
- Coriander
- Cumin
- Dill
- Fennel

AYURVEDA ACTION
Keep a Vata Churna on Hand

In Sanskrit, *churna* means "powder of spices/herbs." Churnas are spice combinations that increase digestive fire and absorption of nutrients and support digestion. The spices in this churna favor the sweet, sour, and salty tastes needed to pacify Vata. Sauté in a little ghee before adding to your dish. Some spices in this blend are fat soluble and some are water soluble, sauté all your spices to be sure they open their intelligence. The spices in Vata churna reduce gas and bloating and calm the nervous system.

- 1 Tbsp cinnamon
- 1 Tbsp (choose as many as you like) coriander seeds, cumin seeds, fennel seeds, turmeric, fenugreek, asafoetida (hing)
- 2 tsp powdered ginger
- 2 tsp mineral salt

Grind the ingredients (as many as you have) in an electric grinder or spice mill. Store in a non-plastic, airtight container such as a colored-glass jar.

NOVEMBER 17
VATA CHUTNEY

Chutneys not only taste delicious, they're also revered for improving digestion and adding nutrition. Fruits, one of the purest food forms in Ayurveda, are a natural supplier of vitamins and minerals, especially vitamins C and A. Fruit is also a resilient antioxidant. Mixing fruits and spices adds high-density nutrients with supportive spices for a powerful digestive aid. You can find many fruit chutney recipes. This one is Vata-balancing.

Dry-roast spices ahead of time, then combine all ingredients in a food processor:

- 4 cups apples
- 3 Tbsp lime juice
- 1/3 cup orange juice
- 1/2 cup fresh ginger root, chopped & peeled
- 1 cup raisins (soak first if too dry)
- 3/4 cup dates, pitted & peeled
- 1/4 tsp hing (asafoetida)
- 1 tsp fennel seeds
- 1 tsp cumin seeds
- 3 tsp coriander, ground
- 1/4 tsp nutmeg
- 3/8 tsp salt

This chutney pacifies Vata and is somewhat pacifying for Pitta. Eat along with your meal.

AYURVEDA ACTION
Moisten Dry Foods to Balance Vata

Dry foods aggravate Vata. But if you love crunch, balance the dryness with good fats. For example, put melted ghee on popcorn, guacamole on tortilla/tostada chips, cashew butter on rice cakes and toast. Another way to add moist crunch to your meals is with lightly toasted seeds—like nutritious sunflower, pumpkin, and sesame seeds.

NOVEMBER 18
PREPARING A VATA PACIFYING BREAKFAST

Tired of the same old breakfast? Start the day with a stewed apple or pear and enjoy many benefits for increasing metabolism and supporting regular bowel movements. Raw, these fruits can aggravate Vata, but cooking them with spices produces ojas (vigor) and pacifies Vata and Pitta.

An apple or pear prepared this way is a light yet nourishing and satisfying breakfast that can increase vitality and aliveness. You can cook on low in a crockpot or other type of slow cooker overnight, covered with 2 inches of water. Or, simply cook in a pot on the stove with 1/4 cup water for 10 minutes in the morning. Not recommended to be eaten at night.

STEWED APPLES: CHANGE UP BREAKFAST AND IMPROVE ELIMINATION

Cooked apples and pears bring a delightful flavor to your first nutrition of the day.

- 1 whole fresh, sweet apple or pear, cored and peeled
- 3 whole cloves or powdered spice blend of cloves, cinnamon & cardamom
- 1/4 cup purified water
- 1 tsp ghee

Core, peel, and slice the apple/pear. Put all ingredients in a covered pot. Cook fruit until soft. Discard the whole cloves if used. Sweeten to taste with raw cane sugar or with raw honey when cool enough to eat.

AYURVEDA ACTION
Eat a Variety of Breakfast Grains

...but especially wheat. Consider oatmeal or rice with cinnamon, ginger, and a small dab of ghee or raw honey on top. Add raw almonds that have been soaked and peeled for crunch and additional nutrients. Wheat products such as cream of wheat, bulgur, couscous, and farina are extra good for balancing Vata. Many wheat sensitivity issues are caused because weed poison is often spread immediately before the crop is harvested to make it easier—so buy organic. If you have gluten sensitivity, try white basmati or jasmine rice.

If you have imbalanced Kapha, avoid wheat as it can increase mucus. Vata needs that moisture; Kapha does not.

NOVEMBER 19
PREPARING A VATA PACIFYING LUNCH/DINNER

The Vata in you probably loves salads, but raw foods should be avoided. A small side salad might appease, but the main part of your meal should be moist and freshly cooked. Lunch should be the largest meal of your day because Pitta time is when digestive fire is naturally the strongest. Consider calling your noon meal dinner and reserve the term supper for your lighter evening meal.

A perfect Vata pacifying lunch/dinner could include some lemon rice or couscous with vegetables such as cooked carrots and peppers in a luscious sauce. Pacify the cold Vata with some black and/or cayenne pepper and season with cardamom, bay leaf, and fresh or powdered ginger. Sauté your spices first in ghee to release the spice intelligence and to moisturize dry Vata. You can add some hing too, which is marvelous at pacifying Vata and I think it gives your food a bit of a garlic flavor.

I also like to toast raw cashews in a black skillet and toss on top of dishes for some crunch. Consider toasted nuts such as almonds or pistachios for some good fats. Top your meal with some homemade vata chutney sauce {Nov 17}. Have a half a cup of hot spice water with your meal and perhaps a small chapati or other unleavened bread.

Rice with veggies is a great meal choice in general for pacifying Vata and even better when prepared in a sauce which offers moisture to the meal. Vary the veggies for interest and with what is in season and check the Vata pacifying diet for a list of vegetables and other food items to favor to pacify Vata.

A favorite go to spot for online recipes is https://www.joyfulbelly.com. You can go to their site and select the diet and recipes tab. Some of the Vata pacifying recipes are:

- Mung dahl kitchari
- Asparagus saffron risotto with lemon
- Sweet potato and spicy pecan crisp

Eating a fresh cooked meal and the largest of your day around noonish can be quite tough. Do what you can and when you can. Check out the Vata Pacifying diet for more ideas {Nov 13}.

AYURVEDA ACTION
Eat Basmati Rice with Lemon for Vata

Most delicate rice is Vata-pacifying. Make it even more so by selecting easily digestible basmati rice and squeezing fresh lemon juice over the rice. The sour lemon pacifies Vata.

NOVEMBER 20
PREPARING A VATA PACIFYING SUPPER

Supper is meant to be "supplemental" and not the main meal of the day. This can be a challenge if the evening meal centers on family or friends. Do the best you can and at least recognize the principle of a light evening meal.

Hearty vegetable soups make a good Vata supper, or kitchari, or a sweet potato with another vegetable. Keep it light; then avoid eating after supper. Let food completely digest until you "break the fast" in the morning. Try to consume meat protein, if you eat it, at midday and skip having meat with supper.

AYURVEDA ACTION
Eat Soup, Soup, Soup

For a heartier broth, consider a squash, carrot, and ginger soup with warmed chapati bread. Although Ayurveda recommends freshly prepared food for its lively qualities, I often make soup I can eat for three days. Heating food that was freshly prepared on a previous day is better than processed.

Each day you heat the soup, add a fresh veggie. For instance, on Day 2, throw in green beans, and on Day 3, carrots. You might want to sauté and spice them in ghee first, so they are about the same doneness as veggies already in your soup.

NOVEMBER 21
VATA BALANCING DRINKS

Vata is drying, and to keep yourself healthy, you might need to drink more water than you imagine is necessary. {Aug 22} Vata does best to sip on hot spice water and warm teas all day long, except for the hour surrounding a meal. Only 1/2 cup of water is advised with a meal.

Dairy is also soothing and balancing for Vata. At bedtime, consider a cup of hot date nut milk, or warm milk with fresh grated nutmeg. A hot, natural-cocao drink in the winter can soothe Vata. If adding sugar, have early enough in the day not to disturb sleep.

But start with the basics—water. Hot water is fabulous for Vata constitution and Vata season—and adding lemon enhances its effect. Lemons have a connection to your lymph system. While lemons are highly acidic, once we ingest them, they become alkaline. Your lymphatic system is responsible for removing toxins, and so needs to be hydrated and working properly. If too many toxins have accumulated, the lymph system is sluggish and unable to do its job, which can lead to illness. Warm lemon water hydrates the system and stimulates toxin elimination.

AYURVEDA ACTION
Splash on Some Sour to Pacify Vata

Many dishes and drinks can be made more Vata-pacifying by adding a sour liquid. Squeeze a bit of fresh lemon or lime juice over foods and in drinks. Use organic lemons or limes. Vinegars also add sour. Balsamic vinegar, in particular, spruces up a salad or other dishes. The sour taste stimulates the senses and awakens the mind. Sour also moistens foods and limits some of their windy/gassy quality.

NOVEMBER 22
VATA DAILY ROUTINE

A HEALTHY DAILY routine is the bedrock for all constitution types, but it is especially essential for Vata. Nothing settles an imbalanced Vata's up-and-down, flighty nature like routine. But you don't need to schedule every minute of your day. Vatas need freedom for creative expression. Put a few good daily habits into your routine and stick with them. If your physiology knows to expect meditation at certain times, or tongue scraping, or a massage, or bedtime, the anticipation brings calm instead of the nervous energy that can arise when Vatas feel uncertain.

Start with a few simple habits. Going to bed by 10 p.m. and arising by 6 a.m. stabilize Vata. Here are things you can do:

- MORNING ROUTINE: Create a self-care morning ritual. Introduce tongue scraping {Apr 20} upon first arising, wash your face, do oil pulling, and meditate. Later you might add yoga, a morning walk, or a pre-breakfast lemon detox drink.
- ALL-DAY ROUTINE: Sip hot spice water. Add in a gentle midday walk or even a short meditation.
- EVENING ROUTINE: An evening routine is precious. Consider stopping all use of media one hour before bedtime and taking two triphala tablets 30 minutes before bed. Bathe or wash up. Once clean, moisturize your face and lightly moisturize your body. Rub coconut oil on your feet. Consider a guided meditation for sleep. When your head hits the pillow, do a walk-through of your activities that day. This brings closure. Acknowledge the blessings of your life.

AYURVEDA ACTION
Hum Like a Bee

BHRAMARI PRANAYAMA—ALSO KNOWN as the bee humming technique—is a lovely way to ground and balance yourself. It is best practiced at night or early in the morning:

1. Sit up straight on the floor or in a chair with a gentle smile.
2. Close your eyes and observe sensations.
3. Place your index fingers on the flap of cartilage to close your ears or put them in your ears and press to seal out external sounds.
4. Make a high-pitched humming sound like a bee.
5. Breathe in and out; continue another three or four times.

NOVEMBER 23
VATA SUPER HERBS

Warming herbs that settle the nervous system are best for Vata. A few stand out as Vata super herbs. If you are stressed (and who isn't?) or you sense your Vata is shaky, consider adding in some of these:

- ASHWAGANDHA—I recommend this often to settle down and nourish Vata. Ashwagandha is also known as Indian ginseng. It has astounding rejuvenative properties, promotes stamina, tones muscles and is grounding and heating. Ashwagandha is known for aiding mental focus and calming the nervous system. Studies show it reduces insomnia and anxiety. Although cortisol has its role, ashwagandha can soothe chronic release of cortisol chemistry. Ashwagandha promotes muscle strength along with healthy joints and a healthy libido. It is said to bestow the strength of a horse and has benefit to seniors in the Vata time of life.
- SHATAVARI—This rejuvenative herb is heavy and unctuous, thus perfect for balancing Vata. Shatavari is often suggested for women as it is known to tonify the reproductive system and libido earning the nickname "100 spouses." Because it is cooling, it is often used in equal amounts with ashwagandha so as not to be too cooling. This herb supports emotional and physical digestion and promotes love and devotion.
- GUDUCHI—This herb is highly prized as an effective nerve tonic. It strengthens the nervous system, boosts the immune system, cleanses and detoxes the physiology. Guduchi also has a strong antioxidant effect. Guduchi taken internally is known to promote healthy skin and a clear, radiant complexion. The heat of guduchi burns up ama in the liver, supporting healthy elimination of toxins.
- BRAHMI—Brahmi soothes the nervous system and promotes divinity. Brahmi can stabilize all three doshas but especially Vata. It increases energy and promotes sound sleep. It promotes memory and concentration and clears the mind. Brahmi means "energy of universal consciousness" and supports the path to higher consciousness.

Remember, start with small amounts of herbs to see if the effect is right for you or consult with an Ayurveda practitioner.

AYURVEDA ACTION
Make a Double Brahmi Tea

There are two forms of the herb brahmi. One form of brahmi, also called bacopa, is good for the nervous system and brain function, especially memory, focus, and clarity. The other brahmi is also called gotu kola and supports skin suppleness in addition to aiding brain functions. It also strengthens the lymph system and the microchannels of the body. Make tea by mixing 1/4 to 1/2 tsp of each in a cup of boiled water. Your brain will thank you.

NOVEMBER 24
VATA WORK AND PLAY

Vata energy is creative, playful, and dramatically energetic. The Vata in you is a great communicator. You hatch large ideas and jump right in, but you must be careful not to burn yourself out. Imagining ideas are exciting, but completion becomes a challenge as you move on to the next cool idea.

Focus on work but avoid multitasking—it just does not serve you (and anyway, it doesn't make you more productive). Work environment is very important to you, so consider adding art pieces or fresh flowers if you can. Put fabric over your bookshelf to soften it up. Warm colors feed your creativity, which is very important to you. If you don't have a job that invites creativity, you might want to consider finding work that gives a deeper sense of satisfaction. Vatas make wonderful artists, designers, teachers, and writers.

Vata is pacified by routine, so develop routines at work. Perhaps you set aside the first hour of the morning to come up with big ideas or make phone calls or check email (although email can suck up all the oxygen). Aim for a regular time for lunch, and a consistent ending time for work each day. Vata energy and interest runs hot and cold, meaning some days you will want to work 10 or 12 hours and then the next day you are exhausted and can't focus. Enjoy the strengths of Vata at work, but keep it pacified with defining routines.

Vatas really like to play. So, have fun! The Vata in you likes being around the playful, unpredictable nature of children. Introduce play that is also stabilizing to balance Vata. Taking methodical strolls, participating in dance classes, or swimming laps can ground Vata—and show it a good time.

AYURVEDA ACTION
Seek Moderation in Work and Play

Vatas can be erratic in both work and play. Seek moderation to get the most from both. If not, you may burn out. Vatas need to walk the line—not too much boredom, not too much excitement. You are an original thinker, so look for creative outlets in work and play. Also, the Vata in you likes to do things you have never done before—maybe things no one has ever done before. Some of this feels good, but don't overdo. Moderation is healthy.

NOVEMBER 25
VATA SKIN – NOURISHING FOR WINTER

A CORE PHILOSOPHY of Ayurveda is that BEAUTY IS AN ESSENTIAL ASPECT OF OUR BEING, AND IT RADIATES FROM WITHIN. The U.S. has a cultural obsession with outer beauty and standards of perfection. Cate Blanchett was praised in blogs some years ago when she appeared on the cover of Intelligent Life, a lifestyle and culture magazine, in a completely non-photoshopped photo. She appeared in working clothes and looking like the mature woman that she was. That made news.

Becoming accustomed to displays of airbrushed perfection that remove wrinkles and resize bodies can make you feel flawed and inferior. Ayurveda unlocks your magnificent, peaceful, and unique radiant beauty and reveals the depth of wholeness. As you live and grow, beauty is formed from the maturing alchemy of life intelligence, capacities to understand with compassion, personality that drags less baggage into communication, soulful expression, and grace in posture and movements.

The skin's outer shell reflects the body's inner workings. Though diet is primo, you also can nourish the skin externally. A skin-care principle in Ayurveda is: "If you cannot eat it, do not put it on your skin." The skin ingests nutrients. Each square inch of skin contains 1300 nerve endings that send messages directly to your brain. What messages do you send?

Vata skin runs dry, and the primary skin care strategy is to moisturize, moisturize, moisturize. Start with a Vata pacifying diet of warm, cooked, moist food with plenty of good fats. Drink plenty of room-temperature and hot water each day. *Then* look at what to put on your face.

Many commercial skincare products actually harm your skin. They often contain petroleum-based mineral oil, which pulls moisture from deeper skin-tissue layers to the surface. When surface moisture is washed away, your skin is left even dryer than before. Whatever you apply must be absorbed and digested to nourish your skin and eliminate waste products.

AYURVEDA ACTION
Moisturize with 100% Organic Oils

A SIMPLE WAY to care for Vata skin is to moisturize it with 100-percent natural organic oils. Those best for Vata include heavy oils such as sesame, almond, avocado, and olive. Shea butter is also a treat for dry Vata skin. Pamper your skin frequently with oil, especially after a bath or shower while skin is damp. The oil seals in moisture. During the day, refresh your face by washing gently in cool water and splashing on more oil.

NOVEMBER 26
VATA SPIRITUALITY

VATA ENERGIES ARE the most spiritual force in your energy field. Prana Vata is a primary subdosha of Vata, which governs the nervous system and a rise in consciousness. A healthy Ayurveda diet increases prana capacities and provides the basic health that allows you to hold the vibration of higher energies. You can't run high current through old, shabby wiring.

A strong Vata constitution leads you to be spiritually perceptive. As you play with air and space that move through, you perceive the nature of the universe. The caution with Vata spirituality is that, according to Dr. Gabriel Cousins, you should "not try to force Yogic practices or other spiritual practices."[74] Overdoing always aggravates Vata, even in the spiritual realm. Slow and steady are best.

Vata is the force behind all movement in the universe. If you are blessed with a healthy Vata constitution, you have your finger on the pulse of the pranic life force. You have an infectious enthusiasm for life that draws you to others, and you can serve as spiritual inspiration.

You are particularly sensitive to sound and touch, so enjoy the sensory pleasures of Nature—her sounds and her textures. Take it in!

AYURVEDA ACTION
Be in Nature

VATAS ARE HAPPIEST when in touch with Nature and the outdoors. This is essential to ground Vata, especially apana Vata. Spend time outdoors regularly, even if it is cold, snowy, or wet. We need the sun's vitamin D, and this is how Vatas are most in tune with their spirituality. My dog, Tilo, gets me out in the snow for daily walks when I might find numerous excuses. I cannot resist her enthusiasm and the head-tilting that is her way of asking, "Is it time for our walk—yet?"

Don't have a dog? Think of winter as a time for mindful walking. When it is quiet outside, what do you see in Nature that you might not see at other times of the year? If you are walking in the city, what is alive and buzzing?

NOVEMBER 27
VATA LOVE AND RELATIONSHIPS

VATAS ARE PRONE to worry and anxiety. When imbalanced, the need for attention and reassurance emerges. If this is you, understand this and take measures to keep worry in check. If you love a Vata, you can help by nourishing their need for grounding.

Vatas need to express themselves, so they may need to "talk it out." It might feel like a rehash of the same stuff, but Vatas need to get it. They love cuddling and hugging as a regular exchange. This may include sex, but too much sex is unsettling for Vatas.

One of Vatas' favorite ways to exit the present moment in a relationship is to manage lots of activity, such as errands, events, and planning for the future. If this is going on in your relationship, see if you can settle into more experiences that bring fulfillment rather than distracting activities.

Vatas like the cuddling and reassurance, and they also need freedom to express and to move in and out of the relationship. As creatives, they require some alone time. They need time to take off in a new direction and then freedom to desert it without judgment or repercussion when it no longer holds their interest.

If you are mostly Vata, understand your needs and be sensitive to how those in relationship with you have needs of their own. Relationships are messy spaghetti tangles at times, yet love is the primal force of the Universe.

AYURVEDA ACTION
Find What Brings Joy—Then Do More

IT'S EASY TO get into a relationship humdrum—same old, same old. Relationships need some spark. Notice when you are laughing. Who is there, what are you doing, where are you doing it? Learn to create this kind of situation more often—but to stimulate your Vata, never quite do it the same way.

NOVEMBER 28
VATA CHILDREN

Vata children may tend toward thinness, if they eat properly. Consuming wrong foods and sugary treats can put on excessive weight. The Vata child tends toward restlessness, as Vata is comprised of air and space, the elements of movement.

Vata children will grasp new ideas quickly, especially if they require imagination. They may forget what they have learned quickly as well. They tend toward larger ideas and may not do well on memorization tasks. With strong verbal skills, Vatas often respond best to auditory learning cues rather than visual or kinesthetic.

Skin issues may be a problem, from dry skin to eczema. Dry skin may even be present in the lining of the intestines, leading to constipation, which is very important to remedy immediately. Elimination gets rid of wastes and toxins, and you do not want that material to be reabsorbed. One bowel movement a day, usually in the morning, is most typical.

Sleep can be an issue, as worry and stress can make it difficult for Vata children to settle down. Children and adults benefit from shutting down media at least one hour before bedtime, but it is a particularly important ritual for Vata children.

Vata children may seem high maintenance because they are sensitive, and they might appear vulnerable to other children who can be ruthless with teasing and bullying. Adults in the life of Vata children should help insulate them from being overwhelmed by stresses and aggressive behaviors.

A diet of warm, mostly cooked food helps, as does routine, even if they fight you on this. Have a regular time for media shutdown and bedtime. Establish daily rituals in the morning and evening. Regularity will help your Vata child to stabilize while navigating the unpredictable and harsh realities of childhood. Help your child feel satisfaction in what they do. Give them language for appreciating their Nature. You might be surprised at how much they can understand what it means to have a Vata constitution. Each doshic Nature has its own strengths and vulnerabilities.

AYURVEDA ACTION
Teach Vata Children to Do Abhyanga

Vata children can be their best when they have some routine in their life. Try to stick with regular meal times and bed times. Vata children also need creative, out-of-routine experiences. But if they have enough dependable structure, they will enjoy their less predictable creative experiences more. They may be nervous, shy, and dry. Show them how to do a self-abhyanga {Dec 6} oil massage to soothe them and nourish their skin.

NOVEMBER 29
VATA AROMAS

VATAS HAVE A particularly rich sensory life. They are influenced by the aromas around them, good or bad. Vatas are all about thoughts and emotions, and smell is the most primitive way to connect to memories and emotions. When you take in a smell, you are absorbing molecules. So, the smell becomes part of you—thus, paying attention to smells is important. Enhance your environment with pleasing aromas.

According to Deepak Chopra, "Linking a particular smell to an emotional state is known as neuro-associative conditioning."[75] This conditioning can activate our inner pharmacy to increase our healing response.

With a little knowledge, Vatas can use helpful aromas, particularly from essential oils, to brighten their day and balance Vata. Even if Vata is not strong in your constitution, this Vata time of the year can benefit from adding aromas to stabilize the Vata external forces.

Aromatherapy from essential oils, herbal extracts, and incense is an integral part of Ayurveda healing. Singular aromas are helpful—but even more so are aromatic, synergistic blends that have an effect greater than the sum of their parts.

AYURVEDA ACTION
Add Essential-Oil Aromas to Work & Home

VATA-BALANCING AROMAS ARE generally sweet, warming, and grounding. Aromas to consider include sweet orange, frankincense, basil, rose and rose geranium, clove, and ylang ylang. You can use these essential oils in a diffuser or put about 10 drops in a saucer of hot water. Try mixing some of these listed for a nice synergistic blend. Add to carrier oils such as jojoba, grapeseed, or olive to moisturize your skin.

NOVEMBER 30
RECAP AND WHAT'S AHEAD

In November, we set the foundation of how to pacify and nourish Vata doshic and seasonal influences. Vata—with air and space elements—is prone to an anxious nervous system and dryness in the body. You need to pacify with grounding foods and activities. Among the best grounding foods for Vata pacifying are freshly prepared brothy soups. They are warm, wet, and nourishing. Just what Vata needs. Vatas like salads, but they are raw and cold and should be avoided or restricted to a side salad.

When Vata is out of balance, your nervous system is wired and you are prone to extremes. Travel toward the middle path to avoid burnout. Balanced Vata is creative and spiritual—a force to behold.

In addition to moist foods, Vata is pacified when skin is moist and supple. Lay on the oils. Sesame oil is a good one to warm your skin. Hydrate a lot. Drink sufficient water.

Vata spices are mostly heating, like cinnamon, cumin, cardamom, cloves, salt, and ginger.

WHAT'S NEXT?

In December, we will delve into deep nourishment of the body and soul. We will get into the aspects of joy and bliss and how to overcome habits of mind. Also, look for some Ayurveda understanding of arthritis and UTI (urinary tract infection) and how to get to core healing of those conditions, which are exacerbated by excessive Vata.

And with December holidays, we often eat sugary foods, travel more, and are a bit stressed. So, we'll mix up some DIY recipes for colds and flus. See you next month.

MONTHLY REFLECTION TIME

What actions did you try? What was your experience? Did the new action feel worthwhile? Did you like it? Did you have adverse reactions? Put a check in the third column for actions you plan to incorporate daily, weekly, monthly, seasonally, or on occasion.

What New Actions This Month?	*Your Experience?*	*Habit Worthy?*
....	....	☐
....	....	☐
....	....	☐

DECEMBER 1
COMMON CONDITIONS FROM IMBALANCED VATA

AYURVEDA NEVER TREATS the conditions that present, nor does it automatically associate particular conditions with a particular imbalanced dosha. Ayurveda attends to the root of the problem, identified first through assessment and then by determining ways to balance doshas.

That being said, some conditions do commonly arise from particular imbalanced doshas. Vata emerges from air and space—with tendencies toward dryness, coldness, and brittleness—imbalances often lead to conditions that arise out of those qualities. Common Vata imbalanced conditions are:

- Anxiety and neurological conditions
- Pain
- Constipation
- Dry, chapped skin
- Arthritis
- Restless-sleep issues
- Jaw pain
- Headaches
- Large-intestine disorders
- Gas and bloating
- Emaciation
- Pneumonia
- Mental confusion
- Tendency toward addictions

If you have such issues, consider that a Vata imbalance is in play. If you are in your senior years, pay attention to Vata imbalance to prevent these conditions from arising. Ayurveda treats the person and their imbalance and not the condition per sé, but it is particularly outstanding at preventing issues.

AYURVEDA ACTION
Consider Ashwagandha for Your Daily Herbal Ritual

ASHWAGANDHA IS SUPERBLY beneficial to many Vata imbalance issues. It is my go-to herb for the Vata in my tri-doshic constitution, especially since I am in the Vata time of life. Ashwagandha is the most prominent of the rasayana herbs. This herb mitigates stress and calms the adrenals while giving us strength. Consider a dose of 1/4 to 1/2 tsp daily. I like to take mine in warm raw cow's milk. If you can't get that, try milk alternatives.

If you take at bedtime, ashwagandha can invite sleep. And here is the seemingly opposite bonus: it can restore libido. Because of the sedative effect, do not take if you are taking other sedatives.

DECEMBER 2
VATA TEAS

Much more than the other two doshas, Vata needs to be hydrated. Made of the elements air and space, Vata is vulnerable to dryness and cold. Drinking hot drinks with Vata-pacifying spices is a valuable strategy to keep your Vata in check.

Here are two Vata teas you can easily make. Always use organic spices.

- Equal parts powdered ginger, cumin, coriander
- Equal parts powdered licorice, cardamom, cinnamon, plus a slice of ginger or ground ginger

AYURVEDA ACTION
Decorate Your Table

Liven up the months with less light by bringing some delight to your dining table with perhaps flowers, candles, or gems. A little beauty invites calm eating and thus good digestion. Plus…it's just sweet.

DECEMBER 3
STRESS AND WEIGHT GAIN

By *Nature's design* the body stores fuel-packed fats, minerals, and vitamins to support you through the winter. When it comes to storing fat, it can be easy to overdo. In the winter, many people feel an extra thickness around the middle, and notice their clothes getting tighter. They may also experience unstoppable cravings or low energy. Losing weight can feel like a formidable task. Ironically "dieting" itself, along with a stressful lifestyle, can lead to overweight issues.

HOW DO STRESS AND DIETING IMPACT WEIGHT GAIN?

The human body is designed for survival. The stress response sends an emergency signal to store fat. Triggers could be, but are not limited to:

- worrying about weight loss
- food deprivation
- eating on the run
- eating in a state of emotional unrest
- extreme exercise
- taking mostly short, shallow breaths into the upper lobes of the lungs

Dieting can stress the body because weight-loss diets often are based on either food denial or hyper-focus. One diet approach, for example, would be to cut carbs and increase protein. Eventually the body will rebel from lack of balance and complete nourishment, resulting in craving and bingeing.

The Ayurveda approach to healthy weight is based on living closer to Nature and eating with the seasons. The focus is on what you eat, but also how you eat and when you eat. Winter is cell-building time and you need to eat more to get more nutrients. When spring approaches, Nature's plan is to detox winter reserves.

AYURVEDA ACTION
Slow Down Eating & Speed Up Metabolism

When you are stressed, you might eat quickly, which can lead to eating more. The brain needs sufficient time to get the message of satiety. Help yourself by taking small portions to begin with. Don't think about how hungry you are at the start of the meal—know that by the middle, you will be filling up. Try that age-old trick of chewing your food thoroughly. Wait until you have completed chewing and swallowing the bite you are on before getting the next bite ready.

DECEMBER 4
HEALTHY HAPPY HOLIDAYS!—PART 1

Holiday celebrations proliferate this month and next. That can mean doing many things we enjoy—more gatherings, more food, more travel. More stress can be a side effect, which could lead to eating too many of the wrong foods.

When energy intensifies, polarities in daily life may become more pronounced. See and accept the reality of this. Ahhh. Seeing and accepting life as it is, brings you peace, even in a hectic holiday season. Now, what other strategies can you employ?

KEEP HOLIDAY EATING HEALTHY (FOR THE MOST PART)

Stress, rich foods, and irregular schedules around the holiday season means ama, the waste product of digestion, can accumulate. Ama clogs body channels and weakens the immune system, which can invite post-holiday illness. You have seen these before, but as the holidays approach, here are Ayurvedic prevention tips.

1. Enjoy Your Main Meal at Noon

Your digestive fire is strongest at midday, so use this to your advantage. Although you need more substance for tissue-building in winter, try to not overeat. A large meal late in the evening can interfere with sleep. Good sleep requires energy, and if energy is being directed to digestion, well, you see how that ends.

2. Don't Snack

The holy grail of Ayurveda is perfect digestion. Between-meal snacking keeps the digestion process constantly "on." If you must snack, choose watery, easily digestible fruits like grapes and oranges, a flavorful herbal tea, or soaked raw nuts.

3. Support Your Digestion

I have hammered the importance of hot spice water throughout this book. Make a tea of hot water with 2 parts fennel seeds to 1 part cumin seeds and 1 part coriander seeds or drink fresh ginger tea. Or eat a slice of fresh ginger with salt and lemon juice.

4. Eat "Intelligently," Avoid "Dumb" Foods

In Ayurveda we go for the intelligence in food to give the physiology quality operating orders. Consume fresh, organic, colorful, unprocessed foods. They are full of prana.

AYURVEDA ACTION
Slow It Down

Eating slowly helps. A practice I have used, when I remember, is setting my fork down between every bite. This is challenging, but it makes for a more mindful meal.

DECEMBER 5
HEALTHY HAPPY HOLIDAYS!—PART 2

Holidays are lovely and challenging. As best you can, find ways to stay close to your center to better handle energetic extremes when they show up. Mindful Ayurveda practices can help you stay balanced at this time of the year. Here are more ways to balance mind, body, and spirit. (continued from Dec 4)

5. Stay Hydrated

People often mistake thirst for hunger. Keep hydrated. When you arrive at a gathering, ask for hot water, with lemon if available. Drink only about 1/2 cup of water right before and during a meal, otherwise you will dowse your digestive fire.

6. Watch the Sugars

This is so hard at the holidays. Once I have a little sugar, I start to crave more. If you're going to eat sugar, go for homemade treats with natural sugars instead of processed sweets with highly addictive fructose. Start with a small serving of a sweet—you can go back for more if you must. Eat sweets slowly, so the feeling of fullness can register.

7. Exercise

With travel and celebration, exercise routines sometimes get shoved to the side. If you are not near your gym or your yoga equipment, maintain some form of daily exercise, like a walk.

8. Keep Routines

Vata loves routine, so as best you can, keep Vata calm with regular rising and bedtimes. Eat at regular times. Continue good daily habits, like tongue scraping {Apr 20} and self-massage.

AYURVEDA ACTION
Treat Yourself to Healthy Hot Cacao

If you really want a holiday treat, make it a healthy one.

- 2 Tbsp raw organic cacao powder
- 1/2 Tbsp maple syrup
- 1/2 tsp organic vanilla extract
- 1 cup almond, coconut, or raw cow's milk
- Spices: 1/2 tsp organic Ceylon cinnamon, 1/8 tsp cardamom, 1-inch fresh ginger (grated)

Stir ingredients while heating. Serve warm.

DECEMBER 6
ABHYANGA—DIY MASSAGE

Abhyanga is a luxurious self-massage with warm oil. Vatas get the most benefit, and it grounds every dosha during Vata season. Abhyanga dissolves accumulated stress and toxins in the mind and body. On days when you do not do a full abhyanga, at least apply a small amount of oil to your skin after each bath/shower.

Abhyanga benefits:

- Restores balance to doshas
- Increases circulation
- Lowers heart rate
- Tones muscles
- Reduces skin dryness and heals cracking
- Lubricates joints
- Increases alertness
- Stimulates internal organs
- Releases and removes toxins
- Invites deep sleep
- Grounding, especially for Vata

Instructions:

1. Warm your chosen oil (see Action below). Put oil in a mug or small glass bottle and use a coffee-cup warmer to heat it up. The amount you warm should allow you to be generous in oil application.
2. Apply oil to crown of your head in circular strokes. Deep-massage to stimulate marma points {Aug 27} and invigorate lymph system in the brain.
3. Massage your face and ears with circular strokes and neck with long strokes.
4. Use long strokes on limbs and circular strokes around joints. Massage toward the heart.
5. Massage the abdomen and chest in broad, circular, clockwise motions. Massage your back as best you can.
6. Massage feet. Spend some time there doing deep massage.
7. Sit with the oil for about 10 minutes. Use this time to floss, brush teeth, or clean nails. Sometimes I also do a facial exfoliation/cleanse.
8. Take a warm shower. You do not need soap; oil is cleansing. The oil pulls toxins from the skin to the surface where they are washed off. Other toxins are relaxed into the lymph system and eliminated. Blot skin dry.

AYURVEDA ACTION
Use Oils to Pacify Doshas

- Vata—sesame or almond oil daily
- Pitta—coconut or sunflower oil 3-4 times a week
- Kapha—try dry-brushing daily and safflower oil 1 or 2 times a week
- All doshas—jojoba oil is good

DECEMBER 7
NUTRIENT DENSE FOODS

Nutrient-dense foods have a lot of nutritional value in ratio to food calories. Generally, nutrient-dense foods contain a lot of water and fiber, take longer to digest, and are more filling.

You do need more energy in winter, but at this time of year, craving (and eating) high-calorie foods with low nutrient-value (processed sugary and fat foods) is tempting. Without sufficient nutrient-dense foods, overeating can result in weight gain, and particularly belly fat.

To be healthy, select high- and low-calorie nutrient-dense foods over high-calorie, low-nutrient foods.

Ayurveda focuses on the positive. Rather than thinking of depriving yourself, what can you add to your daily diet? Adding nutrient-dense foods is likely to curtail cravings, because you are satisfying your body's seasonal need to be nourished.

AYURVEDA ACTION
Add Nutrient Dense High- and Low-Calorie Foods

High-calorie, nutrient-dense foods include small portions of:

- dried fruit
- avocados
- nuts
- seeds
- eggs
- dairy
- meats

Also, eat more low-calorie, nutrient-dense choices that are filling and satisfying. Most fresh fruits, vegetables, and whole grains fit in this category.

DECEMBER 8
FIRST BREATH—
HONORING PRANA VATA

All the world's cultural traditions describe breath in a spiritual manner because it brings and sustains life. Many traditions say the soul enters the body with that first rush of air in the lungs. When someone dies and the life force departs, we say the person has expired. When someone experiences increased energy and creativity, we say that person is inspired. Both words are formed from "spiritus"—breath.

In Ayurveda and yoga, *prana* is the most subtle and enlivening unit of energy. It is the field that underlies your physical/mental structure and functioning. With each inhalation, you breathe in prana, and spirit enters, making higher levels of consciousness possible. Breath is the vehicle for pranic life force.

Such possibility and beauty from breath—and yet, breathing often reinforces your identification with smallness, or *minima*. Breathing and emotion are directly connected. You feel it when you are sobbing in grief, breathing erratically with anger, or holding your breath from fear or pain. Habitual, unnecessarily shallow or jerky breath can keep you in a loop of fear, panic, and anxiety. Unlike involuntary functions, you can consciously control breathing and set a new normal.

"Breathe on me, breath of God"

This hymn is based on a prayer inscribed on the walls of a monastery in Belgium dating back to the 8th century.

> *Breathe on me, breath of God,*
> *Fill me with life anew,*
> *That I may love what Thou dost love,*
>
> *And do what Thou wouldst do.*
>
> *Breathe on me, breath of God,*
> *Blend all my soul with Thine,*
> *Until this earthly part of me*
> *Glows with Thy fire divine.*

AYURVEDA ACTION
Breathe Deeply

Right now, take a deep, full, smooth breath down to your diaphragm. Release stuck emotions and begin the day all over again with new vitality, increased prana, and infusion of spirit. A morning ritual or practice could offer your first deep breath to spirit and recognizing that you can live this day "inspired." As you move through your activities, periodically stop and breathe deeply and mindfully.

DECEMBER 9
ARTHRITIS—*LIFELONG HEALTHY JOINTS!*

Joints take a pounding. Joint issues, in the Ayurveda view, primarily result from ama (toxin) build-up and, on occasion, injury or genetic predisposition. Just as you floss teeth for oral health, joints need to be clean to function well. Pain-free joints will carry you through a lifetime.

If you have no joint issues now, marvelous! You can prevent future issues. If you have joint limitations or pain, Ayurveda offers treatments that go beyond pain management, offering healing at the source of the issue.

Arthritis is characterized by stiffness, inflammation, pain, redness, swelling, and incapacity of basic function. The word arthritis derives from the Greek word "anthron" for joint and "itis" for inflammation. According to the Arthritis Foundation, about 21 percent of adults have been diagnosed with some form of arthritis. About half of adults over age 65 have received the diagnosis. Some 300,000 youngsters (under 18) have an arthritis diagnosis, the second-most diagnosed illness in the U.S.

Arthritis is on the rise and yet remains "a medical mystery," according to naturopath and prolific researcher/author Case Adams. Although Western medicine provides pain management for arthritis, the condition has not been curtailed or reversed. A new perspective comes from the ancient roots of Ayurveda.

AYURVEDA ACTION
Know the Types of Arthritis and Doshic Imbalance Source

Specific types of arthritis can have unique characteristics.

Osteoarthritis

The most common, and usually affects fingers, wrists, elbows, shoulders, hips, knees, ankles, and/or spine. Usually forms from Vata imbalance.

Rheumatoid arthritis

A chronic recurring inflammation, with joints inflaming symmetrically on both sides of the body, e.g., both knees. It is often diagnosed when people are in their 30s or 40s. Associated with Pitta imbalance.

Gout

Technically not arthritis but can cause it. With gout, increased uric acid leads to deposits of crystallized acid in the joints and the kidneys. Associated with Pitta imbalance.

Lyme disease

A reactive arthritis, Lyme bacteria can infect the synovial fluid, which lubricates joints. More likely a Kapha imbalance.

DECEMBER 10
AYURVEDA AND WESTERN VIEW OF ARTHRITIS

WESTERN AND AYURVEDIC views have similar understandings of the conditions of OSTEOARTHRITIS, the most common form of arthritis. For instance:

- Articular cartilage thins
- Subchondral bone ends thicken and begin to rub
- Gaps and cracks appear in the cartilage, allowing synovial fluid to leak
- Fibrin (tough fibrous protein involved in blood clotting) builds up and stimulates immune-system responses to protect and heal the area
- Result: pain, inflammation, stiffness, redness, swelling and other symptoms meant to be temporary immune system responses

Western medicine considers that arthritis is caused by inflammation around the synovial membrane from cartilage breakdown through wear and tear over time. A biochemical cascade ensues, resulting in chronic inflammation. In a typical Western approach, halting this cascade is seen as the solution. But this treats the symptoms.

THE CRUX OF THE AYURVEDA EXPLANATION OF ARTHRITIS

AYURVEDA SEES THE root cause of arthritis as toxins in the joint. With arthritis, cartilage or synovial cells have been damaged by micro-organisms or oxidative radicals from toxins. Case Adams suggests that as we delve into the true causes of arthritis, we will find "toxic joint syndrome rampant."[76]

Unless joints are cleansed of toxins, the immune system will continue to be overwhelmed.

In summary, the Ayurveda explanation of arthritis is about toxins in the system that reside in the joints. Healthy diet and lifestyle choices, limiting exposure to toxins, regular detoxification, and continuing doshic balancing create the solution.

AYURVEDA ACTION
Reduce Joint Inflammation with Frankincense

FRANKINCENSE IS THE most recognized name of boswellia. This aromatic resin can be taken as a powder and is revered in Ayurveda for its capacities against inflammation, the cause of the painful aspects of arthritis. Boswellia is thought to block cytokines, the substances that increase inflammation. It has been identified as a defender against cancer and autoimmune diseases. Increasingly, modern scientific research is being conducted to back up time-tested Ayurveda treatments.

DECEMBER 11
HERBS FOR ARTHRITIS

THE FIRST LINE of defense for arthritis is eliminating toxins with daily and more-intense cleansing. If you have been doing this and believe your system is fairly clear, consider herbs that can support healthy joints.

Pharmaceuticals are isolated chemicals with one primary ingredient. Botanical solutions, through herbs and food, keep the active ingredients in their home, with dozens or hundreds of natural buffers and balancers as well as enhancers—called constituents.

Whole herbs and foods have intelligent healing effects without the side effects caused by isolated active ingredients.

Herb recommendations for arthritis from the sciences of Ayurveda and Naturopathy:

- Anise
- Ashwagandha
- Basil
- Boswellia/frankincense
- Cardamom
- Cayenne
- Dandelion
- Fennel
- Feverfew
- Garlic
- Ginger
- Goldenrod
- Guggulu
- Hops
- Nettle
- Oregano
- Rosemary
- Turmeric
- White willow bark

Triphala guggulu is a revered formula for daily cleansing of toxins, especially for reaching in to clear ama from joints. Pukka is a lovely-tasting detox tea with anise seed, fennel, and cardamom. Both reduce the conditions that give rise to arthritis.

AYURVEDA ACTION
Learn the Science of Sesame Seeds for Knee Osteoarthritis

GOOD NEWS: 4 tablespoons of sesame seeds daily beat out Tylenol plus glucosamine for reducing pain intensity for those with knee osteoarthritis, according to a study published in the *International Journal of Rheumatic Diseases*.[77] You can chew them or sprinkle them over food.

DECEMBER 12
AYURVEDA TRAVEL TIPS

Travel can easily agitate your Vata, composed of the elements air and space. The movement of travel unsettles Vata because you are moving faster than Nature intended. An unsettled Vata leads to unsettled emotions and anxiety.

Here are travel tips to keep Vata grounded, moist, and calm.

DRINK HOT SPICE WATER

No matter how I travel, I always take a thermos of Ayurveda hot spice water {xvi}. When flying, I take about a teaspoon of the dry-seed mix in a thermos and add hot water after I get past security checkpoints.

REDUCE JET/TRAVEL LAG

When you arrive, adjust to the activities of the time zone you are in. If daytime, go in the sun for at least 20 minutes to reset your time clock and release melatonin.

EAT FOODS THAT ARE GROUNDING

Avoid dry foods and eat warm, moist cooked foods. Hot brothy soups are especially good. Avoid salty foods, which can make your ankles swell. Take your own snacks when you travel—fresh fruit or raw nuts.

MASSAGE

Give yourself a sweet self-massage at bedtime. This will calm your nervous system and restore moisture to your skin. Consider taking a neti pot to rinse sinuses.

AYURVEDA ACTION
Try These Travel Herbs

I commonly recommend triphala as a daily herbal formula to clients because it is so effective at supporting healthy digestion. It is especially good for travel. Use the powder to make a bedtime tea by steeping 1/2 teaspoon in a cup of boiled water. Steep for 7–10 minutes. Or take 1–2 capsules.

Ashwagandha is great for calming the agitations of Vata that get exacerbated by travel. Make tea with 1/2 teaspoon of powder or take 1–2 capsules. Ginger, cardamom, and cinnamon teas can keep your energy and circulatory channels open, and they are calming for travel.

DECEMBER 13
MAKE A CLEARING

Vata is born from the elements air and space, but air and space are not the same. Space is emptiness. Sometimes space is thought of as the Zen concept of empty bowl. Air has movement. We feel air as pressure on our skin. Air can move us.

How are you holding space of this time of year? Are you holding it with sacredness and clarity? Or are you allowing Vata winds to blow mental chatter and physical clutter into your space?

This is an especially good time to make a clearing so your experience of expanded space is healthy. Otherwise, you may notice that your mind is chattering more than ever with worry and anxiety. Don't worry about your worrying—it can happen this time of year.

In Vata season, you can accumulate physical toxins because Vata is dry. A dry system is like the lint screen of your clothes dryer. It needs to be cleared. This is a good time to add simple, daily, cleansing strategies to your diet to avoid accumulating toxins this season. Consider clearing out a room in your home this month. Begin, affirm, or expand your meditation practice to honor sacred space. Clearing space in your mind, body, or environment opens energy flow, celebrates expanded Vata space, and leads you to a healthy version of Vata.

CLEARING THE BODY FOR COMPLETE DIGESTION

Herbs and spices are a diet mainstay for sustaining health in all cultures except the U.S. Here spices might be used for taste, but the value of spices goes much deeper. In addition to making food inviting, Ayurveda uses herbs and spices to awaken digestive juices, promote complete digestion, build strong immunity, and restore compromised health.

AYURVEDA ACTION
Eat Spices that Promote Complete Digestion

Most spices enhance digestion and remove ama (toxins), but these are great:
black pepper, cardamom, cayenne, cinnamon, coriander, cumin, fennel, ginger, mint, nutmeg, and turmeric.

Interested in weight loss? Complete digestion is a winning strategy.

DECEMBER 14
WINTER OJAS AND CELL/TISSUE BUILDING

THE HUMAN BODY has hundreds of different cell types and 50 to 75 trillion cells that comprise your inner intelligence. In the world of cells, information must flow, and ama blocks information flow.

Winter is a wonderful time to build ojas. Ojas is a Sanskrit word meaning "that which invigorates." According to Ayurveda, a high level of ojas brings bliss and happiness. Ojas is the vital life force energy that courses through your mind-body. According to Ayurveda wisdom, ojas is the most refined state of physical matter, but it has not yet been discovered by modern science.

Ojas is what is extracted from perfectly digested food. What you eat nourishes your body and emotions. Ojas at its full potential creates energy in all you do. When depleted, your immune system is compromised and you experience physical and emotional breakdowns. Radiant living—balanced in a way that is pure and close to Nature—increases ojas.

AYURVEDA ACTION
Eat More of These to Build Ojas

ENJOY THESE INTELLIGENT foods:

- Boiled raw cow's milk
- Avocados
- Bananas
- Grapes
- Dates
- Figs
- Leafy greens
- Sweet potatoes
- Turnips
- Yams
- Zucchini
- Nuts (especially almonds)
- Mung beans
- Tofu
- Whole grains

DECEMBER 15
CONSCIOUSNESS OF THE COOK

COOKING IS SACRED. The act of preparing food for yourself and others is life-giving. Ayurveda believes the consciousness of the cook is conveyed through the food consumed. Fruits and vegetables raised organically with care begin the journey to your table. You go to the market and find the most vibrant selections to bring home—bright, brilliant, fresh. In Ayurveda terms, that means choosing foods with lots of ojas, the juice of life.

In food preparation, you wash with care and chop with rhythms that seem timeless in a modern kitchen. If you are at peace, settled, and loving, you're like a tuning fork sending vibrations that make the meal sing. You might set a beautiful table with colorful dishes, linens, and candles, including perhaps a few leaves and a special serving dish passed down through your family.

As you sit to enjoy the meal you prepared, as guests move toward their places at the table, take a moment to be grateful. The lively food prepared with love will fulfill the cook's intention to nourish physically, emotionally, and spiritually. The holiday season especially offers you many moments to honor the everyday sacred.

AYURVEDA ACTION
Delight in Movies About Conscious Cooking

THE CONSCIOUSNESS OF the cook has been a theme in some lovely films. Here are a few titles that might be of interest:

- "The 100-Foot Journey" stars Helen Mirren. An Indian family seeking asylum sets up a restaurant 100 feet from an upscale French restaurant. Cultural and gastronomic exchanges delight.
- "Chocolat" with Juliette Binoche is delightful. She opens a chocolate shop and changes people's lives.
- "Babette's Feast" is a classic Danish movie from 1987. Babette prepares a feast of gratitude.
- "Big Night" is a story of two brothers save their failing Italian restaurant by creating a big spread for a famous musician.
- "Tortilla Soup" is a romantic feel-good movie about a Los Angeles restaurateur and his three headstrong daughters. This is a U.S. remake of the fine film by Ang Lee called "Eat, Drink, Man, Woman."
- In "Like Water for Chocolate," the youngest daughter in a patriarchal family learns she can transfer her emotions through the food she prepares. In Spanish.

DECEMBER 16
CRANBERRIES, EFFECTIVE FOR UTI?

ARE CRANBERRIES EFFECTIVE for urinary tract infections? D-mannose is a naturally occurring sugar in cranberries. We can metabolize small amounts of D-mannose. More than small amounts are excreted promptly into the urine.

E. coli (not the strain associated with unsanitary food) is the bacterium responsible for 90 percent of bladder infections. This strain of E. coli is part of the normal microflora of the intestinal tract. But when E. coli moves into the bladder or urinary tract, it can cause trouble. The cell walls of each E. coli are covered with fingerlike projections called lectins. The tips of these "fingers" stick to the bladder's interior walls and the urinary tract and cannot be rinsed out by urination. D-mannose sticks to E. coli lectins even better than E. coli sticks to human cells.[78]

When you drink large quantities of D-mannose via 100% cranberry juice, most spills into the urine through your kidneys and coats the E. coli so they can no longer stick to the walls of the bladder or urinary tract.

Consult with your physician concerning assessment and treatment for persistent UTIs.

AYURVEDA ACTION
Make Cranberry Bliss Balls

A DELICIOUS, HEALTHY Ayurveda dessert alternative. This recipe makes 20 Bliss Balls.

- 1 cup pine nuts
- 1 cup sunflower seeds
- 1 cup cashews or almonds
- 1 cup dried cranberries (or dried fruit of your choice)
- 8-10 large Medjool dates
- 1 tsp vanilla extract
- 1 tsp ground nutmeg
- 2-3 Tbsp maple syrup or coconut oil (reduce if too soft)
- 1/2 cup coconut flakes

Place all nuts/seeds in a food processor and pulse until coarsely ground. Add cranberries and dates; pulse a few seconds and add vanilla and nutmeg. One teaspoon at a time, add maple syrup. Continue to pulse until the mixture sticks together: You want a firm consistency for making balls. Taste for sweetness and add more maple syrup if desired. Place coconut flakes in a shallow bowl. Form the nut/fruit mixture into 1-inch balls and roll them in the coconut. Store in an airtight container and place in refrigerator to firm up.

DECEMBER 17
WHAT, WHEN, AND HOW YOU EAT

WHAT YOU EAT

E AT FOODS THAT are good for you rather than restrict those that are not good for you. Ayurveda recommends eating foods in season. In December, this could be winter squashes stored in a cold cellar, dried beans, nuts, grains, and seeds. Eat warm, cooked foods that are freshly prepared. You can choose foods to pacify your imbalance and also do some pacifying of Vata in this season.

WHEN YOU EAT

EAT THREE MEALS a day with no snacking (for weight loss) or limited "healthy" snacking (for weight maintenance). The largest meal should be consumed at noon when digestive fire is highest. Supper should be the smallest meal. Eat at regular times and have supper by 6 p.m. Eat only when hungry. Skip breakfast or supper if you are not hungry, but don't snack to make up for it.

Note: Between meals, you burn stored fat. When you snack, there is no call for the body to burn stored fat. (If you have hypoglycemia, do what is best to take care of yourself.) A cup of tea could reduce a need to snack between meals. Add a bit of honey if you like.

HOW YOU EAT

SLOW DOWN, RELAX, enjoy the meal.
Be at peace when you eat.
You will digest much better if you eat without watching TV, doing email, or arguing.
Note: If you relax when you eat, you will not signal your body to store fat and will digest and utilize the energy of the food. You will feel full when you have eaten enough to nourish you.

AYURVEDA ACTION
Combine Calm Environment & Time to Properly Digest

AS YOU ATTEND to when, how, and what you eat, pace yourself. Do not strain or your body will see the act of eating as a stressful emergency and store fat. Realize how essential eating proper foods and complete digestion are to your health and effectiveness. Eating your lunch in five minutes will not save you time if your concentration dips and your health suffers.

DECEMBER 18
BALA = STRENGTH

Bala is the Ayurveda word for immunity. Bala includes physical immunity as well as psychological and spiritual immunity. After cleansing, Bala is the vitality principle that imparts firm integrity to the muscles, fortifies motor sensory actions, and enhances intellect to perform natural functions. If your bala is stronger, you are stronger.

In Ayurveda, bala is intimately connected to digestion. When appetite is good and digestion is optimum, immunity is strengthened. Whatever weakens digestion weakens immunity. Bala is also an herb used to promote immunity.

Note: The herb bala is used to strengthen the body and encourages weight loss. There are some issues with this, and the FDA prohibits herbs for consumption that contain ephedrine alkaloids. The rule also states that it "does not affect the use of ephedra preparations in traditional Asian medicine." The Ayurveda Bala herb is an entirely different species than ephedra but contains a small amount of these ephedrine alkaloids. Bala is widely used in massage oils to tone muscles and calm the nerves.

AYURVEDA ACTION
Make Bala-Infused Massage Oil for Muscle Toning

I prefer the cold-infusion method to infusing herbs into hot oil. It takes much longer, but I believe the result is more beneficial.

1. Clean and sterilize a glass jar.
2. Pack jar full of dried bala herb (or a different one).
3. Use a carrier oil of your choice, such as cold-pressed sunflower or sweet almond.
4. Pour oil over the herb, ensuring it is completely covered.
5. Fill the jar almost to the rim with oil. Air gaps promote oxidation and spoilage.
6. Gently push a spoon handle or chopstick around the jar's edge to release any air bubbles.
7. Top with a non-metal lid.
8. Store undisturbed for six weeks in a dark cabinet.
9. After six weeks, strain the jar's contents through cheesecloth.

DECEMBER 19
SPIRITUAL JOY AND BLISS

WHEN YOU TOUCH your innermost spiritual center, you are contacting your field of bliss and joy. Through unbounded awareness, you experience Self, sometimes called Soul or Source, so that the light of bliss can shine through your personality. Your ego might feel reactive or compliant—but your Soul is trying to mentor you to light and creative expression.

As you may recall, Ayurveda offers guidance to strengthen the physical, energetic, mental-emotional, intuitive-wisdom, and bliss koshas {Sep 8} (sheaths around us like Russian stacking dolls) to release old formations so that the light of pure consciousness can shine through!

According to Dr. John Douillard, "the cause of all disease is when the mind and emotions overshadow the experience of the heart."[79] In other words, when you react to life through the filter of fear and anger rather than love and compassion.

The purpose of Ayurveda is to help balance and detoxify the body so it is less dense—to regain the clarity necessary to choose love and compassion rather than anger and fear. Through upgrading practices, you can welcome happiness and increase your capacity to generate, sustain, and share happiness. Joy is your creation.

Nothing brings joy and bliss like radiant health. Optimal health is the foundation for the pursuit of happiness. This is a virtuous cycle. Joy brings health and health brings joy. Although joy may be seen as a spontaneous, sudden experience and happiness a more long-lasting, stable state of mind, in Ayurveda, joy or bliss can be a sustained state that represents your inner nature.

AYURVEDA ACTION
Create/Recognize Bliss as Your Nature

WHAT YOU SEE, you become. For three days, expose yourself to immersive visual and auditory stimuli. Take walks in nature, listen to classical music. This might be easier to do at first when you have extended time off. But then also try it in your everyday home life. You can live a sattvic life. It starts with choosing what you allow to surround and hold you.

DECEMBER 20
SOUL

We are physical, energetic, spiritual beings—all of it. Your deepest nature, though, is your Soul—the infinite self—the most subtle aspect of who you are. Your soul often gets covered over and becomes unavailable in daily life. You want to be more authentic, but how do you clear a path to your real self and claim it as the strongest, most influential part of your identity?

Because of compulsive thinking, unhealthy diets, as well as social and relational tensions, "sludge" develops between daily expression and the infinite self. That Self, or Soul, is always present but gets overloaded and becomes inaccessible.

Life's pains lock you up with neuroses, issues, and patterns. Yogis call this the prison of the ribcage. The Soul is the prisoner. You clench and become unavailable. Gradually, through radiant health and spiritual practices, you become more available, happier, more vulnerable, and more loving. As you live closer to the identity of your soul, you gain authentic confidence in living from the experience of who you truly are.

AYURVEDA ACTION
Clear the Path to the Perfection of Your Soul

You can clear the path to the perfection of soul in three ways:

1. Consistently clean and clear your physical/energy body.
2. Learn about, align to, and live in the knowledge of higher consciousness.
3. Build your life-force energy to be more effective in your journey.

DECEMBER 21
COLDS AND FLU

Depending on where you live, December may be a time when bitter, freezing weather moves in. Cold weather does not specifically cause colds and flu; that happens when viruses are transmitted from person to person. However, a relationship between cold weather and susceptibility to viruses does exist.

Severe weather requires physiological resources to be mustered to keep you warm. This process can siphon energy needed for your immune system. If the cold weather causes you stress, or you eat sugary foods, or move less, or sleep less, it takes a toll on your immune system.

Scientists have found that cold and flu viruses replicate and thrive when the temperature inside the nose is cooler than normal. A cold nose suppresses the localized immune system in that area. If the lungs have also become cooler, the body is vulnerable to a virus settling, replicating, and becoming a cold or lung infection. In this limited sense, cold temperatures can cool the body, allowing it to be a better host for viruses.

AYURVEDA ACTION
Prevent the Conditions for Colds

How to prevent getting a cold or the flu? In the short run, bundle up when you go outside in cold weather, including protecting your nose with a scarf. Exercise and eat properly. Be vigilant about covering your mouth and nose when coughing and sneezing, of course, and wash hands and face frequently in cold season.

Continue to include Ayurveda diet and lifestyle practices in your daily routine to strengthen your immune system. And if you take ill (it happens!), try one of the elixirs in the next two entries to shorten the virus's impact. You need to add heat to strengthen the immune system and weaken the virus. These remedies bring on the heat!

DECEMBER 22
FIRE CIDER FOR COLDS AND FLU

Fire cider is a natural, traditional antibiotic. The cider is a powerful antimicrobial and decongestant. It also boosts circulation and the overall immune system. Vary the ingredients with what you have available. Dosage is typically 1 tablespoon per day for prevention and up to 3 tablespoons daily if treating a cold or flu. This remedy is heating, so be cautious or do not use if your Pitta is high. Also refrain if you have reaction to the ingredients, such as the peppers or if you are pregnant or nursing.

Once it is made, let the cider brew for a month at room temperature in a dark cupboard to allow all the goodness of the ingredients to be extracted. A little shake each day helps, too. You can use it right away if you need to and add apple cider vinegar to replace what you are using. It just won't be at full power for a month.

- 2-3 cloves garlic
- 1/2 cup onion sliced
- 1/2 cup fresh ginger, peeled and sliced
- 1/2 cup horseradish, peeled and sliced
- 2 pieces turmeric root peeled and sliced, or 2 tbsp turmeric powder
- 1/4 tsp cayenne pepper
- 4-5 hot peppers (jalapeño, habanero, sliced)
- 3 slices lemon
- 2–3 black peppercorns
- raw organic apple cider vinegar to fill quart jar
- raw honey to taste (optional) or add when you use it

After a month, strain the ingredients. If you prefer to leave them in, keep the elixir in the refrigerator. Once ingredients are exposed to air, they could mold. Herbalists say this can last up to a year; use your judgment. And certainly, strain first if you are keeping this for a while. See ACV Precautions. {Oct 8}

AYURVEDA ACTION
Start Your Morning with a Little Fire Cider Tea

Some people take a tablespoon of fire cider by itself. I take mine as a morning tea with hot water. This remedy has been miraculous for me. After air travel, I avoid colds by taking fire cider and elderberry syrup remedies at the first sign of symptoms. Bam. Immune system fortified. Health restored!

Not only does fire cider strengthen your immune system, the ingredients are also great for stimulating metabolism and digestion capacity. This is a very healthy start to your morning.

DECEMBER 23
ELDERBERRY SYRUP RECIPE

Traditionally, elderberry has been used as an herbal remedy for colds, coughs, and mild flus because of its virus-fighting, immune-stimulating, and anti-inflammatory effects. Elderberry syrup is flavorful and a good source of vitamin C.

INGREDIENTS

- 2/3 cup dried, organic black elderberries or 1-1/3 cups fresh or frozen
- 3 1/2 cups water
- 2 Tbsp fresh or dried ginger root
- 1 tsp cinnamon powder
- 1/2 tsp cloves or clove powder
- 1 cup raw honey

INSTRUCTIONS

1. Add elderberries, water, and spices to pan.
2. Bring to a boil; then cover and reduce to a simmer for 45 minutes to an hour until the liquid has reduced by almost half.
3. Mash the berries using a spoon or other flat utensil.
4. Pour through a strainer into a glass jar or bowl. Mash the berries again against the strainer.
5. Cool to lukewarm, add honey, and stir well.
6. Pour syrup into a clean quart-sized mason jar. Use right away or refrigerate up to 1 month.

AYURVEDA ACTION
Take Elderberry Syrup Daily in Cold & Flu Season

The dosage is 1/2 to 1 tsp for kids and 1/2 to 1 Tbsp for adults. If you have a cold, take a dose every 2-3 hours. Always test a bit first to make sure it is good for you. You can find dried organic elderberries online if you are unable to find them locally.

DECEMBER 24
VITAMIN D AND COLDS

The best way to get vitamin D is daily exposure to the sun. Try to take a short walk outside every day unless there is subzero weather. As the Scandinavians say, "There's no bad weather, only inappropriate clothes." But if wild weather keeps you inside, take a high-quality vitamin D3 supplement.

There are varied reports and studies on how much vitamin D supplement to take. Do your own research. But it's important to take a vitamin D supplement when you cannot get daily sunshine. It is not nearly as good as sun but is a helpful support.

Opportunistic cold and flu virus pathogens are always around, but our susceptibility increases in winter. According to Dr. Mercola, the immune system is compromised in winter because people congregate indoors and spend less time outside, depleting vitamin D levels.[80]

AYURVEDA ACTION
Keep Nose and Nasal Sinuses Healthy

Nasya oil

Keep nasal passages moist and healthy by rubbing a little massage or medicated nasya oil in each nostril daily.

Neti pot

I recommend doing a neti pot only when you have excess mucus in the nasal sinus area. While some recommend daily neti-pot use, it can unnecessarily dry out your nasal passages {May 28}. You can find videos online for using a neti pot.

Determine a routine that works for you and your nose!

DECEMBER 25
WHOLEHEARTED LIVING FROM DEEP WORTHINESS

Courage, compassion, connection. With those whom we feel close to, two sentiments are worth sharing: "I am sorry" and "You are welcome." It's inevitable to rub up against one another's often subconscious raw spots (sorry). When this happens, we may act in unskillful ways without full awareness of who we are and how we are showing up in the moment. You can also do things daily that hold others warmly and softly in love (you are welcome).

Connection is why we are here. Connection with others gives meaning and purpose to life. According to researcher and storyteller Dr. Brene Brown, in her famous TED Talk on "Vulnerability," truly connecting with others takes courage and compassion.[81] It's not for wimps!

Dr. Brown studied those who have a real sense of worthiness, love, and belonging and found that they possess one fundamental difference from those who do not. Simply, those who have a strong sense of love and belonging "BELIEVE THEY ARE WORTHY" of love and belonging.

The thing that can lead you to enjoy connection is a belief that you are worthy. Underneath it all, according to Dr. Brown, is the courage to be vulnerable. It takes vulnerability to be seen and known authentically by another.

Connection requires compassionate kindness for yourself and your imperfections. In turn, connection requires compassion for those with whom we connect and their imperfections. It takes courage and compassion to be authentic. Letting go of who you think you should be allows you to be who you are. Simple—and yet the work of your life.

AYURVEDA ACTION
Make Food Preparation Sacred

Food preparation is important in Ayurveda. Meals cooked with love and sweet intention nourish the soul and the body. Whatever emotion you put into cooking will be mixed into the food being prepared. Cook with reverence, gratitude, appreciation, and love, and those good things become a part of what is ingested during meals.

While preparation is important, presentation is also important. What can you do to enhance the presentation of a meal that you have prepared?

Here are examples to get your creativity blazing: Play inspiring music during meal preparation, place potted or cut flowers on your dining table, use a tablecloth and cloth napkins, say grace with mindfulness and gratitude, or add a colorful and healthy addition to your meal, like pomegranate seeds.

DECEMBER 26
AN UNCOMMON LIFE — SAMSKARAS

This time of the year inspires life review as you begin to think about resolutions for the upcoming year. Leaving bad habits behind and adopting healthier habits are great, but be wary of a resolve for perfection, taking on too many changes at once, or choosing changes not deeply aligned to who you really are.

If you really want to make changes, understanding how habits form and finding ways to establish better-serving habits aligned with your deepest Nature is important. In yogic philosophy, the habits of mind, good or bad, are called "samskaras." With every experience, a psychological imprint is wired in your subconscious mind. The stronger and more recurring the experience, including recall, the deeper the impression and the stronger the habitual thinking. Some of our deepest impressions are accompanied by or associated with fear. These impressions get well-worn over time and subconsciously direct behaviors even when there's no real reason to be afraid.

Meditation is a healthy way to retune samskaras. When you meditate on a mantra, for instance, each time a thought surfaces to awareness, you return to the mantra. During meditation, the mantra sound and vibration stops subconscious pathways from completing. The sound of the mantra crumbles the edges of the constructed samskaras over time, and clarity aligns to the positive samskaras.

Another strategy is to set new habits that are compelling enough to override "negative" samskaras. What makes a new habit compelling? If the new habit is aligned with who you are in the deepest place of your soul, you will be drawn to it naturally. Making changes is returning to the pure aspect of soulful identity.

AYURVEDA ACTION
Build Healthy Ayurveda Habits for Soul Identity

These are suggestions to build internal fires that support you as you stop feeding your egoic structures and lay down paths to your soul identity. This is a lifetime journey.

- Meditate and/or pray daily—most powerful!
- Set morning and evening routines to steady mind and energies.
- Spend time in Nature. You need this to resonate to her frequencies.
- Associate with individuals, groups, and organizations that offer loving experiences and an opportunity to build positive, powerful samskaras.
- Enjoy classes, artistic events, or outdoor activities to build positive pathways.
- Live in the moment. See reality rather than your expectations of it. Live with gratitude.

DECEMBER 27
AN UNCOMMON LIFE — SANKALPA

A COMMON LIFE is tossed by reactive and protective habitual patterns that form our ego identity over time. Most of us are engaged this way. Sometimes you know reactivity is in your dynamic with another person and sometimes you don't. Either way, you may feel immature or unskillful when these patterns are engaged.

In addition to our ego identity, you have a soul identity that is the pure, essential nature of who you really are. For those on a spiritual path, the aim is to identify more with soul nature so it can shine through egoic expression. A soul-identified life is uncommon, but is your birthright.

Unlike a New Year's resolution that is related to ego identity, a Sankalpa is a sacred intention that aligns with your deepest Self. When you act on that intention, you are building and strengthening a pathway to soul identity.

SIMPLY PUT, A RESOLUTION IS A COMMITMENT TO WHAT YOU WILL DO. A SANKALPA IS ABOUT WHAT YOU INTEND TO BECOME. A New Year's resolution may be to lose 15 pounds. A Sankalpa may be to honor the sacred energy of food sources on this planet. In that state of being, you recognize that energy supplied by eating organic, high-quality food helps to serve a sacred purpose. You might support growing and labeling organic foods. You might choose to pray over food before taking it in. You will be in a different relationship to food because of a different understanding of its true nature and yours. Any number of new behaviors could emerge from that new state of being.

AYURVEDA ACTION
State Your Sankalpa—Your Intention

A SANKALPA RECOGNIZES that you are already perfect. You are simply listening to the deepest, wisest part of yourself to learn how you align with this deeper identity.

What is your Sankalpa? What is the wise one within asking you to enliven? Is it a year for more clarity of mind, for more loving experiences, for more compassionate connection with others, for more service to those in need?

When you state a sankalpa, you are more likely to make small choices to enliven it.

The *art* of an uncommon life is to be attentive to your deepest Nature and to connect with it in a devotional and loving way. The *science* of an uncommon life is to apply the knowledge of how Nature works to your own life: this is Ayurveda.

DECEMBER 28
AN UNCOMMON LIFE—TAPAS

Tapas is the discipline and work to move toward intention—your sankalpa. "Tap" means "to heat." When new intentions, or sankalpas, rub up against old habits, samskaras, the resulting friction from competing patterns produces heat—tapas. The discomfort of change and conflict is the heat needed to burn up the impurities of negative samskaras.

Recognize that this discomfort serves a beautiful purpose if you are on the spiritual path. I believe that every experience is either my joy to celebrate or to benefit my growth. I return to this belief often and have formed a positive samskara. This belief rarely informs my first reaction to anything "negative," but I usually get there eventually.

Ayurveda knowledge can help you make good choices about diet and lifestyle actions that create even more heat, the purification needed to support alignment with soul.

The reason I work with clients on diet and lifestyle is so that they can prepare their physical and emotional forms to receive higher spiritual energies. There is a higher purpose for a healthy diet and lifestyle, which can fortify commitment and foster success for the deepest changes you want to make.

AYURVEDA ACTION
Meet Your Intentions with Tapas & Mercy

When you engage tapas, your intention is stronger than the obstacles you face. You make choices to sidestep old patterns. Tapas is bringing heat to your conditioned responses and burns them up so that your gentler Nature can be revealed. Typical tapas practices include yoga, meditation, or making ethical choices.

Start with one intention and focus. Just one. Maybe your intention is to halt your daily consumption of sugary treats. When you see a cookie, you want to relieve the pressure by eating it. Instead, ride the wave of the experience of desire. What does it feel like to want that cookie? How do you imagine it will taste? Become absorbed in witnessing desire, so you do not become controlled by it. Have mercy and recognize the resistance as habit and not your true Nature. Each time you have a little success, you are rewiring the brain and the grip of the old pattern loosens.

DECEMBER 29
MEDITATION — TRANSFORMING THE MIND

MEDITATION IS A powerful tool to relieve or mitigate stress and put you in pure-bliss consciousness. When you meditate regularly you transform your mind to serve your heart.

Consistent meditation leads you to become more Self-referral (capital S indicating the Soul or Atman) and identified with your infinite Sattvic soul. Additionally, the small sense of self, the reactive, protective defenses formed in childhood, is restricted. This small mind is also called the conditioned mind or ego mind.

Mantra meditation breaks up and releases old stresses from the reactive, conditioned mind. As you develop resilience for the present moment, you're better able to deal with what life delivers. As you identify with Transcendental Self, known as Atma, life's challenges can be handled with more talent, wisdom, and resourcefulness.

I enjoy many forms of meditation but have found mantra (Sanskrit sound) meditation most effective as a daily practice. When you gently and silently say or sing the mantra, the sound carries you to pure consciousness until thoughts and habitual conditions become silent. Quieting mental activity allows the mind to rest, while the nervous system stays in inner wakefulness. The plant of consciousness is being watered, and it naturally grows.

Don't try to expand consciousness—trying doesn't help. Just meditate. Remember that thoughts during meditation are natural. As you bump into constructions and conditions during meditation, you will be pushed to the level of thought. The content of your thoughts likely will not relate to the construction, which is slowly crumbling. You don't need to know how this works. But as you become aware of thoughts, you can become the witness instead of being swept up in the drama. As the witness, you can choose to return to the sound of the mantra. Dr. Paul Dugliss, my meditation teacher, says, "A good meditation is the one that you do." You may wish to visit his site at www.heartbasedmeditation.com/ and for more information and opportunities.

AYURVEDA ACTION
Listen for Your Mantra

I LIKE TO experience the mantra as listening and hearing rather than speaking. But the sway of saying or even singing it first helps you get to a receptive arena of simply listening for its presence. Saying or singing your mantra is like an on-ramp, so that eventually you're constantly in the mantra vibration as you are silent. Once in sync, the omnipresent mantra vibration will pick you up and carry you to pure consciousness. Listen for your mantra. Let it find you. It is always there.

DECEMBER 30
CONSCIOUSNESS ALWAYS

We end this year where we began—with an intention to find pure consciousness. When you experience inner wakefulness without conditions and impressions you have constructed over time, that is consciousness. When you "transcend" during meditation, or when you are transported by a piece of music, the beauty of Nature, or the birth of a child, that is consciousness. When you go beyond the thinking, conditions, and impressions of the mind, you experience the clarity of pure consciousness.

All creation arises out of an underlying field of energy and intelligence. Both quantum physicists and mystics are delivering the same message. Human consciousness, as well as the intelligence in the carrot we eat, is part of that field.

How does the carrot become a carrot and not something else? Coding comes from the intelligence of the underlying field of energy and information. Physiology works on the codes contained in the food you eat, the water you drink, the experiences you take in, and all inputs. Your brain is a part of this field. You are informed by intelligence beyond a separate identity. You share the field with other humans, animals, plants, and everything else that exists. You may be a wave, but you are also the ocean.

All well-being emerges from the intelligence of the field of pure consciousness. By following a clean, nourishing diet, by doing yoga, by knowledgably using herbs, you receive benefit from the intelligence of the underlying field. Without these practices, the connection to this field is likely to be blocked, resulting in confusion and disease.

Ayurveda practices are important, and they are not an end in themselves. They create conditions for the intelligence of the underlying field to find its way to you through food, energy vibrations, and beauty. When you relax your conditions and provide a healthy vessel, the underlying field of intelligence nourishes you to radiant health, a clear mind, and a happy heart. You will find yourself enjoying myriad benefits of lifelong radiant living.

AYURVEDA ACTION
Drink Saffron Tea to Open Your Universe

Saffron is the most expensive herb on the planet. Drinking saffron tea can seem quite indulgent. Go ahead, indulge yourself once in a while. You only need five or six threads of saffron in a cup of boiled water to impart its wonders. Saffron is credited with opening the mysteries of the Universe. It clears the energy centers and connects you to the oneness of all.

DECEMBER 31
YEAR IN REVIEW

You have arrived at the closure of *365 Days of Ayurveda*. Lifelong, radiant health is about living close to Nature and your own nature. Key word is balance. When a dosha is excessive, you apply opposite qualities to reduce it. What did you claim of Ayurveda wisdom? Did you develop new knowledge-based habits, and let go of mind and body habits that no longer serve? More than anything, I hope you learned about yourself.

As a unique person in an ocean of shared humanity, I hope you have come into Ayurveda in a way that makes you feel a vital part of the whole and that you see yourself clearly as connected to the underlying field of intelligence. Also, I hope that Ayurveda has become a mirror that reflects a sense of joyful reality instead of reactive conditioned responses that limit our view and understanding. I hope you have the health and energy for more authentic experiences and love. I trust that you do.

WHAT'S NEXT?

It's up to you. If you choose to go through this book again, you will start from a new platform, as your understanding of yourself and of Ayurveda will go deeper. Opportunities will continue to come, perhaps with more of a sense of synchronicity than ever. I am happy to have shared this path with you, however you used this book to support your journey. I wish you complete cheer and blessings as you continue.

YEARLY REFLECTION TIME

Reflect back on the year. It can be challenging to see progress day to day, but as you look back, can you see it? What tips did you try? What was your experience this month, and this year? Did the new action feel worthwhile? Did you like it? Did you have adverse reactions? Put a check in the third column if this is an action you plan to incorporate daily, weekly, monthly, seasonally, or on occasion. What new habits did you add in this year? What got squeezed out?

What New Actions This Month?	*Your Experience?*	*Habit Worthy?*
		☐
		☐
		☐

New habits firmly established this year:

....
....
....
....
....
....

Old habits squeezed out:

....
....
....
....
....
....

Habits I am still working to fully establish:

....
....
....
....
....
....

New actions to start the new year—might become a habit for me—I shall see:

....
....
....
....
....
....

ASSESSMENT 1
YOUR CONSTITUTION AND CURRENT IMBALANCE

Your body type, physical characteristics like eye and hair color, and lifelong issues are your best indicators of Prakruti (primal), your Ayurveda constitution. If you think any trait has changed over time, think back to your childhood. Childhood traits are good indicators of your constitutional needs and preferences. Your goal is to restore balance to your Prakruti. Thus, your current imbalance, your Vikruti (variable), is of much greater interest in the quest to rebalance and should be the focus of your strategies.

A full assessment by an Ayurveda Doctor or Practitioner will be more accurate than this self-report, which will give you a general feel for your doshas. An Ayurveda professional would use measures such as pulse diagnosis and tongue analysis, in addition to an assessment interview, to ascertain your constitution and current imbalances within your doshas as well as your seven layers of tissues and doshic energy reserves. A self-assessment, though, is a good start.

Place check marks by items that tend to describe you. Next, tally each column in the Prakruti section to see your totals, suggesting your Prakruti constitution. The highest number is your strongest dosha. Your highest Vakruti number suggests the dosha most out of balance—likely the one to choose to balance first. Low numbers in this area are good.

Note: You can mark more than one column in a row or leave a row blank if it does not apply. This is especially true with your Vikruti; only mark it if it is currently an issue.

	VATA	PITTA	KAPHA
Body Type	☐ thin body frame, light muscles, long legs and arms, lanky	☐ medium build, often muscular	☐ solid, sturdy, large bones and muscles, may be overweight
Chin	☐ thin, angular	☐ tapering	☐ round, double chin
Cheeks	☐ hollow, wrinkled	☐ smooth, flat	☐ round, plump
Eyes	☐ small, dark, often close set or wide set, active, dry	☐ bright, sensitive, sharp, often gray, blue, or green	☐ large, wide, thick lashes and brows, blue or brown beautiful "cow" eyes
Nose	☐ crooked, deviated septum	☐ long, pointed, red tip	☐ short, round, button
Teeth	☐ uneven, stick out, thin gums, space between	☐ medium, tender gums	☐ bold, white, large, strong gums
Lips	☐ thin, dry	☐ medium in size, pinkish-red in color	☐ full, moist, smooth, large, dark
Skin	☐ dry, rough, flaky, thin/visible veins, dark, cold	☐ warm, pale, delicate, ruddy or rosy, may have freckles or moles, prone to acne and rashes, oily	☐ thick, oily, smooth, cool
Hair	☐ dry, brittle, curly, thin	☐ fine, oily, usually straight, may be reddish, sandy, or prematurely gray, hair loss	☐ thick, oily, often dark and curly
Nails	☐ brittle, may have ridges, dry, rough	☐ medium in size, pinkish in color, sharp, flexible	☐ large, smooth, white in color, thick, oily
Chest	☐ flat, sunken	☐ moderate thickness	☐ round, full, expanded
Belly Button	☐ small, irregular	☐ oval	☐ big, deep, round
Joints	☐ cracking, cold, dry	☐ moderate, inflammation	☐ large, lubricated, swelling
Body Weight	☐ low, thin	☐ medium	☐ heavy, gains weight easily
Neck	☐ thin, long	☐ medium	☐ large, folded
PRAKRUTI TOTAL			

Determining Your Constitution—Prakruti

RHONDA EGIDIO, PHD

	VATA	PITTA	KAPHA
Appetite	☐ variable with little consistency day to day	☐ strong, becomes irritable when skipping a meal	☐ Low, lack of appetite
Digestion	☐ irregular, gas, bloating	☐ quick, burning	☐ slow, mucus
Taste Craving	☐ sweet, sour, salty	☐ sweet, pungent	☐ sweet, salty
Thirst	☐ variable	☐ strong, excessive	☐ Little
Elimination	☐ constipation	☐ loose	☐ thick, oily, soft
Psychology	☐ anxious, fearful, nervous, unstable	☐ judgmental, controlling	☐ greed, depression
Relationships	☐ timid, difficulty speaking up for oneself	☐ overly intense, jealous, stubborn, demeaning manipulative, egotistical	☐ attached, greedy, not passionate
Speech	☐ low, weak, prone to hoarseness	☐ argumentative, loud, piercing, direct	☐ slow, silent
Movement Pace	☐ quick, uneven, hyper	☐ forceful	☐ slow, lethargic
Physical Activity	☐ addicted to movement, may have nervous ticks	☐ overdoes vigorous exercise, competitive at sports	☐ slow and lethargic, may lack enthusiasm
Mental Activity	☐ Hyperactive	☐ quick, controlling	☐ slow, sleepy
Emotions	☐ anxiety, fear, nervousness	☐ anger, jealousy, self-critical	☐ attachment, sadness, hoarding
Learning	☐ learns and forgets quickly	☐ competitive and singular, not cooperative	☐ slow to learn, need lots of time and repetition
Intellect	☐ quick but faulty	☐ analytical to the exclusion of other ways of knowing	☐ slow, not creative
Sleep	☐ light or prone to insomnia, difficulty falling asleep	☐ light, early morning awakening	☐ deep sleep, often snores, difficult to get up in the morning
Dreams	☐ quick, active, fear	☐ fiery, violent	☐ water, few or no dreams
Menstruation	☐ irregular cycles with severe cramping and scanty blood flow	☐ regular but may have heavy bleeding or longer period due to internal heat	☐ regular but prone to water retention and clotting
Financial	☐ struggles, spends on trifles	☐ spends easily on luxuries, extravagant	☐ does not easily spend on pleasure, hoards
Foods that Aggravate	☐ cold, raw, rough (salads), dry (beans), light (popcorn)	☐ hot, spicy (chilies, ginger), burning or acidic (vinegar, citrus)	☐ sweet, excessive dairy, heavy (cheesecake), oily, substantial (meat)
Foods that Balance	☐ sweet, sour, and salty tastes, warm, unctuous (oily), heavy, whole grains, squash, grapes, cooked/steamed vegetables	☐ sweet, bitter, and astringent tastes, barley, sweet fruits (not sour like grapefruit), both cooked and raw vegetables, kale, broccoli	☐ bitter, pungent, and astringent tastes, cooked vegetables, astringent fruits like pomegranate, apples
VIKRUTI TOTAL			

Determining Your Current Dosha Balance/Imbalance—Vikruti

ASSESSMENT 2
LOOKING AT THE THREE GUNAS

Check all the boxes that apply to you to assess your guna mental and spiritual state. Total each column. This will help identify your tendency toward the psychological challenges that are likely to arise for you. Be a scout and be prepared. What emerges is your work.

Ahara/Intake

Food	☐ Vegetarian	☐ Some	☐ Heavy meat-daily
Water and Beverages	☐ Pure water, teas, and juices	☐ Mixed	☐ Alcohol
Air	☐ Good quality	☐ Medium	☐ Poor quality/polluted
Sensory Impressions	☐ Calm, pure	☐ Agitated	☐ Dark, violent
Emotions	☐ Peaceful	☐ Disturbing	☐ Dark
Information	☐ Spiritual	☐ Mixed	☐ Material
Ideas	☐ Spiritual	☐ Worldly	☐ Few or none
Associations	☐ Spiritual	☐ Egoistic	☐ Deluded, confused

Vihara/Activity

Sleep	☐ Good	☐ Disturbed	☐ Poor
Eating Habits	☐ Regular	☐ Irregular	☐ Excessive
Sexual Desire	☐ Low	☐ Medium	☐ Excessive
Exercise	☐ Good	☐ Medium	☐ Low or none
Speech	☐ Calm and peaceful	☐ Agitated	☐ Dull
Work	☐ Selfless	☐ For personal goals	☐ Lazy

Negative Emotions

Anger	☐ Rarely	☐ Sometimes	☐ Frequently
Fear	☐ Rarely	☐ Sometimes	☐ Frequently
Desire	☐ Little	☐ Some	☐ Much
Pride	☐ Modest	☐ Some ego	☐ Vain
Depression	☐ Never	☐ Sometimes	☐ Frequently
Attachment	☐ Little	☐ Some	☐ Much
Greed	☐ Little	☐ Some	☐ A lot

Yoga Practices of Yamas and Niyamas

Non-violence	☐ Always	☐ Mainly	☐ Rarely
Truthfulness	☐ Usually	☐ Partly	☐ Never
Right use of Sex	☐ Always	☐ Mostly	☐ Rarely

RHONDA EGIDIO, PHD

Yoga Practices of Yamas and Niyamas

Non-stealing	☐ Always	☐ Sometimes	☐ Rare
Non-coveting	☐ Always	☐ Sometimes	☐ Never
Self-discipline	☐ High	☐ Medium	☐ Low
Surrender to God	☐ High	☐ Medium	☐ Low
Cleanliness	☐ High	☐ Medium	☐ Low
Contentment	☐ High	☐ Medium	☐ Low

Main Yoga Practices

Asana	☐ Good	☐ Medium	☐ Low
Pranayama	☐ Good	☐ Medium	☐ Low
Concentration	☐ Good	☐ Medium	☐ Low
Meditation	☐ Good	☐ Medium	☐ Low
Samadhi	☐ Frequent	☐ Occasional	☐ Never

Yogic Qualities

Devotion	☐ High	☐ Medium	☐ Low
Compassion	☐ High	☐ Medium	☐ Low
Self-Knowledge	☐ High	☐ Medium	☐ Low
Service	☐ High	☐ Medium	☐ Low
Yoga Practice	☐ High	☐ Medium	☐ Low
Internal Peace	☐ High	☐ Medium	☐ Low

Mental Qualities

Discrimination	☐ High	☐ Medium	☐ Low
Detachment	☐ High	☐ Medium	☐ Low
Memory	☐ Good	☐ Moderate	☐ Poor
Will Power	☐ Strong	☐ Variable	☐ Weak

Ayurvedic Considerations

Dosha Accumulation	☐ Low	☐ Medium	☐ High
Ama Accumulation	☐ Low	☐ Medium	☐ High
Agni (Digestive Fire)	☐ Balanced	☐ Erratic	☐ Low
Dhatus (Tissues)	☐ Good quality	☐ Medium	☐ Poor quality
Malas (Waste materials)	☐ Low	☐ Medium	☐ High
Channel systems	☐ Clear	☐ Disturbed	☐ Blocked

Total	SATTVA	RAJAS	TAMAS

Chart reprinted with permission, Frawley, D., & Kshirsagar, S. (2016). The art and science of vedic counseling. Twin Lakes, Wisconsin: Lotus Press.

CHART
THREE DOSHAS-AT-A-GLANCE

The doshas are the three organizations or bioenergies that govern the unique psychophysiology of the individual. They are present in every cell, tissue, and bodily system. Changes in diet, habits, external forces (environmental, stressors) and in one's life (personal, relational, emotional, spiritual or physical) may result in one or more of the doshas going out of balance. Doshic imbalances become evident in certain signs and symptoms.

It is important to correct these imbalances before they progress to disease stages. The principle of opposites can be used to balance aggravated doshas and brings radical healing. Like attracts like and opposite qualities can facilitate balance.

	VATA	PITTA	KAPHA
Function	Transportation Movement Communication (talking & nervous system)	Metabolism Digestion Transformation	Lubrication Structure Strength/immunity
Keyword	Changeable	Intense	Relaxed
Composed of elements	Air & Space	Fire & some Water	Earth & Water
Governs	Colon, Nervous System, Inside Bones	Small Intestine, Stomach, Liver, Skin	Chest, Low Back
Qualities	Light, Dry, Rough, Dark, Changeable, Movable, Subtle	Hot, Sharp, Pungent, Intense, Flowing (but grounded), Oily, Liquid, Light	Unctuous (oily), Cold, Heavy, Sticky, Slimy, Moist, Stable, Strong, Soft, heavy, dull, static, gross
In Balance	Enthusiastic, alert, flexible, creative, talkative, strong communicator, artistic, adaptable, emotionally sensitive, perceptive, spiritually inclined, spontaneous, heightened intuition, compassionate	Loving, content, highly intelligent with penetrating ideas, articulate, courageous, focused and goal oriented, confident, courageous, willful, funny, joyful, high achiever, natural leaders, emotionally observant, sharp memory	Affectionate, steady, high stamina, resistant to illness, graceful, capable of vigorous exercise, steady desire for sex, sleeps deeply and feels rested upon awakening, thick hair, smooth skin, speech slow and deliberate, sweet personality

	VATA	PITTA	KAPHA
Out of Balance	Restless, fatigued, constipated, anxious, underweight, lives in past (attachment) or future (imagination), easily bored, variable appetite, muscle cramping, addicted to movement, wide variation in sexual desire, prone to insomnia, fast and erratic speech, dry/flaky skin, dry/brittle hair, flighty and uncommitted in relationships.	Perfectionistic, frustrated, angry, irritable, premature gray or early hair loss, strong appetite, irritable when skipping a meal, digestion easily affected by spicy foods, soft loose stool, too competitive at sports, overly strong sexual appetite, light sleep with early morning awakening, loud, sharp, piercing speech, delicate oily skin, prone to acne and rashes, manipulative, jealous, egotistical.	Dull, prone to oily skin, prone to allergies, possessive, oversleep, overweight, overly sentimental, low appetite, often not hungry when awakening, digestive fire often weak, oily coat on stool, tends to avoid physical exertion, often snores, oily skin and hair. Attached and greedy in relationships.
Aggravated by (avoid)	Wind, caffeine, traveling, irregular routine, irregular meals, cold dry weather, excessive mental work, dry foods, multi-tasking.	Heat, alcohol, smoking, pressure, stress, excessive spicy (pungent) or salty foods, excessive activity, skipping meals or fasting, vigorous forms of exercise. Onion, garlic, tomato, beets. Chiles, cayenne, mustard seeds, cloves.	Cold, damp, oversleeping, overeating, heavy foods, too little variety in life. Snacking. Sweet, sour and salty foods. Fatty fried foods. Meat. Wheat, dairy products, avocado, banana, lemons, plums and salt.
Seasons—adjust for global locale	Fall and early winter, November- February Cold and dry	Summer and early fall, July-October Hot	Spring and early summer, March-June Cold and wet
Time	2-6 am and pm	10-2 am and pm	6-10 am and pm
Common disorders	Arthritis, high or low blood pressure, cracking joints, urinary infections, muscle stiffness, dry skin, headaches, IBS, insomnia, constipation, dizziness, tinnitus, gas and bloating, premature aging, chronic fatigue, food allergies.	Sensitive skin—sunburn, hives, rashes, eczema, heartburn, hot flashes, psoriasis, ulcers, inflammation, canker sores, diarrhea, liver disorders, bad breath, bloodshot eyes, food allergies to nuts, excessive hunger and thirst.	Slow metabolism, overweight. Emotional eaters, diabetes, colds and coughs, yeast conditions, lymphatic system disorders, water retention/bloating, asthma (some types), sinus congestion (some types), low thyroid function, congestive heart failure.

	VATA	PITTA	KAPHA
Practices to Balance (favor)	Moisture, good sleep habits, regularity, warm weather, touch, soft music, soft colors like soft orange yellow and white (avoid black, brown grey), spiritual books, mantra meditation, do one thing at a time, abhyanga, drink water, lavender and sweet orange essential oils, walk, go to bed by 10pm with hot milk and pinch of nutmeg, do gentle exercise like yoga	Stay cool (both physically and mentally), downtime, cool bath or swim, walk in moonlight, healthy daily elimination, take warm showers instead of hot, protect skin and eyes from sun, drink cool water, swimming and aquatic exercise, go to bed by 10pm and up by 5 or 6am, rub coconut oil on scalp and soles of feet at bedtime. Use cooling colors like white, green, and blue (avoid red and black).	Warmth, daily physical and mental activity, warming spices. Challenge oneself. Work hard and rest less. Early to rise is good. Skip breakfast if not hungry. Practice detachment. Eat larger lunch, small dinner. Liquid fast once/week. Go for a walk when getting the urge to eat between meals. Scrape tongue daily. Dry massage before a shower. Wear hot vibrant colors—bright red, orange, golden yellow (avoid white, pink, pale blue or pale green).
Foods that balance	Eat sweet, sour, and salty tastes, warm cooked foods. Eat root vegetables and nuts for grounding, hot soups, warm cereals, carrots, asparagus, sweet potato, zucchini, cooked leafy greens, basmati rice, ghee and olive oil. Dairy is good. All nuts good especially walnuts and almonds. Basmati rice and wheat good. Reduce beans. Favor sweet, sour or heavy fruits like oranges, bananas, avocados, melons, berries, mangoes. Use natural sweeteners in moderation like turbinado sugar, raw honey, whole cane sugar, molasses.	Eat sweet, astringent, bitter tastes, cool foods/salads in summer, warm foods good in winter. Dairy-milk and ghee good (not sour cream and cheese). Eat sprouts, asparagus, broccoli, cauliflower, leafy greens, peas, zucchini, potato, cucumbers, green beans, celery. Reduce hot peppers, onions. Cilantro is very cooling. Eat most ripe fruits but not citrus. Favor sweet fruits like grapes, cherries, melons, avocados, pomegranates. Barley, oatmeal, cream of wheat, basmati rice, mung beans, chickpeas, soybeans. Coconut, sunflower and olive oil. All sweeteners but not honey and molasses.	Eat bitter, astringent, and pungent foods, light, warm, spicy foods. Use small amounts of ghee to kindle the agni fire. Eat fruits—apple, pear, apricot, berries, cherries, pomegranate. Avoid bananas, melons, avocados. Eat vegetables—asparagus, cooked beets, bitter gourd, broccoli, Brussels sprouts, cabbage, cooked carrots, leafy greens. All vegetables are good except tomatoes, cucumbers, potatoes, and zucchini. Grains—barley, corn, millet. Clear vegetable soups with beans or lentils. Raw honey is recommended sweetener. Reduce all nuts.
Herbs/ spices that balance Note: consider precautions such as pregnancy	Heating spices are good for Vata, especially salt and ginger. Drink ginger tea (especially when traveling). Use black pepper, hing, cumin, cayenne (in moderation), mustard seed, clove cardamom, cinnamon.	Use cooling spices—coriander, cinnamon, cumin, dill, fennel, cilantro, cardamom, saffron, small amounts of fresh ginger. Take amalaki, triphala, warm milk with a pinch of cardamom at night. Avoid hot, pungent spices.	Hot pungent spices—ginger, cumin, black pepper, cloves, turmeric, mustard seed, cayenne, cinnamon, fenugreek (weight loss). Limit salt. Hot herbal teas—green tea, ginger tea, or cinnamon tea. Hot water with juice from 1/2 lime and 1/2 tsp honey.

REFERENCES

1. Cousins, G. (2005). *Spiritual nutrition: Six foundations for spiritual life and the awakening of Kundalini.* Berkeley, CA: North Atlantic Books.
2. https://www.cdc.gov/chronicdisease/center/index.htm
3. https://adaa.org/about-adaa/press-room/facts-statistics
4. Dugliss, P. (n.d.). Transform the health of the world through the wisdom of Ayurveda. Retrieved from https://www.newworldayurveda.com
5. Dugliss, P. (2007). *Capturing the bliss: Ayurveda and the yoga of emotion.* Ann Arbor, MI: MCD Century Publications.
6. Tsunetsugu, Y., Park, B., & Miyazaki, Y. (2009). Trends in research related to "Shinrin-yoku" (taking in the forest atmosphere or forest bathing) in Japan. *Environmental Health and Preventive Medicine, 15*(1), 27-37. doi:10.1007/s12199-009-0091-z
7. Kshirsagar, S. (2018). *Change your schedule, change your life.* (3) New York: HarperCollins.
8. Kshirsagar, S. (2018). *Change your schedule, change your life.* (12) New York: HarperCollins.
9. Harvey, A. & Saade, C. (2017). *Evolutionary love relationships: Passion, authenticity, and activism.* Toronto: Enrealment Press.
10. Douillard, J. (2018, January 30). The difference between brahmi and bacopa. Retrieved from https://lifespa.com/benefits-differences-brahmi-gotu-kola-bacopa
11. Douillard, J. (2013, May 11). Why do kids make mucus for a living? Retrieved from https://lifespa.com/why-do-kids-make-mucus-for-a-living
12. Douillard, J. (2018, July 19). 3 Ayurvedic pillars of effortless exercise. Retrieved from https://lifespa.com/ayurvedic-exercise-training-tips
13. Douillard, J. (2004). *Perfect health for kids: Ten Ayurvedic health secrets every parent must know.* Berkeley, CA: North Atlantic Books.
14. Maharishi Ayurveda (2017). Be your best this new year: Tips for an Ayurvedic lifestyle. Retrieved from https://www.mapi.com/ayurvedic-knowledge/seasonal-health/tips-for-living-an-ayurvedic-lifestyle.html
15. Douillard, J. (2014, May 6). 15 benefits of breathing through your nose during exercise. Retrieved from https://lifespa.com/15-benefits-nose-breathing-exercise/
16. Mercola, J. (n.d.). One in three Americans have or will get diabetes—are you one of them and don't know it? Retrieved from https://www.mercola.com/ebook/diabetes-symptoms.aspx
17. Ji, S. (2018, February 28). Is the cure for diabetes a humble root? Retrieved from http://www.greenmedinfo.com/blog/cure-diabetes-humble-root
18. Douillard, J. (n.d.) John Douillard's LifeSpa. Retrieved from https://lifespa.com
19. GreenMedInfo. (n.d.). Turmeric. Retrieved from http://www.greenmedinfo.com/substance/turmeric
20. *The truth about cancer.* (n.d.). Retrieved from https://thetruthaboutcancer.com
21. Shaw, N. E. (2013, Aug. 8). Why an alkaline approach can successfully treat cancer. Retrieved from http://www.greenmedinfo.com/blog/why-alkaline-approach-can-successfully-treat-cancer
22. Novak, S. (2011, May 14). CDC confirms oil of lemon eucalyptus as effective as DEET. Retrieved from https://www.treehugger.com/lawn-garden/cdc-confirms-lemon-eucalyptus-oil-as-effective-as-deet.html
23. Fowler, J. H., & Christakis, N. A. (2008). Dynamic spread of happiness in a large social network: Longitudinal analysis over 20 years in the Framingham Heart Study. *BMJ, 337,* 1-9. doi:10.1136/bmj.a2338
24. Maharishi Ayurveda (n.d.). Your Ayurvedic lifestyle guide for a healthy, energized, renewed you. Retrieved from https://www.mapi.com
25. DeBow, M. (2014). Dynamic of light. Retrieved from http://www.medicallightassociation.com/?q=node/68
26. Esposito, L. & Kotz, D. (2018, July 18). How much time in the sun do you need for vitamin D? Retrieved from https://health.usnews.com/wellness/articles/2018-07-18/how-much-time-in-the-sun-do-you-need-for-vitamin-d
27. Environmental Working Group (n.d.). Retrieved from https://www.ewg.org/
28. Douillard, J. (2014, May 6). 15 benefits of breathing through your nose during exercise. Retrieved from https://lifespa.com/15-benefits-nose-breathing-exercise/
29. Mercola, J. (n.d.). The low-down on cholesterol: Why you need it—and the real methods to get your levels right. Retrieved from https://www.mercola.com/ebook/how-to-lower-cholesterol.aspx
30. Mercola, J. (n.d.). The low-down on cholesterol: Why you need it—and the real methods to get your levels right. Retrieved from https://www.mercola.com/ebook/how-to-lower-cholesterol.aspx
31. Mercola, J. (n.d.). The low-down on cholesterol: Why you need it—and the real methods to get your levels right. Retrieved from https://www.mercola.com/ebook/how-to-lower-cholesterol.aspx
32. Environmental Protection Agency (n.d.). Colony collapse disorder. Retrieved from https://www.epa.gov/pollinator-protection/colony-collapse-disorder
33. Brach, T. (2014, October 15). Part 1: Happiness [Video blog post]. Retrieved from https://www.tarabrach.com/part-1-happiness
34. The Chopra Foundation. Gratitude studies. Retrieved from https://www.choprafoundation.org/education-research/past-studies/gratitude-study/
35. Kshirsagar, M. (2015) *Enchanting beauty: Ancient secrets to inner, outer, & lasting beauty.* Twin Lakes, WI. Lotus Press.
36. Atreya. (1998). *Practical Ayurveda: Secrets for physical, sexual, & spiritual health.* York Beach, ME: Samuel Weiser.
37. Kshirsagar, M. (2015) *Enchanting beauty: Ancient secrets to inner, outer, & lasting beauty.* Twin Lakes, WI: Lotus Press.
38. Douillard, J. (2015, Feb. 14). Become the source of love. Retrieved from https://lifespa.com/become-source-love
39. Environmental Working Group (n.d.). Retrieved from https://www.ewg.org

40. Farr, B. (n.d.) How to make an all-natural sunblock. Retrieved from https://www.instructables.com/id/How-to-Make-an-All-Natural-Sunblock
41. Environmental Working Group (2019). Shopper's guide to pesticides in produce. Retrieved from https://www.ewg.org/foodnews
42. Maharishi Ayurveda (n.d.) Tender loving coconuts: Ayurveda plant for cooling. Retrieved from https://www.mapi.com/ayurvedic-knowledge/plants-spices-and-oils/coconuts-and-ayurveda.html
43. Ji, S. (2018, Dec. 3). Coconut water: Far more than just a refreshing beverage. Retrieved from http://www.greenmedinfo.com/blog/coconut-water-far-more-just-refreshing-beverage
44. Ji, S. (2013, April 4). MCT fats found in coconut oil boost brain function in only one dose. Retrieved from http://www.greenmedinfo.com/blog/mct-fats-found-coconut-oil-boost-brain-function-only-one-dose
45. Adams, C. (2013, Jan. 8). How much water should we drink? Retrieved from https://www.realnatural.org/water-research-confirms-needs-for-healthy-water-consumption
46. Donald, B. (2013, Aug. 27). Willpower is in your mind, not in a sugar cube, say Stanford scholars. Retrieved from https://news.stanford.edu/news/2013/august/willpower-study-sugar-082713.html
47. Adams, C. (2009). *Pure water: The science of water, waves, water pollution, water treatment, water therapy and water ecology*. Wilmington, DE: Logical Books.
48. Merriam-Webster. (n.d.). Intercept. Retrieved from https://www.merriam-webster.com/dictionary/intercept
49. Maharishi Ayurveda (n.d.) Ten Ayurvedic dietary must-do's. Retrieved from https://www.mapi.com/ayurvedic-knowledge/ayurvedic-diet/nine-ayurvedic-secrets-to-a-healthy-diet.html
50. Mischke, M. (2019). Love your liver: An Ayurvedic guide to fostering liver health. Retrieved from https://www.banyanbotanicals.com/info/ayurvedic-living/living-ayurveda/health-guides/love-your-liver
51. SLUCare (n.d.). Liver disease facts. Retrieved from https://www.slucare.edu/gastroenterology-hepatology/liver-center/liver-disease-facts.php
52. Douillard, J. (2016) Alcohol, Ayurveda herbs, and your liver. Retrieved from http://everydayayurveda.org/alcohol-ayurvedic-herbs-and-your-liver
53. Keltner, D., & Haidt, J. (2003). *Approaching awe, a moral, spiritual, and aesthetic emotion. Cognition and Emotion*, 17(2), 297-314. doi:10.1080/02699930302297
54. Centers for Disease Control and Prevention (2017, Aug. 23). Heart disease fact sheet. Retrieved from https://www.cdc.gov/dhdsp/data_statistics/fact_sheets/fs_heart_disease.htm
55. Sai Ayurvedic College (2018, Feb. 12). Ayurveda: Benefits of drinking from a copper vessel. Retrieved from https://saiayurvediccollege.com/ayurveda-benefits-of-drinking-from-a-copper-vessel
56. HeartMath Institute. (n.d.). The mysteries of the heart [Infographic]. Retrieved from https://www.heartmath.org/resources/infographic/mysteries-of-the-heart
57. Environmental Working Group (2019). Dirty dozen. Retrieved from https://www.ewg.org/foodnews/dirty-dozen.php
58. Douillard, J. (2016, March 14). The brain-lymph connection for better mood and memory. Retrieved from https://lifespa.com/brain-lymph-connection-better-mood-memory
59. Douillard, J. (2016, March 14). The brain-lymph connection for better mood and memory. Retrieved from https://lifespa.com/brain-lymph-connection-better-mood-memory
60. Douillard, J. (2019, March 19). At-home SAN (sagittal sinus abhyanga nasya): Cleanse your sinuses + emotional baggage. Retrieved from http://lifespa.com/how-to-clear-your-sinuses-and-emotional-baggage
61. Pert, C. B. (1999). *Molecules of emotion: The science behind mind-body medicine*. New York, NY: Scribner.
62. Douillard, J. (2018, Oct. 16). How to release unwanted emotions with Ayurveda. Retrieved from https://lifespa.com/cleanse-toxins-and-emotions-right-out-of-your-fat
63. Cloudmind. (n.d.). Health: Benefits, dosage and side effects of apple cider vinegar. Retrieved from https://cloudmind.info/health-benefits-dosage-and-side-effects-of-apple-cider-vinegar
64. Lin, H. H., Tsai, P. S., Fang, S. C., & Liu, J. F. (2011). Effect of kiwifruit consumption on sleep quality in adults with sleep problems. *Asian Pacific Journal of Clinical Nutrition, 20*(2), 169-174.
65. Maharishi Ayurveda (n.d.). Sleepless in America. Retrieved from https://www.mapi.com/ayurvedic-knowledge/sleep/cure-insomnia-with-ayurveda.html
66. National Institute for the Clinical Application of Behavioral Medicine. (2011, July 25). 7 ways inadequate sleep negatively impacts health. Lecture. Retrieved from https://www.nicabm.com/
67. Stanford Medicine (2004, Dec. 6). Stanford study links obesity to hormonal changes from lack of sleep. Retrieved from http://med.stanford.edu/news/all-news/2004/stanford-study-links-obesity-to-hormonal-changes-from-lack-of-sleep.html
68. National Institutes of Health (2011, Oct. 17). Prostate cancer risk from vitamin E supplements. Retrieved from https://www.nih.gov/news-events/nih-research-matters/prostate-cancer-risk-vitamin-e-supplements
69. Artemis, N. (2013). *Holistic dental care: The complete guide to healthy teeth and gums*. Berkeley, CA: North Atlantic Books.
70. Martino, J. (2013, July 11). Is baking soda a good alternative to toothpaste? Retrieved from https://www.collective-evolution.com/2013/07/11/is-baking-soda-a-good-alternative-to-toothpaste
71. Peedikayil, F., Sreenivasan, P., & Narayanan, A. (2015). Effect of coconut oil in plaque related gingivitis—a preliminary report. *Nigerian Medical Journal, 56*(2), p. 143. doi:10.4103/0300-1652.153406
72. Banyan Botanicals. (2019). Dosha-balancing yoga. Retrieved from https://www.banyanbotanicals.com/info/ayurvedic-living/living-ayurveda/yoga/intro-to-dosha-balancing-yoga
73. Mercola, J. (2018, Oct. 31). Ninety percent of sea salt contains plastic. Retrieved from https://articles.mercola.com/sites/articles/archive/2018/10/31/sea-salt-plastic.aspx
74. Cousin, G. (2017, Sept. 26). The vata dosha. Retrieved from http://treeoflifecenterus.com/Vata

75. Chopra Center (n.d.). *How to balance your vata with aromatherapy*. Retrieved from https://chopra.com/articles/how-to-balance-your-Vata-with-aromatherapy
76. Adams, C. (2009). *Arthritis: The botanical solution*. Wilmington, DE: Logical Books.
77. Ji, S. (2013, Nov. 10). *Eating sesame seeds superior to Tylenol for knee arthritis.* http://www.greenmedinfo.com/blog/eating-sesame-seeds-superior-tylenol-knee-arthritis
78. Beerepoot, M., & Geerlings, S. (2016). Non-antibiotic prophylaxis for urinary tract infections. Retrieved from https://www.ncbi.nlm.nih.gov/pmc/articles/PMC4931387
79. Douillard, J. (2010, Nov. 25). Eliminate emotional pain. Retrieved from https://lifespa.com/eliminate-emotional-pain
80. Mercola, J. (2009, Dec. 3). How to prevent the flu—as easy as 1, 2, 3. Retrieved from https://articles.mercola.com/sites/articles/archive/2009/12/03/how-to-prevent-the-flu-easy-as-1-2-3.aspx
81. Brown, B. (2010, June). The power of vulnerability. Speech presented at TEDxHouston, Houston. Retrieved from https://www.ted.com/talks/brene_brown_on_vulnerability

GENERAL INDEX

Abhyanga 12/6
Agni 2/5-10, 2/22, 3/19, 4/17, 6/28-29, 7/2, 8/9, 8/30
Ama 1/26-29, 2/9, 2/22, 3/15, 4/3, 5/9, 10/16
Amalaki 5/8, 9/14
Apple cider vinegar 10/8, 10/9, 12/22
Arjuna 5/15, 6/23, 8/30, 9/20
Aromas 3/29, 7/29, 11/29
Arthritis 12/9, 12/10, 12/11
Ashwagandha 2/4, 2/25, 4/13, 5/15, 6/23, 11/23, 12/1
Bacopa 3/5, 7/5, 7/23, 9/27
Bala 12/18
Barberry 9/14
Bhumyamalaki 9/14
Brahmi 2/25, 3/5, 4/9, 5/14, 7/5, 7/23, 9/27, 11/23
Breath 1/12, 3/14, 3/26, 4/18, 4/28, 5/22, 6/11, 6/29, 8/13, 9/24, 9/26, 10/13, 11/4, 12/8
Cancer 5/16, 5/17, 5/18
Cholesterol 5/16, 6/13-15
Children 3/9, 3/28, 7/28, 11/28
Chyawanprash 10/18
Chutney 3/17, 7/17, 11/17
Cleaning, natural 4/14, 4/15, 4/29
Cleansing 2/9, 3/20, 3/30, 4/1-4/5, 5/8, 5/9, 9/29, 10/16-17, 10/19, 10/26-27, 12/13
Clearing Mind and Clutter 4/26-27, 12/13
Coconut 1/18, 6/25, 7/10, 8/8, 8/12, 8/15-8/20, 9/4
Colds and Flu 12/21-24

Conditions 3/30, 7/30, 12/1, 12/16, 12/21
Consciousness 1/1, 1/11, 1/21, 4/6, 5/19, 5/29, 9/17-18, 9/21, 9/24, 12/15, 12/20, 12/25-30
Cough 2/24
Depression and Sadness 5/14, 5/21
Detoxification 3/11, 4/1-5, 10/17
Dhatus 1/18
Diabetes 4/22-24
Digestion 1/21, 1/26, 2/5-6, 4/13, 5/8, 7/2, 8/9, 8/29, 10/26, 12/17
Digestive spices xvi, 1/7, 5/5
Dinacharya (daily routine) 1/30, 3/22, 7/22, 9/5, 11/22
Disease 4/12, 10/1-10/7
Doshas x, 1/2, 1/12, 1/22-25, 2/13, chart at end
Dosha diet 3/13, 7/13, 11/13
    Dosha breakfast 3/18, 7/18, 11/18
    Dosha lunch/dinner 3/19, 7/19, 11/19
    Dosha supper 3/20, 7/20, 11/20
Drinks 3/21, 7/21, 8/8, 8/18, 8/29, 11/21
Ear health 8/26
Elements 1/2, 1/12-1/17
Emotions 3/6, 5/14-15, 6/10, 6/1-2, 6/26, 7/6, 8/7, 8/30, 9/8, 9/29, 11/6, 12/19, 12/25
Eyes 8/25
Exercise 6/11
Ghee 5/11
Ginger 1/29, 2/4, 3/19, 3/23, 5/25, 9/9
Greens 4/21, 5/4-6

Gotu Kola 3/5, 9/27, 11/23
Guduchi 9/14, 11/23
Guiding principles 1/8-1/11
Gunas (tamas, rajas, sattva) 1/20, 5/7, assessment 2
Habits/Change and Spiral Learning vi 1/4, 1/30, 4/5, 9/1, 9/7, 12/26-28
Hair 6/25, 8/27
Haritaki 5/8
Health 4/13, 12/17
Heart health 9/19-9/23
Herbs and Spices 4/6-10, 5/25, 9/9
Honey 6/16-6/19
Hydration 8/10, 8/22, 8/28-29, 9/2-3
Immune system 2/25-2/28, 5/3, 9/15-16, 10/28, 12/18
Inflammation 5/16, 6/13, 6/14, 6/15, 8/19, 9/3, 12/9, 12/10
Kappikachu 6/26
Kapha 1/23, all of March
Liver 9/11-13
Love 2/11, 6/26
Malas (waste products) 1/19
Men 6/23
Meditation 4/28, 12/29
Mind 3/5, 4/28, 6/20, 7/5, 9/27-28, 11/5
Nasya/Nasya oil 9/28
Neti pot 5/28
Oil pulling 5/20, 10/23
Ojas 1/21, 5/19, 12/14
Pitta 1/23, all of July
Prakruti 1/22, 8/21
Pre and probiotics 6/7-9
Principles 1/8-11
Protein 5/23-24, 10/20
Qualities 1/6

Relationships 2/11, 3/27, 7/27, 11/27
Ritucharya (seasonal routine) 2/2, 3/7, 7/7, 11/7
Seasons 1/25, 3/7, 7/7, 10/30, 11/7
Shatavari 2/4, 7/23, 11/23
Sitopladi 3/28
Skin 3/25, 5/13, 6/21, 6/25, 7/25, 8/4-8/6, 8/10, 8/23-24, 8/27, 11/25
Sleep 6/27, 10/10-10/15
Spices 2/22, 3/16, 3/23, 7/16, 7/23, 9/9, 11/16, 11/23
Spirituality 3/26, 7/26, 11/26, 12/19-20, 12/25-30
Sunshine 6/3-6/6, 8/12, 12/24
Tastes (six) 2/12-2/21, 3/12, 5/5, 7/12, 11/12
Teeth 10/21-24
Time of day/life 1/25, 3/8-9, 7/8-9, 11/8-9
Tongue 5/21
Tongue scraping 4/20
Travel 12/12
Trikatu 2/17
Triphala 4/3, 4/9, 4/19, 5/8, 7/22
Turmeric 5/16
Underlying Field 1/1-3, 1/7, 1/11, 5/2, 12/30
Urinary Tract Infections [UTI] 12/16
Vata 1/23, all of November
Vikruti 1/22, 1/24, assessment 1
Vitamins 6/3-6, 10/8, 10/18
Weight 3/15, 4/16, 4/18-19, 4/26-27, 7/15, 8/11, 11/15, 12/3
Women 4/25
Yoga 7/4, 8/13, 11/4

RECIPES & NATURAL FORMULAS INDEX

CLEANING

Cleaning, natural 1/28, 4/14, 4/15
Drain Cleaner 4/15
Toilet Scrub 4/15

DRINKS

Healthy Hot Cacao 12/5
Hot Spice Water {xvi}
  With ginger 1/2
  With licorice root 2/14, 7/16
  With a punch 4/1
  Vata Water 10/29, 11/7
Lassi, Digestive 8/29
Lassi, Sweet 8/29
Ojas Drink 5/30
Pitta Mocktail 9/3
Warm milk with add-ins 10/15

FOOD

Chia Seed with Coconut Oil 10/19
Chutney, Kapha- 3/17
Chutney, Pitta 7/17
Chutney, Vata 11/17
Cilantro-Mint-Coconut Chutney (Pitta Pacifying) 7/17
Cranberry Bliss Balls 12/16
Ghee, How to Make 5/12
Ginger Pickle 3/19
Kitchari 3/19
Liver-Cleansing Soup 9/14
Mint-Coconut Sauce 9/4
Mung Bean Soup 3/20
Stewed Fruit for Heart-Healthy Breakfast 9/23, 11/18

REMEDIES

Bath, Healing 8/19
Cold remedies 2/23, 12/21, 12/22, 12/23, 12/24
Cough remedies 2/24, 8/21
Elderberry Syrup 12/23
Fire Cider 12/22
Honey Formulas 6/18
Sore-Throat Gargle 8/9

SKIN

Bala-Infused Massage Oil 12/18
Cleanser-Toner-Exfoliator 5/13
Dark Circles 8/5
Deodorant 6/12
Face Mask 8/5
Insect, Bite treatment 8/4
Kapha Skin 3/25
Lip Balm 10/25
Moisturizer 6/25, 8/6, 9/4
Mosquito Spray 6/22
Pitta Skin 7/25
Repellent 5/26, 5/27, 6/22
Rosewater 7/7
Tick Preventative 6/22
Sun Block/Screen 6/4, 8/12
Vata Skin 11/25

SMOOTHIE

Ayurveda Style 5/6
Coconut 8/8
Watermelon 7/21
Spiced Coconut Smoothie 7/8

SPICE BLEND

Churna, Kapha 3/16
Churna, Pitta 7/16
Churna, Vata 11/16
Emotional Balance 6/2
Healthy Skin 6/21
Immunity Spice Mix 2/27

TEAS

Ama Busting Tea 1/29
Ayurveda Detox Tea 4/1
Cleansing Tea 3/30
Cold Soother Tea 9/6
Detox Tea -Tri-Doshic 6/28
Fall-Blend Tea 10/30
Kapha Balancing Tea 3/21
Kapha Warming & Cleansing Tea 3/30
Lemon Detox Drink 1/26
Lemon Detox/Weight Loss Tea 1/27
Lemon Water 2/15
Milk Thistle Tea 9/12
Mucus-Softening Tea 3/2
Pitta Pacifying Teas 7/16, 7/21, 8/11
Pungent Tea 4/7
  Turmeric Tea 5/16
  Vata Sleep Tea 4/13
  Vata Teas 12/2

WHAT OTHERS ARE SAYING

"Living an Ayurvedic lifestyle is a daily practice that produces subtle, yet powerful results. Take it one day at a time with this beautiful book."

—Lissa Coffey, bestselling author of *What's Your Dosha, Baby?: Discover the Vedic Way for Compatibility in Life and Love*

"Learn to THRIVE one day at a time, balancing mind, body and spirit with the wisdom of the ages applied to our Western way of life."

—Susan Niedzielski BS, MA, RYT, AAPNA, yoga teacher & Ayurveda Practitioner

"One-of-a-kind, heart-filled gem of daily Ayurvedic wisdom to guide you to an awakened life."

—Meena Puri, E-RYT500, RAP, author of *Healing Your Relationship With Food: The Ayurveda Answer*

"*365 Days of Ayurveda* translates the ancient wisdom of Ayurveda into exquisitely practical, day-by-day ways to integrate its benefits into modern life. The book's laser focus on healthy mind, body, and spirit is truly a recipe for radiant living."

—Maren Showkeir, coauthor of *Yoga Wisdom at Work*

ABOUT
THE AUTHOR

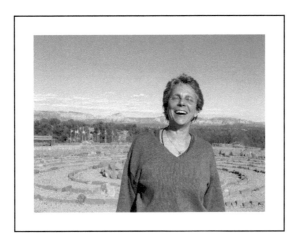

RHONDA EGIDIO, PHD, is Founder of Radiant Life Ayurveda through which she offers workshops, consultations, and free educational content via an e-newsletter. Home base is Kalamazoo, Michigan, U.S.. Rhonda served as an educator at Michigan State University (E. Lansing, Michigan) from 1983 to 2012. As a Professor of Education, she lovingly taught graduate courses related to personal and organizational development and adult learning and development. For decades, she also worked globally with Ministries of Education on large-scale education reform projects and designed eLearning environments for rehabilitation counselors.

Rhonda believes that knowledge and healing come from the *Underlying Field of Consciousness* and our connection with Divine Source. As a lifelong practitioner of yoga, Rhonda was introduced to Ayurveda in 2003. Ayurveda taught her that when the body is relatively clean and well-functioning, we can operate from a higher consciousness and positively impact our life-view and behaviors.

Rhonda completed her Ayurveda Health Practitioner training in 2010 and is a Registered Advanced Ayurvedic Practitioner. She is honored to study with Paul Dugliss, MD, Founder and Academic Dean of New World Ayurveda and a renowned, prolific author who is shaping modern Ayurveda from the ancient principles. She has been in private practice ever since, helping people transform their lives using the time-tested mind-body-spirit principles and practices of Ayurveda.

For personal consultations, workshops, and free monthly newsletter:

Visit http://radiantlifeayurveda.com

Printed in Poland
by Amazon Fulfillment
Poland Sp. z o.o., Wrocław